THE
WELLNESS
GUIDE

Thunder Bay Press
An imprint of Printers Row Publishing Group
9717 Pacific Heights Blvd, San Diego, CA 92121
www.thunderbaybooks.com • mail@thunderbaybooks.com

Printers Row Publishing Group is a division of Readerlink Distribution Services, LLC. Thunder Bay Press is a registered trademark of Readerlink Distribution Services, LLC.

Correspondence regarding the content of this book should be sent to Thunder Bay Press, Editorial Department, at the above address. Rights inquiries should be addressed to HarperCollins*Publishers*, 1 London Bridge Street, London SE1 9GF. www.harpercollins.co.uk.

Thunder Bay Press
Publisher: Peter Norton • Associate Publisher: Ana Parker
Editor: Dan Mansfield

Produced by HarperCollins*Publishers*
Editor: Sarah Vaughan • Designer: Rosamund Saunders
Authors: Rachel Newcombe, Claudia Martin, C. Norman Shealy, Anthea Courtney, Barbara Currie, Christina Feldman, Stewart Michell, Lesley Ackland
General Editors: Rachel Newcombe and Claudia Martin
Cover and interior images © Shutterstock
Illustrations (pages 112-117): Joe Bright

Library of Congress Control Number: 2022939172

ISBN: 978-1-6672-0084-2

Printed in Bosnia-Herzegovina

26 25 24 23 22   1 2 3 4 5

THE
WELLNESS
GUIDE

General Editors:

Rachel Newcombe and Claudia Martin

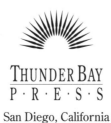

THUNDER BAY
P·R·E·S·S

San Diego, California

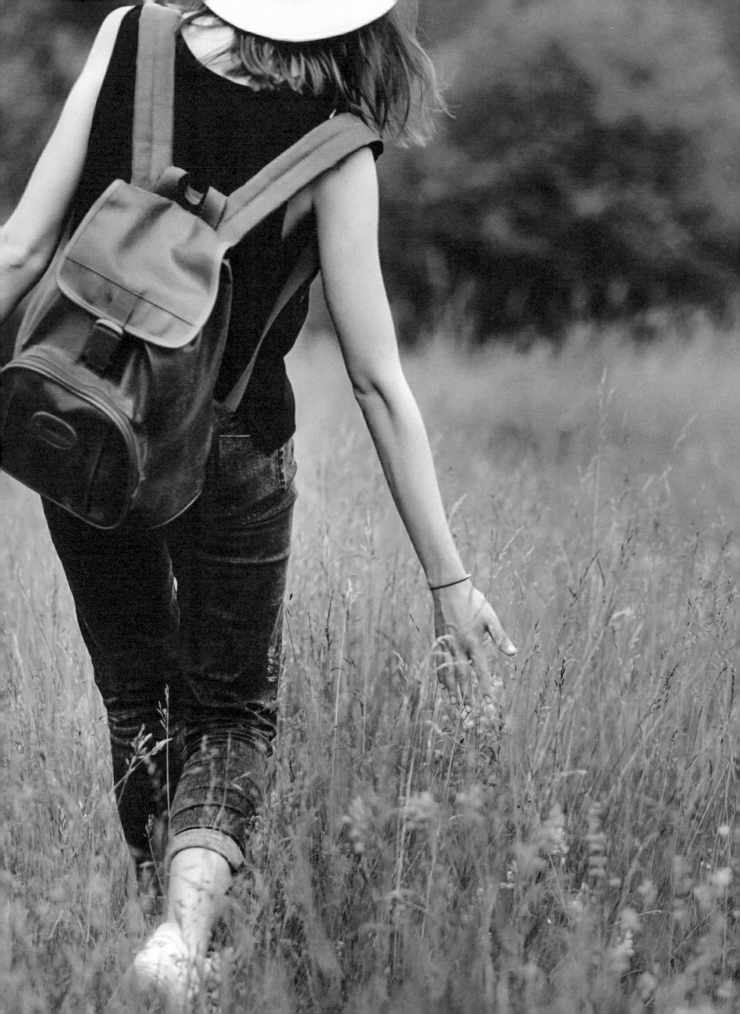

CONTENTS

Part Two: Mental Wellness

Part Three: Emotional Wellness

Part Four: Work–Life Wellness

FOREWORD

The term "wellness" was rarely used before the 1950s, when the American health statistician Halbert L. Dunn defined and examined the difference between good health—not being ill—and what he termed "high-level wellness." He described wellness not as a static state of being but as a movement, or process, in which the individual travels toward a higher level of functioning, happiness, and fulfillment. Since the 1950s, the concept of wellness has become mainstream, among ordinary people as well as among conventional health-care providers and public-health strategists. Today, the "wellness" industry is valued at trillions of dollars.

Yet why was "wellness" rarely discussed until after World War II? Why did the term become mainstream—a buzzword— only toward the end of the twentieth century? Perhaps the answer to this question is purely that better health care and diets led us to have higher expectations of our lives. Perhaps longer life spans, as well as the all-important introduction of weekends free from work, simply gave us more time to examine our health and happiness.

The full answer to these complex questions may be approached by examining an interesting case study. A few years ago, there was a small international stir when it was noticed that the Greek island of Ikaria had a higher than usual percentage of centenarians. In fact, Ikarians live around ten years longer, on average, than people in North America and the rest of Europe. A third of Ikarians live into their nineties, while suffering lower rates of heart disease, cancer, dementia, and depression.

Scientists and journalists descended on Ikaria to find out

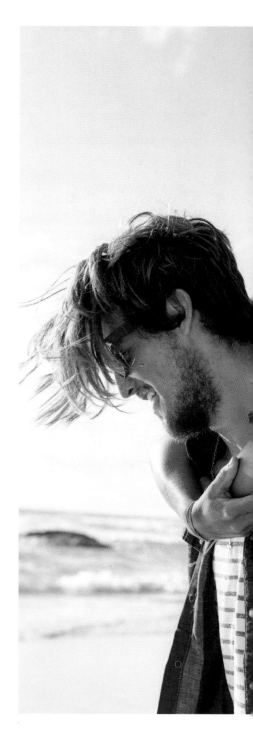

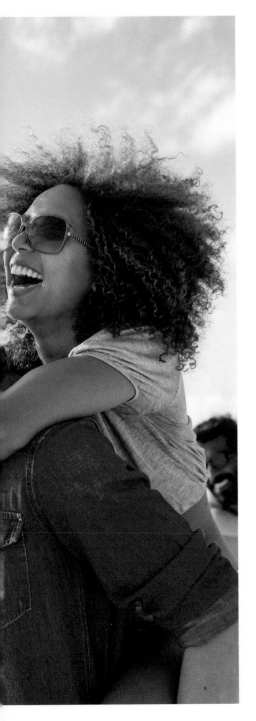

what was going so right—what was making so many islanders so well? The researchers discovered that, on their isolated island, most Ikarians have an excellent, varied diet with plenty of homegrown vegetables and little sugar, although no shortage of red wine. The older generation of Ikarians have stayed physically active through middle age and into old age, due to the necessity of tending their fields and walking up and down the island's steep hills to the nearest café. Ikarians are rarely alone, their friendships spanning a lifetime, and multiple generations enjoy each other's company constantly. Most important of all, the scientists concluded, most Ikarians seemed happy.

The modern world has brought many of us freedoms and opportunities, yet it has also brought losses, most notably in community and our closeness to the natural world. We can be sure that the majority of older Ikarians do not spend their working day behind a desk or in a factory line. They do not spend their evening snatching a packaged meal as they scroll through their friends' social media feeds. While we would be very wrong to believe that Ikarian life has never been backbreaking or heartbreaking, the Ikarian case study sheds light on the links between happiness, connection, purposeful work— and wellness.

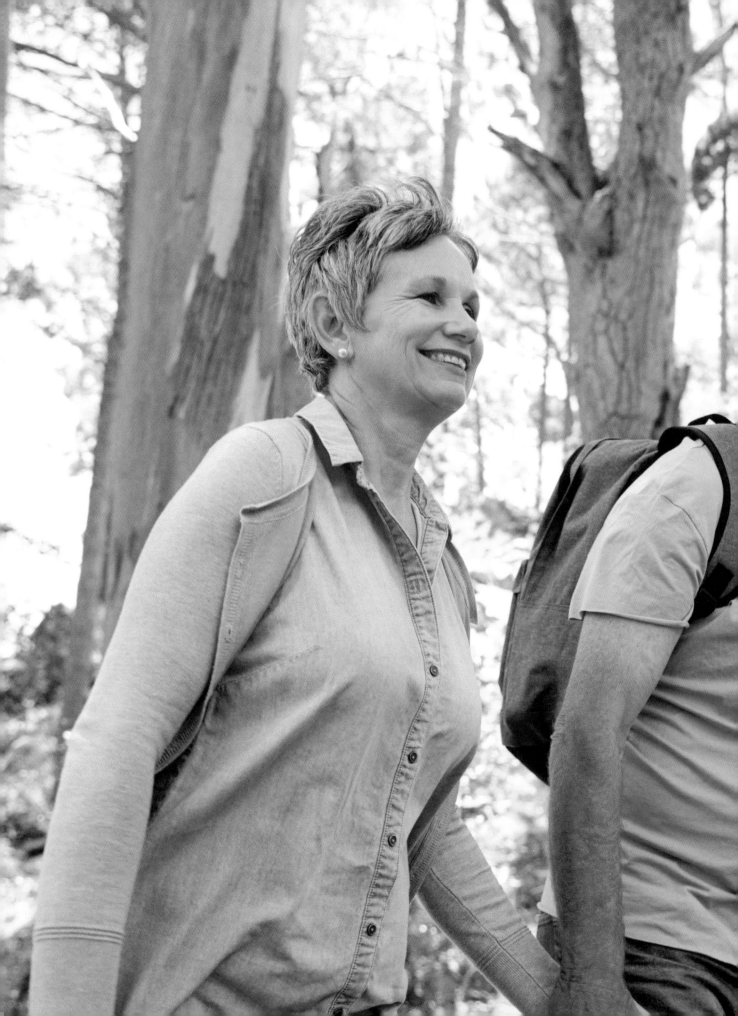

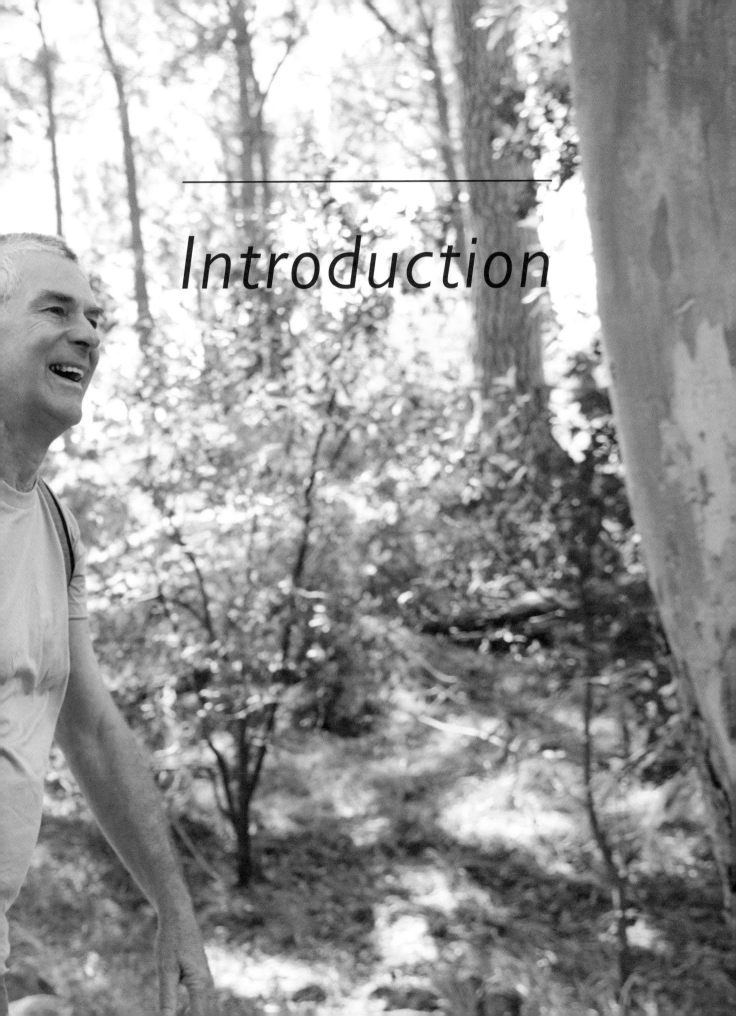

Introduction

WHAT IS WELLNESS?

Wellness is about so much more than having good physical health. True wellness is rooted in mental, emotional, social, occupational, financial, and physical well-being. Wellness is fed and watered by practicing healthy—but simple—habits that allow us to grow and blossom. For those living with chronic illness or challenges to their mental or emotional health, true wellness may seem intangible, even impossible. Yet for all of us, however difficult our circumstances, the wellness journey is one infinitely worth taking, with even the smallest steps—particularly if those small steps are all we can take—rewarded by great joys.

Wellness and well-being

The word "wellness" is often misunderstood. When we talk about "wellness," it is often physical health at the forefront of our minds. We hear someone told they look "well" when they have lost weight, toned their abs, or dyed their hair to hide the gray. We link "wellness" with physical activities: running, weight lifting, eating healthily. Above all, we link the possibility of achieving "wellness" with the mental strengths and decision-making that can bring about physical changes in the body—or maintain the body in peak condition—such as the willpower needed to diet, run marathons, or hit the gym every day.

In contrast, when we talk about "well-being," we rarely mention physical fitness or appearance. We talk about emotional states of being, such as happiness and peace of mind. If asked to visualize well-being, we may imagine resting in a tranquil garden, enjoying an ocean view from a sunlit terrace, or sharing a meal with family and friends. We link "well-being" not with the ability to bring about physical changes but the ability to enjoy the moment, to view the past with pride, and to face the future with equanimity.

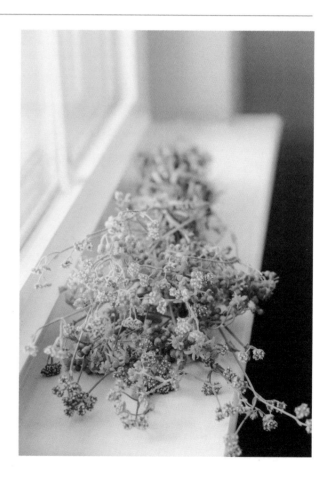

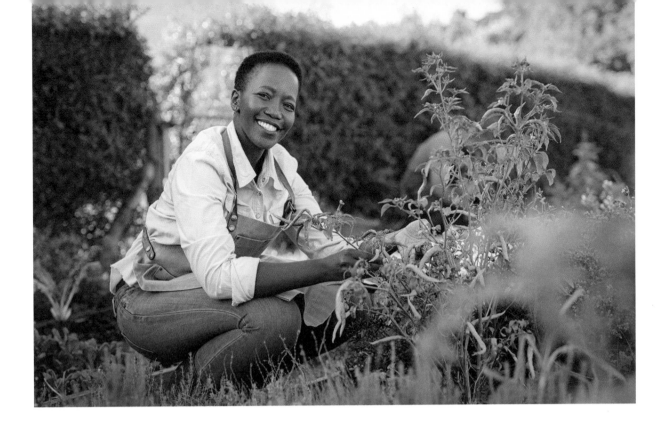

True wellness

Yet true wellness is well-being and true well-being is wellness. True wellness is based in physical, mental, and emotional health. It recognizes that physical health is not irrevocably linked with physical appearance. By freeing our minds from the chains of this self-defeating link, we can also break free from crash dieting and from exercising only so we can lose a few pounds. Instead, we can focus on truly feeding our physical health by building lasting habits of good sleep, sustainable exercise, and rounded nutrition. There may indeed be a need for willpower to set up those habits. However, that willpower will gain more fire from self-worth than from the desire to change ourselves. The habits of eating well and exercising regularly are best sustained by the key components of emotional well-being: enjoyment and peace of mind.

Likewise, our emotional and mental health cannot be separated from our physical health. Feeling sick or exhausted can challenge our enjoyment even of that tranquil garden, as those living with chronic pain or illness know well. Yet, for all of us, it is our connections with others that can sustain us through even the greatest challenges. The habit of mindfulness—focusing one's awareness on the present moment, while accepting our emotions, thoughts, and physical sensations—can allow us not only to enjoy that garden but to plant it and grow it in our own minds. Our emotional and mental well-being are the greatest resources we have for physical health, just as our physical health is a foundation of mental and emotional health.

In short, true wellness is the physical, mental, and emotional ability to enjoy life to the fullest. True wellness is the physical, mental, and emotional freedom to be our best self—loving, kind, generous, helpful, creative. True wellness is the self-esteem that grows not from how good we look to the world, but from being able to give a kind word, help a friend, and do a little good in the world.

WHY IS WELLNESS IMPORTANT?

Our wellness shapes every aspect of our daily lives, from our family lives to our social lives to our working lives. It affects our feelings, choices, and actions. Wellness is our ability to live a healthy, enjoyable, fulfilling life, as well as our ability to connect with and care for the people around us.

Aspects of wellness

We can identify ten aspects of our lives—all closely interconnected—on which our wellness impacts and which in turn impact on our wellness. By examining these ten areas more closely, we can not only identify areas in which we feel challenged, but note how one aspect of our lives affects every other. We may note how chronic illness is shaking our social wellness or, in contrast, how our emotional and intellectual wellness is bolstering our occupational and financial wellness. By examining our personal and specific needs, we can move toward a holistic approach to our wellness.

• Physical wellness: Physical health gives us the energy and freedom from pain to enjoy our work, family, and leisure time to the fullest. Common issues with

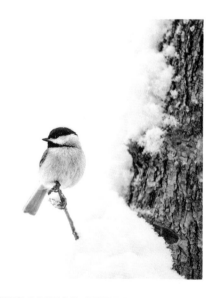

physical wellness include fatigue, insomnia, headaches, body aches, and digestive problems.

• Mental wellness: Mental well-being allows us to make the most of our abilities, to face life's stresses, and to build a life that boosts our self-worth. At the most fundamental level, mental wellness impacts on all areas of our lives. Everyone will find their mental health challenged at some point during their life, with depression, anxiety disorders, and eating disorders among the most common conditions.

• Emotional wellness: When we feel emotionally well, we are able to manage our emotions and feel resilient in the face of change and challenge. Feeling emotionally overwhelmed may lead to stress, depression, strains on social relationships, and impacts on physical health such as insomnia and increased blood pressure.

• Social wellness: Closely linked with emotional wellness, social wellness is the feeling of having strong relationships that meet our need for belonging and connection. These relationships offer companionship, advice, and support. The sense of lacking these vital connections can lead to loneliness and low self-esteem, impacting on our emotional, mental, and physical wellness.

• Intellectual wellness: This aspect of wellness is based on feeling intellectually stimulated. This feeling can be gained both at work and in leisure time through learning, engaging in creative and enriching hobbies,

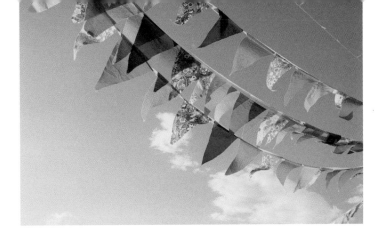

and sharing knowledge with others. Intellectual wellness builds happiness, self-esteem, and fulfillment, while a lack of it can make us feel frustrated, bored, and listless.

• Occupational wellness: Occupational wellness may be closely bound with intellectual wellness, but it is also centered on feeling respected, trusted, and safe in the workplace. For most people, occupational wellness also depends on feeling financially rewarded and on achieving a sufficient balance between work and leisure time. Occupational wellness impacts on all other aspects of our lives.

• Financial wellness: Financial wellness is feeling that we have enough money to meet our needs and to allow us to enjoy life. It is about feeling financially secure because we are in control of our day-to-day finances and able to prepare for the future. Financial worries can impact on our physical and mental health and stand in the way of social and intellectual wellness.

• Environmental wellness: Our surroundings have an immense effect on our bodies and minds. We all need safe, quiet, comfortable spaces—free from allergens and pollution—in which to sleep, relax, work, and eat. For many of us, being able to access leafy green spaces in which to exercise and wind down is also key to our mental, emotional, and physical well-being.

• Cultural wellness: For many of us, a key aspect of our wellness is being aware of and able to maintain our culture, express our sexuality, and be respected for our gender or abilities. Our cultural wellness resides in celebrating our own culture, ethnicity, or sexuality as well as taking joy in celebrating all the other cultures, ethnicities, lifestyles, genders, abilities,

and ages in our community. For many of us, cultural wellness is closely bound with emotional, social, and spiritual wellness.

• Spiritual wellness: Spiritual wellness is having beliefs, morals, or values that give a sense of the meaning of life. Spiritual wellness may give a feeling of being connected to something greater than ourselves. For believers, spiritual wellness may be found in communal worship and discussion. For others, spiritual wellness may be gained through meditation, yoga, volunteering, or travel. It can be boosted by activities as diverse as singing in a choir, keeping a gratitude journal, and joining a climate-change protest.

Personal wellness assessment

A useful step in a wellness journey is to carry out a personal wellness assessment, examining how wellness—or our need for it—is impacting on the ten key areas of our lives listed here. Unless you instinctively lean toward a more fluid approach, you may find it useful to give each aspect of your wellness a score of 1 through 10, then note which specific areas are troubling or rewarding you. You may note that the areas you have awarded lower scores are interconnected, such as your financial and occupational wellness or your social, spiritual, and cultural wellness. From this mindful vantage point, you are one step closer to formulating a plan and achieving your wellness goals (see pages 26–27).

THE WELLNESS CONTINUUM

The concept of the illness–wellness continuum was proposed by American physician John Travis in 1972. It has since gained widespread acceptance among practitioners of alternative and conventional medicine, as well as among public health strategists and businesspeople. The wellness continuum is a sliding scale between illness and wellness, on which we all move backward and forward constantly. Key to the continuum is the understanding that physical, mental, and emotional wellness are inextricably linked.

A neutral midpoint

At the midpoint of the wellness continuum is a neutral point, where we have no symptoms of illness but also no symptoms of wellness. Central to our understanding of this midpoint is the fact that wellness has both physical, mental, and emotional dimensions, so the absence of physical pain or discomfort does not make us "well" any more than it makes us feel fulfilled. In terms of physical health, we might name this midpoint "freedom from pain." In mental health terms, we might label it "coping" or "getting by."

Toward illness

The left side of the continuum represents degrees of illness. If we find ourselves on the left side of the continuum, we are in need of professional care or advice. Medicine can treat our disease, condition, or injury, nursing us back to the midpoint on the continuum. In mental health terms, we might give different names to the stages on this side of the continuum. We might replace "symptoms" with "struggling." We might replace "illness" with "in crisis." Just as with physical illness, appropriate help, advice, or support can nurture us toward a neutral point.

Yet we are never merely passengers on this journey toward wellness, as it is recognition of our symptoms and the bravery to seek and embrace help that are essential. Importantly, it is our own inner resources and positive attitude that keep us facing toward the right-hand side of the continuum, ready to make our way toward wellness.

Even those enduring chronic or terminal illness can face toward the right-hand side of the continuum. Our position on the continuum is less important than the direction in which we are looking. However, awareness of the continuum should never compel anyone who is seriously unwell to feel that they must "put on a brave face" or that "a positive attitude is all that matters." In these instances, the continuum is ideally a guide for loved ones and caregivers, a reminder that even the worst situations can be alleviated.

ILLNESS ▶ SYMPTOMS ▶ NEUTRAL ▶ ENRICHMENT ▶ WELLNESS

Toward wellness

The journey from a neutral point toward true wellness is mental, emotional, and physical. To move toward "enrichment" and on toward supreme "wellness," we must first be mindful of our current position on the continuum so that we can identify our needs. We can then embrace a holistic approach to wellness, choosing ways in which to build physical, emotional, social, or occupational health and resilience, one day and one step at a time. A first step toward "enrichment" may be simply taking a walk. It may be practicing yoga, trying a talking therapy, or starting a crochet class.

Again, in mental health terms, we might give different names to this side of the wellness continuum. We might replace the word "enrichment" with "thriving" and the word "wellness" with

"excelling." Yet both "wellness" and "excelling" mean the same thing: joy, fulfillment, and realizing one's full potential.

The wellness continuum is a fluid and dynamic process, so our standing start for the journey need not be—and rarely will be—a point of neutrality. We may begin from a point where we feel fighting fit and happy, or we may begin from a point when we are injured, either physically or mentally. There is one thing that all journeys toward wellness have in common: trying to face in the right direction by moving hopefully. That hope may be for good sleep and a strong body, for happiness, for creative success, for connection with ourself and others—or anything else you dream of.

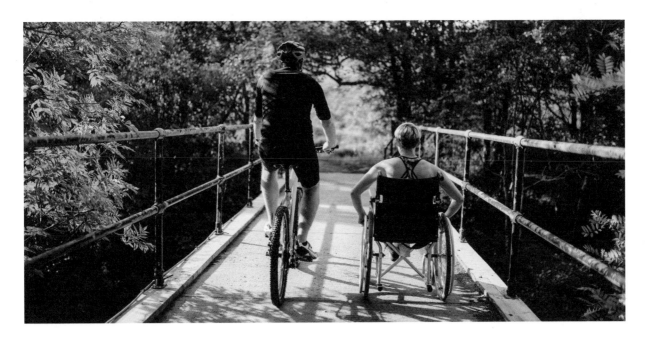

WORKING TOWARD PHYSICAL WELLNESS

Physical wellness is the ability to enjoy life without exhaustion, pain, or physical stress. Whatever our physical condition, physical wellness depends on the same factors: preventive medical care, healthy diet, exercise, sleep, and relaxation.

Seeking medical advice

The cornerstone of physical wellness is knowing when to seek medical advice. Key to this is listening to your own body and having the confidence and bravery to seek help when something does not seem right. In addition, we must learn to be careful with ourselves, by protecting ourselves from injury, by avoiding reliance on substances that damage the body or impair judgment, and by having regular checkups. Physical wellness means taking control of our sexual health, as our bodies change through time.

If you are worried about your physical health, make an appointment to see your primary care provider. If you find it hard to talk to health-care professionals or fear that you will not be listened to, take along someone to support you, such as a relative, friend, or professional advocate. Before going, you may find it useful to make some preparations so that you can get the most out of your appointment. Write down the things you want to discuss, then check them off while you are in the office. Also note down a list of your symptoms. You may find it helpful to write a list of questions. When you are in the doctor's office, do not be embarrassed to ask questions about anything you do not understand, including any uncommon words the doctor uses.

Exercising

For optimum fitness, doctors recommend we do some form of physical activity every day. Just making sure we are physically active once or twice a week will reduce the risk of negative physical outcomes such as heart disease and stroke. If you have not exercised in a long time or are recovering from illness, injury, or pregnancy, seek your health-care provider's advice on exercise that is right for you.

Experts advise that we do muscle strengthening activities at least twice a week. These activities could be yoga, Pilates, tai chi, working with weights or resistance bands, gardening, or pushing a wheelchair or stroller. In addition, we are advised to do at least 150 minutes of moderate-intensity exercise every week, or 75 minutes of vigorous-intensity exercise. Moderate-intensity activity includes fast walking, cycling, dancing, and in-line skating. Vigorous activities include aerobics, running, swimming, cycling uphill, team sports, skipping rope, and martial arts. The key to making exercise into a habit is to make it a fun, stress-free, and rewarding part of life. You will find tips on doing so in Part One.

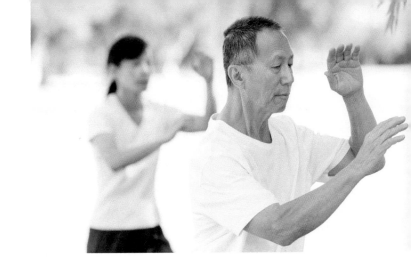

Eating healthy food

Physical wellness depends on feeding ourselves with a wide range of fresh, wholesome foods. Our physical wellness does not benefit from fad or crash diets but from building long-lasting, positive eating habits. Most important, wellness depends on eating without guilt and stress. For many of us, rules and restrictions around food (unless they are advised by our health-care providers) can lead to more guilt, stress, and disordered eating—even if they can offer short-term success with dropping pounds. As with maintaining a healthy exercise routine, the key to maintaining a healthy diet is to make good food a fun and rewarding part of life. For tips on achieving this, turn to Part Two.

Sleeping well

To feel well, alert, and calm, most of us need eight hours' sleep, as unbroken as possible. Good sleep comes easily to some, while for others it is always longed for and never reached. As with exercise and diet, building positive habits is a large step in the right direction. It is helpful to go to bed at the same time each night, in a calm, quiet place. Falling asleep is easier still if we avoid caffeine, screen time, and working immediately before bed. Yet most of us will experience sleep disturbances when we are worried, stressed, or troubled by trauma, guilt, or regret. Sleep is a nightly demonstration of the link between physical, mental, and emotional well-being. For advice on mental and emotional wellness, turn to Parts Two and Three.

Making time to relax

Finding the time to relax is key to all areas of our wellness. There is no one right way to relax. For some, it is a night on the couch with a favorite show, while for others it involves reading or knitting. For those who find it difficult to wind down, massage or meditation may be the key to relaxing muscles and soothing a rushing mind. Stepping out into nature—gardening, hiking, cycling, or surfing—can open the mind and heart, while at the same time exercising the body and encouraging the brain to release mood-boosting endorphins. For advice on wellness in your day-to-day life, turn to Part Four.

Help with addictions

An addiction is defined as not having control over doing, taking, or using something to the extent that it could be harmful to you. An addiction to smoking, alcohol, or drugs impacts not only our physical health but every other aspect of our lives. Substance abuse may be a way of blocking out difficult issues in our lives. Some studies show that we are more at risk of becoming addicted if we have family members with addictions. All addictions are treatable. No one has to face addiction alone. The first step is to get help, by making an appointment with your primary health-care provider. See Resources on page 296 for services that can also provide help with addictions.

WORKING TOWARD MENTAL WELLNESS

We all experience periods when our mental wellness is challenged, during times of stress, change, loss, or loneliness. Many of us face ongoing mental health problems. Knowing that we need to seek professional help is the single greatest step toward wellness. Yet even when we are not under stress, bolstering mental wellness is a key aspect of self-care, no less important than remembering to brush our teeth.

Taking steps

If you decide to seek support from a mental health professional or someone trained in complementary or alternative therapies, it is helpful to know what different professionals can offer and what treatment options are available. The below is a starting point rather than a definitive list. Your primary care provider can offer advice on which options may suit your needs. Licensed mental health professionals have received extensive training, usually at a postgraduate level, and are required by law to uphold ethical standards.

To start a course of complementary treatment such as hypnotherapy or acupuncture, a good starting point is a referral from your primary health-care provider. If you are considering a therapy for which there is less clinical evidence, such as aromatherapy, your health-care provider is less likely to offer a recommendation, so you will need to vet qualifications, training, and experience for yourself. However, you can try many beneficial therapies, from sketching to meditation, whenever you want, in the privacy of your own home.

PSYCHIATRIST: A psychiatrist has the medical training of a general medical practitioner, as well as several years' training in the diagnosis and treatment of psychiatric conditions, such as

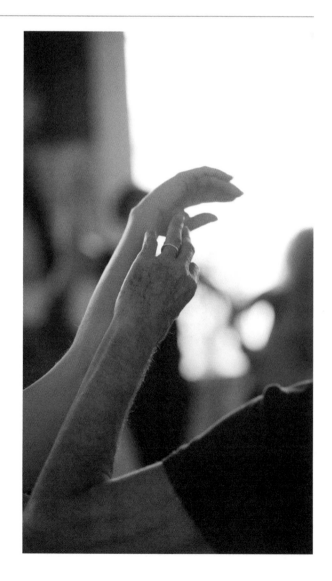

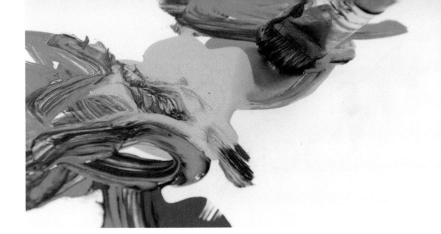

depression and bipolar disorder. Psychiatrists can prescribe medication and may also offer counseling (see "Licensed counselor") and talking therapies (see "Psychologist"), although some refer their patients to psychotherapists for this support.

PSYCHOLOGIST: A psychologist's lengthy training focuses on human behavior and development, while also including counseling (see "Licensed counselor") and talking therapies such as cognitive behavioral (CBT), interpersonal, and psychodynamic therapy. Cognitive behavioral therapy focuses on challenging exaggerated or irrational thought patterns and their associated behaviors, while offering coping strategies. Interpersonal therapy centers on resolving issues with and within relationships. Psychodynamic therapy is a form of psychoanalysis, aiming to reveal the unconscious content of a patient's psyche and how this may be causing inner conflict. Psychologists do not prescribe medication.

PSYCHOTHERAPIST: Qualifications differ among psychotherapists, so ask about professional memberships, training, and approach. Most psychotherapists have many years' training in the use of psychological methods to help a person change behavior, increase happiness, and overcome problems. Psychotherapists may specialize in a range of therapeutic approaches, such as cognitive behavioral therapy, psychodynamic therapy, or narrative therapy. Narrative therapy helps patients identify their values and skills, then coauthor a new narrative ("story") in which they use these skills to confront problems. Psychotherapists can offer individual, couples, family, and group therapy.

LICENSED COUNSELOR: Counselors are trained to provide guidance and support during difficult times. They do not diagnose or treat psychiatric conditions, but work with patients to manage personal, mental health, and physical issues. Counseling is based on conversation, which the counselor gently directs toward creative problem-solving and the untangling of thoughts and emotions.

ARTS OR CREATIVE THERAPIST: These therapists are trained in the use of painting, music, dance, or drama as a means to express and understand yourself. Most arts and creative therapists have postgraduate qualifications in psychotherapy, with special training in group work and creative therapies. These therapies are particularly useful for those who find it hard to talk about their feelings.

COMPLEMENTARY OR ALTERNATIVE THERAPIST: The clinical evidence for these therapies is not as robust as for the above therapies, yet many people find that they work for them. These therapies may be particularly useful for alleviating depression, anxiety, and sleep problems. Therapies include meditation, yoga, massage, hypnotherapy, acupuncture, herbal remedies, and aromatherapy. When seeking a practitioner, always ask about training and membership of professional organizations. If you are pregnant or breastfeeding, have a physical or mental health problem that could be made worse by the therapy, or are about to have a medical procedure, consult with your primary care provider before beginning treatment.

EMOTIONAL AND SOCIAL WELLNESS

Emotional and social wellness are so closely interconnected that one cannot be truly addressed without the other. Social wellness is founded on our connections with others, our families, friends, and coworkers. Emotional wellness is based on being connected with ourselves. It is about being able to understand and manage our own feelings. By truly understanding ourselves—the whole hoping, hurting, haywire human being—we can understand others, be patient with them, support them, and, the greatest of all blessings, be supported in turn. On a daily basis, we can take steps to nourish our emotional and social wellness in four key ways.

Being mindful

Mindfulness means paying more attention to our own thoughts and feelings, our own body, and the world around us. It means being present in the here and now, rather than worrying about the future or regretting the past. Mindfulness can help us understand ourselves better, by recognizing our own motivations, hopes, fears, and patterns of behavior.

Mindfulness also encourages us to enjoy the moment, appreciating the cup of coffee, the panting dog, or the clear freeway that we can see, hear, feel, touch, and smell right now. Studies have shown that appreciation of the moment not only makes us feel happier in that moment but helps us to see and find more causes for happiness, tomorrow and the next day.

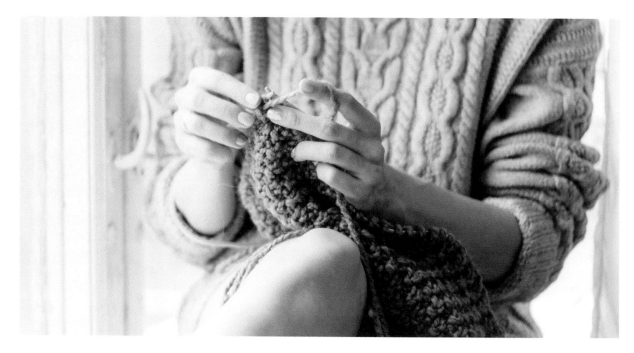

"In the depth of winter, I finally learned that within me there lay an invincible summer." —Albert Camus

Connecting with others

Our relationships give us a feeling of belonging, while giving us the opportunity to express our feelings and receive emotional support. In the digital age, it is key to abandon social media as the main means through which we communicate with others, as we can easily fall into the habit of only texting each other or scrolling through feeds, rather than truly talking. Instead of communicating digitally, we can play a game with our family, have lunch with a coworker, hike with friends, and video-chat with loved ones who live far away.

Giving to others

Many philosophers consider kindness to others an existential necessity, a pillar of religious faith, or a social duty. But numerous scientific studies have shown that acts of kindness can benefit our own emotional and social health, too. Helping others can build feelings of self-worth, purpose, and happiness. It can also help us connect with others. We can give to others in small ways, such as remembering a birthday or listening to a friend who needs support. In addition, we can buy lunch for a harassed coworker, help a neighbor with a DIY project, or volunteer in a local school, hospital, or soup kitchen. Knowing that we might be making our complex world even a slightly better place—one small gesture at a time—is an ideal antidote to sleeplessness, anxiety, and depression.

Learning new skills

Gaining a new skill can build feelings of fulfillment, self-confidence, and hopefulness. Taking a class is also an excellent way to make connections with others. A new skill might be creative, such as writing poetry or painting still lifes. Alternatively, you might choose a practical skill, such as learning a language, a computer program, or a trade such as plumbing or carpentry. You might decide to reawaken an old skill, such as the trumpet, soccer, or performing arts you got so much pleasure from back in high school. If you feel the need of greater fulfillment at work, you could offer to mentor a junior member of staff, raise your hand for new challenges, or ask for on-the-job training. If you do not have the time or desire to join a class or team, learning a new skill can be as simple as downloading information on cooking and trying it at home.

Although learning any new skill might hold the possibility of occupational, financial, or travel opportunities, there is no need for your activities to lead to a qualification, pay rise, or new business! Learning a skill can be for fun, for enjoying the moment, for making new friends, for knitting a pair of booties, or finally finding out how to make a soufflé.

WELLNESS AS SELF-CARE

Self-care is not a new concept, even if today it is a buzzword that you may see regularly on social media and in magazines. Self-care is about more than just looking and feeling good. Put simply, self-care is the act of looking after and nurturing yourself—physically, emotionally, socially, and financially.

Self-care today

In today's hectic and often stressful world, it is easy to forget to focus on yourself and to look after your needs. When life is busy, it is only natural to get caught up in work, taking care of children, rushing from one place to another, and enjoying an active social life. With so many commitments to juggle, it is no wonder that looking after yourself can get overlooked. It is often only when things "catch up" with you, when physical or mental health problems occur, that you realize you matter, too, and you need to stop putting yourself last.

This is why self-care is so important. When you learn to focus on self-care, you can integrate it into your daily life to form part of your regular routine. Self-care is about achieving a better balance in your life and knowing when to give in, stop, and look after yourself. It is learning about your needs, how you cope best in certain situations, and how you can manage difficult issues better. And it is about finding things that you enjoy doing and including them in your life as much as possible.

Ultimately, discovering self-care involves learning to look after and love yourself so that you can experience optimum wellness, physically, mentally, and emotionally, allowing you to live your life as the best version of yourself.

Self-care is not . . .

Self-care is not about being selfish. It is not a selfish act to focus on yourself and to take time to look after you: It is a self-respectful act. Yet, more than that, taking time to look after yourself and keep your physical, emotional, and social wellness in check will give you more energy to focus on your work, friends, loved ones, and commitments. By developing regular self-care practices, you are taking control and empowering yourself.

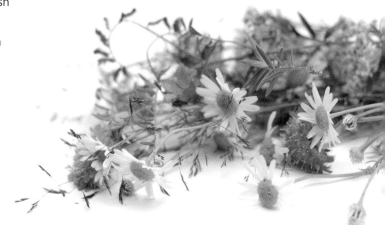

It is also important to learn how to truly relax and develop healthy nighttime routines.

Elements of self-care

The art of developing self-care habits does not involve one single act. Instead, there are multiple elements involved, from improving areas of your physical wellness routine and looking after your emotional health, to taking care of your life balance and achieving a better social wellness. It is incremental and holistic. Developing a self-care routine will not happen overnight. It is a gradual process of finding what works best for you and the areas you most need to focus on. Yet the more you practice self-care, the more it will become second nature, and the happier and healthier you can be.

PHYSICAL SELF-CARE: Physical self-care involves taking care of your body in order to improve your physical wellness. One of the key elements of keeping your body moving and maintaining the energy you need to get through the day is to ensure that you get a good night's sleep. It is also important to learn how to truly relax and develop healthy nighttime routines, giving yourself the best chance for your body to unwind and find deep and restorative sleep. What you choose to eat and drink plays a major role in your physical wellness. This means making healthy choices about the foods and drinks that will make you feel good and give you the right balance of the energy and nutrition you need. Exercising is a vital element of physical self-care, too, and it helps if you can find forms of exercise that not only meet your body's exercise needs but that you enjoy doing and can incorporate into your daily life.

MENTAL AND EMOTIONAL SELF-CARE: Mental and emotional health play an equally important role in physical health, yet they are often overlooked. Mental and emotional self-care practices involve finding ways to take care of your mind, from managing stress and developing emotional resilience, to learning to meditate and exploring new ideas for creative pursuits. Emotional self-care also involves finding out more about your true self and developing skills such as kindness, compassion, and improved communication to help you cope better with challenging situations at home or work.

SOCIAL, OCCUPATIONAL, AND FINANCIAL SELF-CARE: Social self-care involves taking care of your work–life balance and maintaining your relationships with others. You are deeply affected by your support systems and how you communicate with others. Focusing on your social relationships can boost your wellness, allowing for deeper and more nurturing relationships. Your pace of life, time management, and how you deal with money are areas that need deep and focused self-care. When it comes to financial and career wellness, self-care means regularly taking stock of our credits and debits, needs and goals. Self-care may mean seeking advice from accountants and mentors. Above all, self-care means recognizing the conveyor belt we are riding and questioning whether it is fulfilling our own particular needs.

SETTING WELLNESS GOALS

Some of us shy away from setting goals, preferring to grow organically, as a tree sends out searching twigs, which grow stronger year by year with no need for formal measurement. Yet for many of us, goals provide an impetus to change, a route toward change, and a yardstick to measure our achievements.

Being SMART

The mnemonic acronym SMART is helpful to bear in mind when setting wellness goals. The term was first used by business consultant George T. Doran in 1981, but with minor variations his goal-setting framework is as relevant to personal wellness as it is to business growth.

S for specific: When identifying goals, make sure they are specific, clear, and delineated. For example, rather than setting yourself the goal "To get fit," you could set the goal "To jog around the park three times without stopping for breath."

M for measurable: Make sure your goals are measurable, so you have clear aims. For example, you may feel a need to build a stronger relationship with a family member. Yet, as is the case with so many emotional wellness needs, how can we measure "stronger," "better," or "healthier"? Consider how you could set a measurable goal, which will also help you to identify your specific needs. For example, you could try: "To enjoy a date night once a week."

A for attainable: If goals are not achievable, they can lead to disappointment and discouragement. For example, the goal for so many of us is "To eat healthily." Yet if we have a history of disordered or emotional eating, this goal is far from easy. A more attainable goal may be "To eat five portions of fruits and vegetables every day"; "To swap out refined grains for whole grains on at least three nights per week"; or "On weekdays, avoid added sugars."

R for relevant: It may require keen insight and self-knowledge to establish if our goals are relevant to our needs. For example, we may identify a need to take care of our social wellness. The first goal that comes to mind may be throwing a party or going out on more nights each week. Yet will these goals truly meet our social, spiritual, and emotional needs?

T for time-bound or timely: Set yourself a realistic time period for achieving your goal. If your goal is about creating an all-important habit, there can be no time limit, but do ensure your goal is timely, or achievable right now, not after the holiday season or when your kids have gone off to college.

Being focused

You may have multiple goals you would like to work on, perhaps in linked areas such as exercise and diet, or concerning both your social and emotional health. Do not overwhelm yourself by setting too many goals at once. Decide on your priorities so that progress does not become too challenging. Place your goals in order of priority, then focus on the goal (or closely linked goals) that will give you the greatest boost—or

Set yourself a realistic time period for achieving your goal.

even act as a stepping stone to the achievement of your other goals.

Once you have determined a goal, break it down into smaller, step-by-step achievements. You may find it helpful to use a journal to write down a road map toward achieving these steps. Make a note of any preparations that would help you embark on your journey, then check off each element as you achieve it. For example, before you can begin working to achieve the goal "To jog around the park three times without stopping for breath," you may need to book an appointment with your health-care provider, buy a comfortable pair of running shoes, and arrange childcare. You might like to make an additional list of factors or events that could spur you on to achieve your goal, such as enlisting a running buddy or registering for a local fun run.

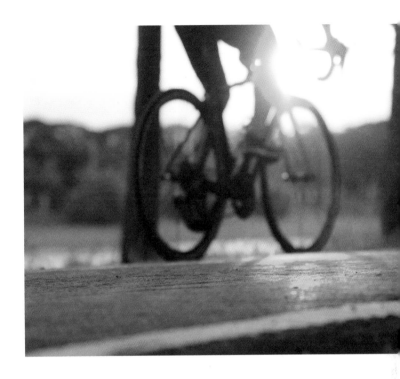

Creating habits not hurdles

As the old saying goes, humans are creatures of habit. We find bad habits hard to break but, luckily for us in our quest for wellness, we find good ones difficult to break, too. As will be discussed throughout this book, wellness is best achieved through the establishment of positive habits. The key to physical wellness is to make healthy eating, regular sleep, and exercise into a habit. Habits do not form overnight. When setting wellness goals and identifying how to reach them, consider ways that you can form habits rather than set yourself short-term goals. For example, the goal "Cycle to work every day" could create a habit, whereas the goal "Compete in a long-distance cycling race" sets yourself a hurdle.

When we have successfully leaped a hurdle, our tendency is to pat ourselves on the back and take a well-deserved break!

Emotional, social, spiritual, and financial wellness may also be based in habits, even if they are less apparent than the habits of physical wellness. The habits of regular mindfulness and gratitude encourage a positive outlook. The habit of taking stock of our financial situation can lead to careful decisions and enhanced financial security. Suitable goals for all these areas of wellness could begin "Every Sunday morning, make time to . . ."

HOW TO USE THIS BOOK

This book is in four parts, which focus on physical, mental, emotional, and work–life wellness. If there is one particular area of your life in need of nurturing, dive straight into that chapter. Yet you may find it rewarding to read other parts of the book, since our happiness in the workplace impacts on our emotional and mental well-being, which will usually find a way to express themselves as physical strain.

Part One: Physical Wellness

This part of the book offers information, advice, and practical tips for building the habits of regular exercise, good sleep, nutritious food, and relaxation. To help you kick-start an enjoyable exercise habit, on pages 40–65 there are Pilates, yoga, and aerobics routines. If refreshing, unbroken sleep is your goal, pages 68–77 offer facts about insomnia and advice on sleep hygiene. To find out the science behind healthy diet, drinks, and nutritional supplements, turn to pages 92–99. On pages 110–117, learn how to use self-massage for relaxation.

Part Two: Mental Wellness

Part Two offers advice and resources for enhancing mental wellness. Advice on choosing and accessing professional mental health support is on pages 188–189. Pages 122–135 offer facts and advice about common mental health issues, including stress, anxiety, and depression. Pages 136–145 provide suggestions and guidance about complementary methods of nurturing mental health, including being in nature, exercising, and enjoying hobbies. On pages 146–151, there is an in-depth guide to meditation. Pages 162–165 explain the wide benefits of mindfulness.

Part Three: Emotional Wellness

In Part Three, there are facts and advice for building emotional intelligence and wellness. After a look at the science behind emotions, pages 196–211 offer support and practical steps for working with common "negative" emotions, such as anger, jealousy, and loneliness. Pages 214–215 are a guide to using meditation for emotional wellness, with guided meditations to enhance positive feelings and resilience. Finally, pages 244–247 supply tips for developing a gratitude habit and exploring creativity and journaling.

Part Four: Work–Life Wellness

Part Four gives guidance on rebuilding or developing social, financial, intellectual, occupational, and environmental wellness. Pages 252–269 are a self-help guide to social wellness, with advice on healthy relationships, self-respect, and finding support. For a practical guide to troubleshooting your finances, turn to pages 272–277. If you feel that your work–life balance or your intellectual and workplace wellness need attention, pages 280–289 offer practical advice. Finally, pages 290–293 will help you to create a relaxing home environment.

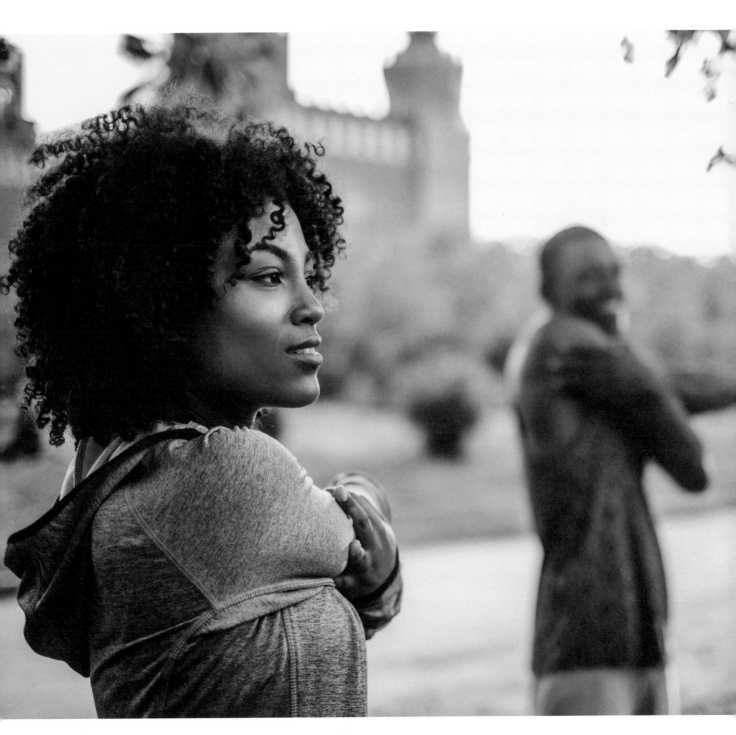

GLOSSARY

AEROBIC EXERCISE
Also known as cardio, aerobic exercise depends on the body's muscle cells generating energy aerobically, by using oxygen. Aerobic exercise, such as running or swimming, is performed by repeating sequences of light- to moderate-intensity activities for an extended time. In contrast, anaerobic exercise—such as strength training—is more intense but shorter in duration. During anaerobic exercise, muscle cells break down glucose without using oxygen.

ALTERNATIVE AND COMPLEMENTARY MEDICINE
Treatments that aim to achieve the healing effects of medicine but stand outside conventional, science-based medicine. Complementary treatments are those that are offered alongside conventional medicine, while alternative treatments are offered instead of conventional medicine. Complementary and alternative therapies include traditional treatments, such as herbalism, that have been proven to work for a limited number of health conditions, as well as treatments that are not based on evidence recognized by the majority of scientists, such as homeopathy.

AMINO ACID
A simple organic compound, gained from eating protein, that the body uses to build muscles, make enzymes that carry out chemical reactions, transport nutrients, prevent illness, and carry out other functions.

ANTIOXIDANT
A substance, such as vitamin A, C, or E, that may prevent cell degeneration and decay.

AROMATHERAPY
A complementary therapy involving the use of essential oils and other aromatic materials.

AURA
A magnetic field, or luminous glow, around a person or other living thing, said to indicate the health of body and soul.

BODY IMAGE
A person's thoughts and feelings about the attractiveness of their own body, usually shaped by social and cultural forces.

BODY POSITIVITY
A social movement based on the acceptance of all bodies and the rejection of social constructs around beauty and desirability.

CARBOHYDRATE
A nutrient, found in cereals, potatoes, and sugars, which the body breaks down into glucose, the main source of energy for the body's cells, tissues, and organs.

CHAKRA
In traditional Eastern thought, one of seven or more centers of spiritual power in the human body (see page 125).

CHANNEL
In traditional Chinese thought, an invisible pathway through which qi (or chi) travels through the body.

COGNITIVE BEHAVIORAL THERAPY
A talking therapy used by trained mental health professionals which focuses on challenging exaggerated or irrational thought patterns and their associated behaviors, while offering coping strategies.

CONVENTIONAL MEDICINE
The science-based practice of caring for a patient to prevent, diagnose, treat, and alleviate physical injury and disease, as well as to promote mental and emotional health through treatment by psychiatrists and psychologists.

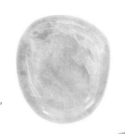
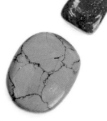
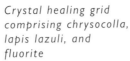
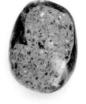

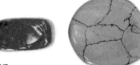
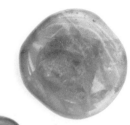
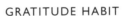

Crystal healing grid comprising chrysocolla, lapis lazuli, and fluorite

COUNSELING
Providing guidance and support through conversation between a licensed counselor and a client.

CRYSTAL THERAPY
A complementary therapy involving the use of crystals and rocks.

EFFLEURAGE
Slow, rhythmic massage.

EMOTIONAL INTELLIGENCE
The ability to understand, manage, and use our own emotions to relieve stress, communicate with others, and overcome challenges.

ENDORPHIN
A chemical made by the brain's pituitary gland to relieve stress and pain.

ENZYME
A protein made by the body to bring about a chemical reaction (causing a change, such as the breaking down of food).

ESSENTIAL OIL
The distilled essence of an aromatic plant.

FATTY ACID
A simple organic compound, gained from eating fats, that is a source of fuel and a structural component of cells.

FLOWER REMEDY
A preparation of the flowers of various plants used as a complementary therapy for emotional issues.

GLUCOSE
A simple organic compound, gained from eating carbohydrates, that is the body's key source of energy.

GRATITUDE HABIT
Taking regular time to be thankful and to return kindnesses.

GUIDED MEDITATION
Entering a state of inner stillness with the help of a guide, such as a meditation teacher, who leads the meditator through visualizations.

HERBALISM
A folk and traditional medicinal practice based on the use of plants.

HOLISTIC
Characterized by the treatment of the whole person, taking into account physical, mental, emotional, and social factors.

HORMONE
A chemical that acts as a messenger in the body, changing the behavior of its target cells to bring about change, such as growth or sleepiness.

INFUSION
A liquid obtained by steeping a herb in hot or cold water.

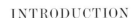

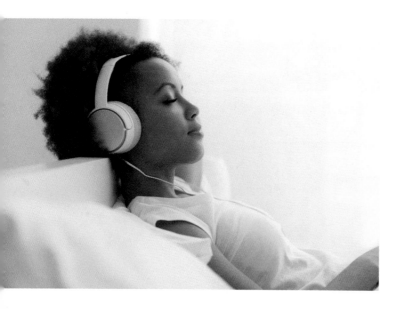

INTERPERSONAL THERAPY
A talking therapy used by trained mental health professionals, focused on resolving issues with and within relationships.

JOURNALING
Writing in a diary or journal, often used as a method of self-expression, self-awareness, and personal growth.

MACRONUTRIENT
A type of food—fat, protein, or carbohydrate—needed in large amounts in the diet.

MANTRA MEDITATION
Entering a state of inner stillness through the repetition of phrases (mantras) to promote focus.

MASSAGE
The rubbing and pressing of muscles and joints to relieve tension or pain.

MEDITATION
A practice in which the meditator uses a technique, such as focusing the mind on a particular thought or place, to focus attention and awareness, thereby achieving emotional calm and mental clarity.

MICRONUTRIENT
A material—such as vitamins and minerals—needed in small amounts in the diet.

MINDFULNESS
Being conscious and fully aware of the present moment, both of one's own mental and emotional state and of one's immediate surroundings.

MINDFULNESS MEDITATION
Entering a state of inner stillness through being focused on what one is feeling and sensing in the moment.

MINERAL
A naturally occurring chemical element, such as calcium or iron, that the body needs in small amounts in the diet to develop and function.

MOTHER TINCTURE
In the complementary therapy of flower remedies, the source remedy, which can be diluted to make therapeutic dosages.

NARRATIVE THERAPY
A talking therapy used by trained mental health professionals, focusing on identifying values and skills, then using these skills to confront problems.

NUTRIENT
A substance that provides nourishment that is essential to the maintenance of life.

OCCUPATIONAL THERAPY
The use of assessment and intervention to develop or recover skills and to help patients engage in activities. Occupational therapists are specially accredited health- and social-care professionals.

PHYSICAL THERAPY
Also known as physiotherapy, physical therapy is the treatment of disease or injury through physical methods

such as massage, heat treatment, and exercise. Physical therapists are specially trained health-care professionals.

PILATES
A system of mind–body exercises designed to improve physical strength, posture, and flexibility.

PRANAYAMA
The yogic practice of focusing on breath.

PROTEIN
A nutrient, found in fish, meat, and beans, that the body breaks down into amino acids, which are themselves used by the body to build materials.

PSYCHODYNAMIC THERAPY
A form of psychoanalysis carried out by trained mental health professionals, focusing on revealing the unconscious content of a patient's psyche.

PSYCHOTHERAPY
The use of regular personal interaction with a psychotherapist, psychiatrist, or psychologist to increase happiness and overcome problems.

QI (OR CHI)
In traditional Chinese thought, a vital life force that circulates through the body's channels.

QIGONG
A traditional Chinese system of exercise and healing that uses meditation, controlled breathing, and movement.

SHIATSU
A form of massage that works on the body's pressure points.

TALKING THERAPY
Talking with a trained mental health professional about thoughts, feelings, and behavior, with the aim of understanding and coping with problems.

TINCTURE
A herbal remedy prepared in an alcohol base.

VITAMIN
An organic compound that is needed in small amounts in the diet to develop and function.

YOGA
A physical, mental, and spiritual practice that originated in India. There is a wide variety of schools of yoga, with one of the most commonly practiced a modern form of hatha yoga, a posture-based physical fitness system that encourages mental strength and relaxation.

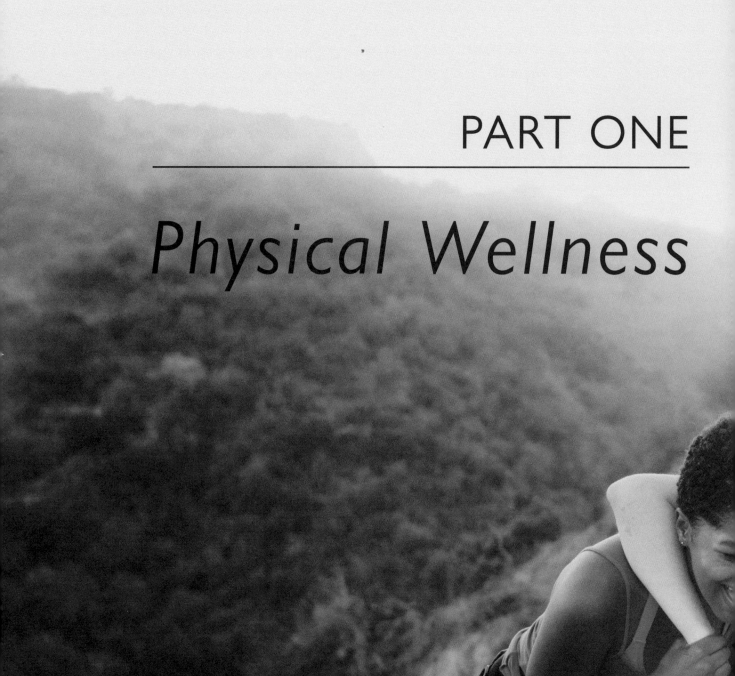

PART ONE

Physical Wellness

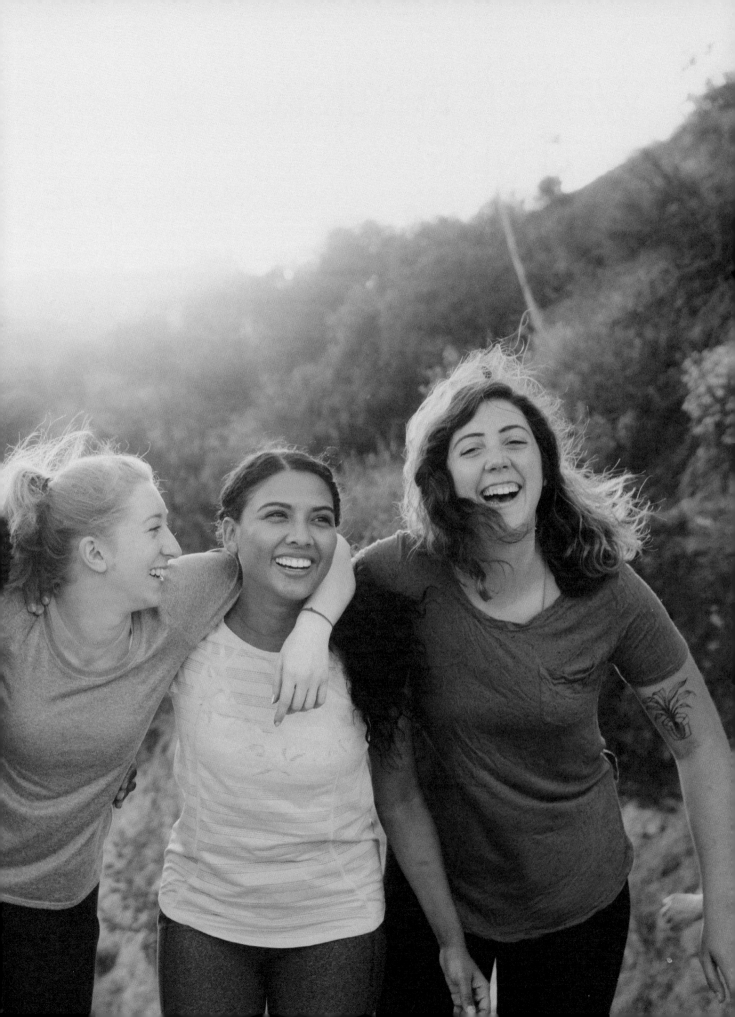

WHAT IS PHYSICAL WELLNESS?

The ancient Greek physician Hippocrates wrote that "health is the greatest of human blessings." We never know the truth of that statement with more certainty than when we are sick, injured, or exhausted. Physical wellness is the blessing that allows us to enjoy our daily life, from work time to family time and down time. Physical wellness starts with listening to, and taking care of, your body. Its foundations are healthy activity, good food, regular sleep, and relaxation.

Being active

For those who have already built exercise into their daily routine, staying active is only a question of maintaining motivation. For others, it is more challenging to make exercise a part of the day. The challenge may be illness or injury. For some, the challenge is finding the time between meeting responsibilities, from deadlines to childcare. However, for many of us, our problems with exercise are linked with our problems about body image.

Whatever our challenges, the key to an active lifestyle is finding exercise that suits both our bodies and our minds. Once we have found activities we can practice and enjoy, it is extraordinary how much more easily they can be slotted into our schedules. Experts recommend we do a mix of moderate-intensity and muscle-strengthening activities. For those who are not natural runners, swimmers, or cyclists, moderate-intensity exercise could be brisk walking or pushing a lawn mower. If weight lifting does not work for you, other muscle-strengthening activities include yoga, Pilates—even giving the kitchen floor a thorough scrub! Just a little activity every day can boost our physical wellness.

Enjoying good food

Later in this chapter, we offer the "rules" of good nutrition, which amount to eating a balanced diet that is rich in fresh, wholesome foods and low in packaged, processed foods. Yet, just as maintaining an active lifestyle is a challenge, so is maintaining a healthy diet. Many of the challenges are the same: lack of time and lack of motivation. It takes time to plan menus, shop, and cook. It takes less effort to eat the food that comes in a package or to stick with the meals we have always cooked. But, for many of us, the greatest challenge of all is our emotional relationship with food, which may have been forged in childhood or during a period of stress or loneliness. When we reach for food, we are often searching for comfort, a desire to assuage more than an empty stomach.

As with exercise, the key to a healthy diet is to enjoy the food we eat. This may involve a little time spent in taste-testing new foods and recipes. More than anything, however, it involves forgiving ourselves, for the times we break the "rules," for the foods we will never enjoy, and for the people we will never be. Then we can enjoy good food, most of the time.

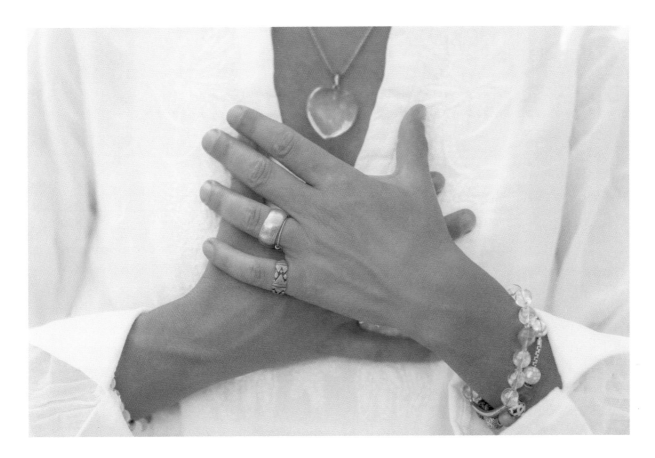

Sleep and relaxation

Sleep and relaxation are closely bound, each necessary to the other. Your body craves the right amount of sleep, regular sleep, and untroubled sleep. Although neuroscientists are still discovering the secrets of sleep, we know that sleep allows the body to recharge and the brain to store new information as memories. Our dreams are the muddled results of our brains sorting through daytime experiences and emotions. Without good-quality sleep, we soon become tired, forgetful, and more emotionally vulnerable. Yet for those who are insomniacs, knowing these facts only worsens the negative cycle of stress and sleeplessness. A bedtime wind-down routine as well as a calm place to sleep are key. More difficult to achieve is the relaxed state of mind that allows us to sleep without our thoughts keeping us awake.

Finding the time to relax—both at bedtime and during the day—is key to good sleep, as well as being in itself essential to mental and physical health. A good book, a good chat, a good movie are all time-honored methods of relaxing. Many find that meditation or massage can untie the physical and emotional knots of the day's stress. For others, it is scrapbooking, crocheting, or carpentry that quietens the racing mind. Whether we are trying something new or trying something old, the key to relaxation is to enjoy our time, without guilt or watching the clock.

GENTLE EXERCISE FOR PHYSICAL WELLNESS

Walking

Walking is one of the most convenient, accessible—and also free—forms of exercise. You don't have to buy expensive equipment (the only thing you'll need is a good pair of shoes) and you can walk almost anywhere, be it in a city or in the countryside.

Walking is a gentle form of exercise, so it's ideal if you haven't been physically active recently. You can walk as fast or as slow as you like and build up your pace over time as you get fitter.

Walking outdoors gives you the chance to breathe in fresh air and enjoy the environment. A simple stroll and a change of scene can help reinvigorate you, boost your mood, and clear your head.

If you're not keen on going out on your own, or you would like to make this an opportunity to connect with other walkers and to try new routes, look for local walking groups you could join. Many communities have walking groups, while some neighborhoods have groups that meet regularly. You could try starting your own; for example, post a notice at your local community center to find others who want to walk. If you're wary of meeting strangers, choose somewhere public for your first outing, such as a park.

Jogging

Like walking, jogging is another convenient and free form of exercise. Once you have a decent pair of running shoes, you can get started straightaway. Again, as with walking, you can pick your pace and enjoy being outdoors and getting some headspace. Local parks are a great place to jog and, if you go frequently or at the same time of day, you may find you begin to spot other regulars, with the added bonus of making it a sociable time as well.

If you don't want to jog on your own, see if any friends or family would like to join you. There are also many local running clubs where new members are always welcome, or you could try out a fun run to meet other like-minded people.

Dance classes

One of the best things about dance classes is that they often don't feel like exercise. You can get so absorbed in the rhythm of the music and enjoying yourself that the time will fly. There are a host of different styles, from ballroom, ballet, tap, and salsa to street dance, swing, Bollywood, jive, and jazz.

If you're unsure what type of dance class would be best for you, see if you can have a taster session. That way you can try out the different methods and see which best suits your fitness level, interests, and ability. Look for details of local dance classes running at community centers or gyms, or ask on social media for recommendations. In most cases you don't need to worry about a dance partner—there will always be someone at the class that you can pair up with if needed.

Gym

If you prefer to exercise inside, going to the gym is the ideal choice. You can use exercise equipment such as rowing machines, treadmills, or exercise bikes, or take advantage of one of the many classes that gyms offer.

Buying a gym membership can help with motivation and encourage you to go regularly. The wide variety of classes on offer also gives you the chance to try out different forms of exercise and helps increase the chance of you finding something that you enjoy, making fitness fun.

When you're looking for a gym to join, find out if they offer free trials, and take advantage of everything that they have. Look for special offers on gym memberships that could save you money.

Exercise outdoors for the combined benefit of fresh air and sunshine.

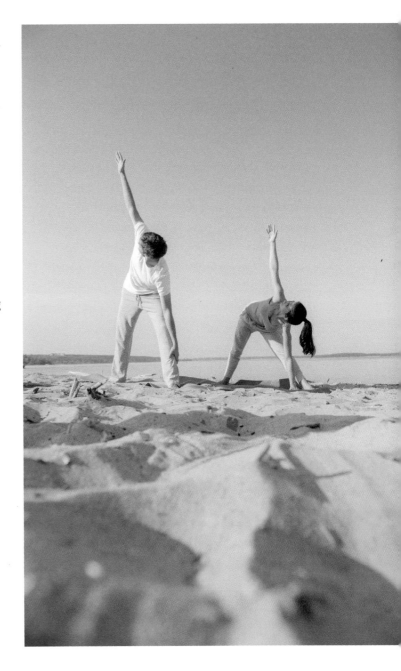

PILATES

The main principle of Pilates is that exercise is essentially a mind—body technique and when you exercise you mentally focus on the muscle groups that you are using. Pilates recognizes that it is only through the synchronizing of thought and action that exercise is truly effective; to create a healthy and fit body you need to integrate the mental, physical, and spiritual spheres.

Mind over matter

It has long been established that the mind has an enormous influence on the health of the body. Research shows that the mind has an infinite capacity to induce positive physiological effects, which have both an internal and external effect. You may have noticed that when you're in a good mood you automatically seem to look and feel better.

Think for a moment how you feel when you are stressed. Not very pleasant. This is because your body produces an excess of "stress" chemicals (e.g., adrenaline and cortisol), which causes your whole system to speed up. Your heart beats faster, your blood pressure goes up, your breathing becomes rapid and shallow. At times, this type of response is necessary. It is what motivates you when you are faced with a crisis. In large doses this type of reaction can, however, be extremely harmful and can lead to all sorts of unpleasant symptoms such as dizziness, shaking, profuse sweating, insomnia, and migraines. Positive feelings of calm and contentment have a much more beneficial effect, as they induce the body to produce health-enhancing, feel-good chemicals (e.g., endorphins and serotonin), which are vital for well-being. They promote a sense of serenity—you breathe more easily and deeply, your heart rate is slower, and your blood pressure lowers. The more relaxed you feel, the less tension you hold in the muscles throughout your body. This has a beneficial effect on your posture and your general bearing.

Mindful exercise

If thoughts are so powerful, it makes sense to try and harness your thinking to bring about positive changes in your body. This is, in fact, the very essence of Pilates. By learning to execute each exercise correctly you are also allowing your mind to exert a greater influence over your body. With Pilates you do only a limited number of repetitions. You do them slowly, so that you can concentrate more clearly on directing your energy toward what it is you are trying to achieve. If you view your body in a negative way, you will need to reverse your direction of thought. Positive thoughts bring about positive changes.

To ensure that an exercise can be of real benefit and bring about changes, for example a strong, straight back, it is necessary to complement each physical action with a mental focus. By practicing creative visualizations regularly, you will gradually develop the ability to internalize the physical changes that you wish to make.

Once you've done this, the external changes will start to appear. As you become aware of your body and its needs, you can consciously start to make changes through exercise. Pilates is based on lengthening and stretching the body to its full potential. This eventually creates a longer, leaner

The more relaxed you feel, the less tension you hold in the muscles throughout your body.

shape, increased flexibility, and a suppleness that promotes a greater ease of movement. These exercises concentrate on strengthening weak muscles and stretching those that are too tight. Initially, it may take a while to fully understand the mechanisms, and if you're new to Pilates, you should expect to do only about 30 percent of what you will eventually be capable of doing. It takes about ten sessions to comprehend the technique. Pilates is a form of exercise that gets progressively more difficult, but the results are worth it. In time, you will look taller, slimmer, and more toned.

Creative visualization

Whatever we create in our lives begins as a basic image in our minds. Many of these images are unconscious. Through creative visualization it is possible to alter these thoughts and pictures. With Pilates, the idea is to create an image in your mind that will help you to focus on the area of the body that you are working. This requires a very deep level of concentration, which does become easier with practice. On a superficial level, many of the exercises appear quite simple. How you physically position your arms and legs, however, is only part of the process. Pilates, unlike many other disciplines, is actually much more complex, as with each movement you must be constantly aware of what your entire body is doing. Even when you are doing a series of movements specifically designed to work a certain group of muscles, such as your quads, you must always remember to be equally focused on the rest of your body. Initially, this can seem quite difficult and using visualization techniques can be enormously helpful.

Understanding how your body should be feeling means it becomes easier to assume the correct position. Eventually, these images will arise naturally through association, without too much effort.

Basic techniques

Anyone can learn to visualize. It helps, though, if you can begin by feeling relaxed. A still mind is more conducive to conjuring up images.

• Spend a few minutes gathering your thoughts. Try to forget about external influences such as work and any worries you might have. This is your time.
• Do some gentle stretches and focus on your breathing. Slow, deep breathing has an instant calming effect because it helps to promote soothing alpha brain waves. Once you are feeling sufficiently relaxed, you can start your exercises.
• As you exercise, focus on each part of your body. How does it feel? With each exercise try to perceive a specific picture. If you are trying to envision yourself on a sandy beach, focus clearly on how this feels. Think of images that will help you to get into exactly the right position.
• Invite each image to emerge with as much intensity as possible, so that you can almost feel it. Once you have created a familiar picture, eventually all you will have to do is to focus on it and your body will automatically respond. The concept of Pilates is to bring about permanent changes. You can hasten this process by using visualization techniques when you are not exercising. These will automatically help you to walk, stand, and sit in the correct way.

PILATES FOR POSTURE AND BREATHING

Perfect posture: how to look instantly taller and slimmer

Not sure if you're standing correctly? Then practice this position for a few minutes daily. After a while it will feel so natural that you no longer have to think about it. Stand with your feet hip-width apart. Imagine that you're standing on sand. Your feet are relaxed. Think of your weight being over the middle of each foot, with your toes gently lengthening into the sand. Close your eyes and make a mental note of the following:

• Don't sink back into your heels or lean forward. Keep your weight evenly distributed over your feet.
• Let your arms fall naturally in front of your body.
• Let your hands hang from the shoulders, totally loose and relaxed.
• Don't lock your knees. They should feel relaxed and not rigid.
• Keep your inside thighs and bottom relaxed.

• Imagine that your head is like a beach ball bobbing up and down on the water. It's not going side to side but resting directly upon your shoulders and rocking gently up and down until it settles into a comfortable, neutral position.
• Think of the bones directly behind your ears. Try to imagine them "reaching" toward the ceiling.
• Pull your stomach in, without tipping the pelvis forward. Think of a piece of string from your pubic bone to your navel. It is shortening as you pull up and in. Feel your tailbone drop—as if it is weighted to the floor. This will seem much easier after you've done more of the stretches to release the pelvic girdle.
• Keep the front of your thighs relaxed. Now your whole body is perfectly aligned—you should feel as if you are floating an inch off the ground.

Breathing

Correct breathing is a very important facet of Pilates. By remembering to breathe properly, you'll find it becomes much easier to exercise. The problem is that most people don't breathe deeply enough. Breathing slowly and deeply is very energizing. It ensures there is sufficient oxygen circulating throughout the body. It may sound obvious, but when you exercise do not hold your breath. It's better to breathe incorrectly than not at all. Practice the following exercise before you start any of the stomach work.

Breathing slowly and deeply is very energizing.

Basic breathing exercise

Lie on your back in a relaxed position, resting your head on a folded towel, with your knees bent.

• Place one hand on your stomach and, very gently, breathe in through your nose. Feel your lungs filling with oxygen, and slowly expand and relax your stomach. Breathe out.

• With one finger on your pubic bone and one on your navel, try to shorten that gap as you breathe out, and flatten your stomach to your spine without tilting your pelvis.

• Breathe in again and feel that gap slightly expand.

• Breathe out. Imagine there is a piece of string or an elastic band that links your pubic bone to your navel. Very gently feel it pulling up and in. This will get all three sets of stomach muscles working, including your oblique muscles, which will tighten your waist. Make sure you breathe slowly and deeply. One of the main rules of Pilates is to breathe out on the point of effort. If in doubt, particularly on the stretches—breathe naturally. When you breathe in, your stomach gently expands. However, it shouldn't swell in an exaggerated way. Try to think of your rib cage expanding gently to the sides so that you're not just breathing into your throat and upper chest.

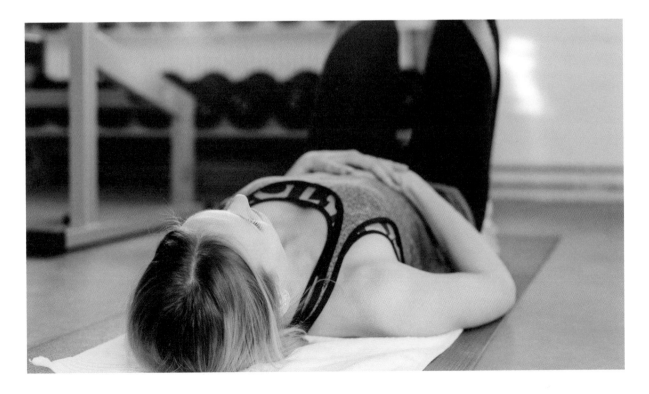

PILATES FOR BETTER BALANCE

If you're worried about slipping, tripping, or not being able to catch objects thrown toward you, your sense of balance is probably poor. What seems to occur, as you get older or as a result of any injury, is that you lose your awareness of balance and your reflexes are no longer as sharp. This can cause feelings of insecurity. Perhaps you begin to worry more about safety. We all know that the simplest of falls might have serious consequences. This is reflected in the body, which becomes stiff and constricted as a result. The easiest way to change this is to practice the following exercises every day. In time, you will start to feel lighter and more confident in the way you move. For each of these exercises, the same rules as the "perfect posture" exercise apply (see the checklist on page 42).

Standing on one leg

• With bare feet, stand on one leg, lift your hands above your head, and imagine you are on a beach with soft sand between your toes. Keep your other leg slightly lifted.
• Count for ten seconds and change legs. Repeat four times, twice on each leg.
• Now, do the same—with your eyes closed. Make sure you have something to hold onto, in case you fall over.

Standing on one leg with a towel

Do exactly the same as above, standing on a flat towel. This gives you a slightly more unstable surface and makes the exercise more difficult. Even if you don't exercise regularly, try to do these every day—especially if you are over 45.

Walking backward

Start in the "perfect posture" position and, with feet approximately an inch apart, start to walk backward. Slowly drag your foot back, so that it never entirely leaves the floor. The easiest way to master this is to imagine that you are trying to remove some chewing gum from under your feet.

Look in the mirror—but do not look down at your feet. This exercise is even more effective if you imagine you are walking on sand.

This exercise is even more effective if you imagine you are walking on sand.

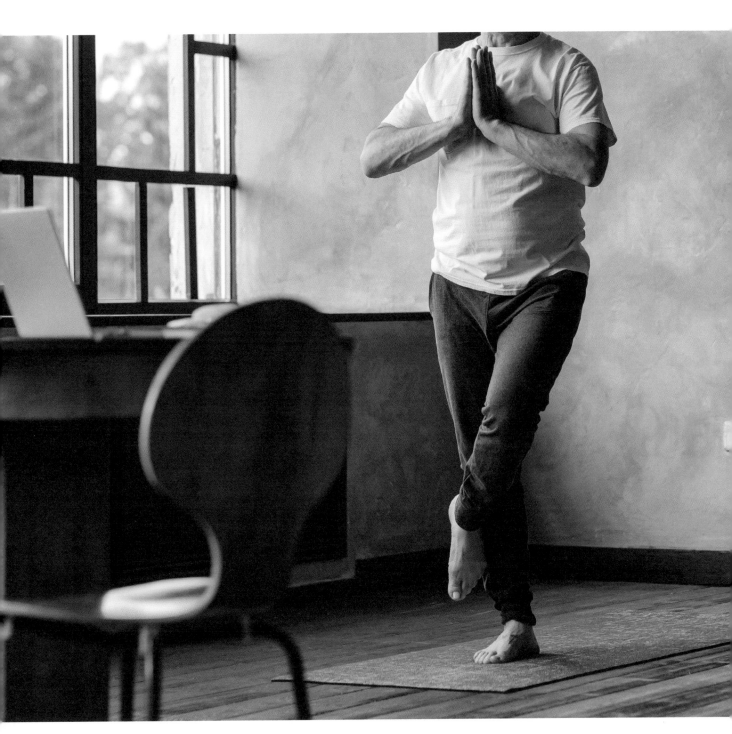

YOGA

The word "yoga" means union of body, mind, and spirit with the universal spirit. The yogis of ancient India realized that for perfect health and inner peace, both body and mind must work together in perfect harmony. Yoga's combination of intricate physical postures, deep breathing exercises, balances, relaxation, and meditation are the perfect discipline to relieve stress, calm the mind, and tone the entire body, both inside and out.

Benefits of yoga

In the quest to earn more, do more, and have more, modern humans subject themselves to increased physical and mental stress. Unfortunately, although medicine has made many amazing breakthroughs in the West over the last hundred years, the focus continues to be on treating diseases and not their causes. This is where yoga can help us all so much.

Yoga's physical movements, combined with deep breathing exercises, will carefully rid the body of tension and stimulate the delivery of oxygen-rich blood to our cells, so providing them with the nutrients that they require. As well as toning all of our muscles, the physical exercises will also strengthen our bones and keep our spine and joints flexible.

Yoga's calming balances necessitate tremendous concentration and so they take the mind off its day-to-day activities, giving it a rest. From breathing exercises to relaxation and meditation, yoga will help calm the mind and help us to achieve the peace we often need and desire. And just as stress inhibits our energy flow, a calm and peaceful mind will lead to abundant energy and that genuine "good to be alive" feeling. Eventually, we stop looking elsewhere for our pleasures and concentrate on "looking within," disciplining our mind to search inside ourselves for our joy and happiness.

Origins of yoga

It is unclear when yoga actually originated, but seals were discovered depicting a yoga posture during the excavation of some ruins in prehistoric India, and revealed a very advanced civilization dating to around 5000 BC. The earliest texts mentioning yoga were the Vedas, and these seem to have spanned from 3000 to 1200 BC. These texts were followed by the Upanishads, written between 800 and 400 BC. The word "Upanishad" literally describes a sitting where the master or guru instructs his pupils. This is how yoga has been passed on from generation to generation over the years. Patanjali's Yoga Sutras, written between 200 BC and AD 200, are a crucial yoga text. Patanjali wrote of a practical eight-part approach to yoga, frequently referred to as the Eight Limbs of Yoga.

These eight limbs were not regarded as a ladder to be climbed one rung at a time, but more the necessary ingredients in the recipe for life. The ancient yogis realized that life can be a difficult and complicated journey, but its careful teachings and disciplines guide us along our path. They had a deep understanding of human nature and of the mind-body connection, and they devised this system to help us obtain happiness and peace of mind, as well as a perfectly toned, healthy body.

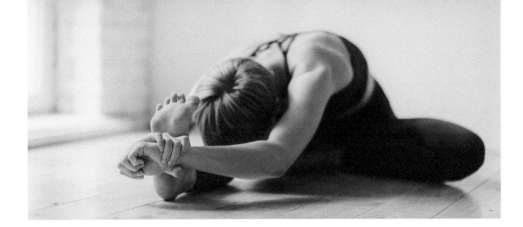

The Eight Limbs of Yoga

1. Yamas

These are moral guidelines and are the basic principles of right living and restraint; they include no violence, stealing, or envy, and command us to be truthful with both others and ourselves. Yoga teaches us that happiness is not in external objects but within ourselves.

2. Niyamas

These are the personal disciplines of daily life. They are cleanliness of mind and body, purity, contentment, study, work, and devotion to God or the universal spirit. A temple of the spirit and keeping the body in perfect condition is our duty.

3. Asanas

These are the yoga exercises or postures. It is said that there are 840,000 of them! These movements work the entire body, freeing it from tension, toning, and firming and strengthening every muscle, internal organ, and gland. The balancing postures teach us the power of concentration and focus. Deep relaxation calms the mind, and meditation trains the mind to achieve stillness and peace.

4. Pranayama

This is yoga's breath control. There are many breathing exercises in yoga to stimulate life-giving oxygen to every cell, to energize the body, and calm and soothe the mind. The word *pranayama* means "controlling the energy flow."

5. Pratyahara

This is the withdrawal of the senses from the external world to the self within to give one peace and calm. This is achieved by practicing the *asanas* and *pranayama*. Most of our daily activities necessitate our concentration and involvement with external objects and thoughts, but by concentrating on our body, and by concentrating on our breathing, the mind and body become peaceful and calm.

6. Dharana

This is the power of constant concentration and focusing of the mind. They discipline the mind to concentrate on just one spot while performing the balances. This skill develops so that eventually one is able to concentrate and focus on a subject of interest even in the midst of turmoil.

7. Dhyana

This is meditation. Meditation is a powerful tool for freeing our minds from the pressures of life, helping us feel peaceful and calm. When this is accomplished, new ideas appear and the way ahead looks clearer.

8. Samadhi

This is the result of our total efforts and is the experience of enlightenment and bliss, living in the present moment, and the realization that we can manifest whatever we wish. The mind becomes full of joy and peace. It is the state of union with the universal spirit or God.

YOGA TODAY

The collective knowledge of these ancient texts began to appear in the West at the end of the nineteenth century, and since then interest in yoga has grown to an all-time high. Students of all ages are pouring into classes to learn yoga, and for many diverse reasons. Some come simply to improve their body shape, some to cure an aching back, some to relieve stress. Whatever the reason, yoga can help you live healthily in this chaotic, exciting, and wonderful modern world.

While hatha yoga remains the most widely practiced form of yoga in the West, other forms include:

- Raja yoga—the yoga of the mind
- Karma yoga—the yoga of action
- Bhakti yoga—the yoga of devotion
- Jnana yoga—the yoga of the intellect

Because of the many approaches to teaching yoga, finding a class to suit you can be very confusing. I often receive phone calls from people inquiring as to what sort of yoga I teach. I suppose that since I have been teaching for over thirty years, by now I have put my individual stamp on the ancient art. Throughout this time, I have tried to make yoga understandable, enjoyable, and available to all. It is my firm belief that everyone can benefit tremendously from yoga practice.

But how can you find a class that will be to your liking? I am afraid that this will be a bit like trying to find everything else—from a plumber to a dentist. Often you have to try several until the perfect one appears. There are some excellent yoga teachers around, so quite simply search for a class until you find one that works for you. As a first move, you can't do better than to search online to find classes near where you live.

Guidelines for practicing

You need very little equipment for your yoga practice, so it is easy to fit in with any lifestyle. Once you have learned your basic movements, you can do them at home or even on vacation. Having said this, there are a few basic guidelines that you should take note of before you start.

- You need a warm, airy room if you are practicing inside, but in warmer climates it is wonderful to do your yoga outside. Never practice in the heat of direct sun.
- You need a mat or blanket to sit on. My preference is for a blanket or thick, warm mat for indoor practice. However, if you are practicing yoga outside, perhaps on a beach, you need a waterproof mat to keep you clean and dry.
- Wear loose clothing, ideally a leotard and leggings for women, or leggings and a close-fitting T-shirt. Jogging bottoms or shorts and a T-shirt are best for men. If you are outdoors in a warm climate, your swimsuit is just fine.
- Bare feet are essential for yoga practice. Always wait at least two hours after a main meal before you practice yoga.
- The golden rule of yoga is never ever to strain.

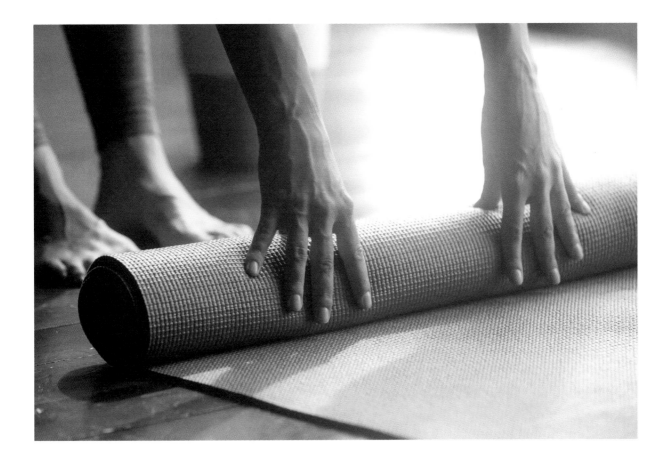

• Don't worry if you are stiff and uncoordinated to start with. This is quite normal. Just persevere, work at your own pace, and you will be delighted at how quickly your body responds to the movements and how much more flexible you are after only a few weeks of practice. You will start to feel better almost immediately and will soon be delighted with your new svelte shape.

• Although yoga is for everyone, if you have any health concerns it is always wise to check with your doctor before you begin. Never substitute yoga for your doctor's treatment. Yoga is good for your health and some movements are particularly beneficial for certain conditions. However, they must never replace medical attention.

• If you are pregnant and have not done any yoga before, then please wait until after your checkup at about fifteen weeks. If everything is OK and your doctor is happy, then you may start to practice yoga very gently, omitting the movements marked unsuitable for pregnancy.

• Following the baby's birth, wait until after your six-week checkup before you recommence your yoga practice. If your doctor is happy for you to restart, then inform your teacher of the nature of your delivery. Go gently and soon you will find your shape and energy coming back fast. In yoga we breathe deeply with every movement to help to stimulate the delivery of oxygen to every cell and energize our entire systems. Breathing is done through the nose. As a general rule, gently allow your abdominals to push out as you inhale deeply through the nose at the start of a posture, and exhale slowly and quietly through the nose as you go into the movement. While in the positions, breathe calmly and peacefully through the nose.

MORNING YOGA WORKOUT

Have you ever watched an animal wake up after a rest? It stretches its body from top to toe. This gets rid of tension and makes sure it is in perfect condition to start the day. This morning yoga workout is an ideal sequence to start your day. It will greatly improve your shape and flexibility, give you bundles of energy, and can be a tremendous help to people with an aching back.

The energizing breath

This is a wonderful breathing exercise. It is a great tonic when done first thing in the morning, but it will also give you that "good to be alive" feeling anytime, anywhere.

1. Stand straight with your feet together. Place your fingertips interleaved under your chin with your elbows together. Inhale slowly through your nose for a count of five. As you do this, bring your elbows up as high as possible. Feel the breath at the back of your throat.

2. Gently let your head drop back and exhale slowly and thoroughly through your mouth. At the end of the exhalation, slowly bring your elbows together as your head returns to its normal position. Repeat this cycle five times to begin with, increasing to ten times as you become used to the movement.

BENEFITS: This stretch is excellent for slimming and toning the midriff and waistline, and releasing tension in the lower back.

NOTE

This movement sounds simple, but standing straight and moving your head back can be quite difficult at first. Please don't worry. Many people have a lot of tension in their necks, but as you progress in yoga you will find it becomes easier. Also, some people feel dizzy or light-headed at first. If so, start by doing the movement only twice and take your head just a tiny way back, gradually building up to five times as you progress.

Sideways stretch

Stand straight with your legs at least 3 feet apart and your toes facing forward. Inhale deeply and lift your right hand in the air. Exhale, gently bend over to the left side, sliding your left hand down your left leg. Don't strain. Breathing normally, hold the position for a count of five, increasing to ten as you progress. Inhale and slowly return to an upright position. Exhale, slowly lower your arm, and relax. Repeat the movement to the other side.

BENEFITS: Because of our sedentary lifestyles, most people use less than one-third of their lung capacity. This wonderful movement helps to increase lung capacity, so increasing the oxygen supply to all our cells. This will give you energy and help to relieve stress.

Because of our sedentary lifestyle, most people use less than one-third of their lung capacity.

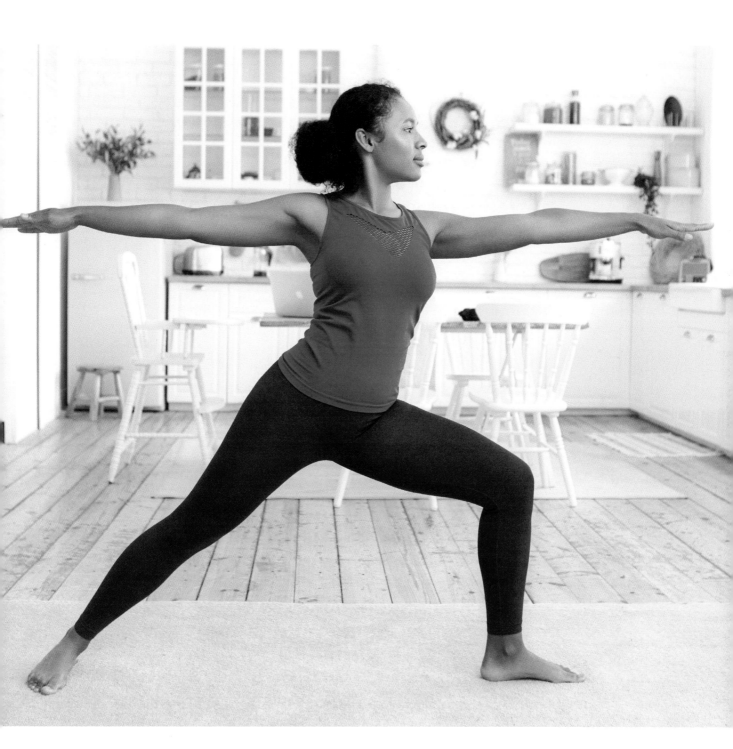

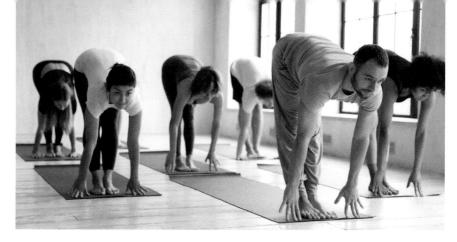

Head-to-knee posture

1. Stand straight with your legs together. Inhale and lift your arms up above your head. Entwine your fingers together and stretch your body upward (A). This is great for helping to realign your spine and release tension from your entire body. As you lower your arms, exhale slowly through your nose. Repeat the movement. Now place your right foot about 3 feet in front of your left foot.

2. Inhale and move your arms behind your back so that your palms meet. As you exhale with your head up, back flat, and legs straight, start to move forward, aiming your chin just past your knee (B). Don't worry if you are nowhere near this position to start with. Just relax in your maximum position and stay there for a count of five, breathing normally. Take note of your maximum stretch on this side.

BENEFITS: This movement helps to correct imbalances in the lower back. It firms the backs of the thighs and calves and the bottom, and slims the midriff and waistline.

(A)

(B)

Forward and backward bend

1. Stand straight with your feet about 1 foot apart and your toes facing forward. Inhale deeply, and slowly lift your arms in the air, stretching them upward. Exhale slowly through the nose as you move calmly and gently forward, keeping your back flat and your legs straight (A). Relax in your maximum position and stay there, breathing normally. Don't worry if your maximum position isn't very far in the beginning. It will improve quicker than you can imagine. Do not strain yourself.

2. Breathing normally, stay in the maximum position for a count of five, increasing to ten as you progress. Eventually your chin will be on your shin (B). Again, this might seem impossible at first, but with practice you'll get there, I promise!

3. Slowly lift your head and, as you inhale, continue to come up slowly into an upright position with your hands stretched up above your head. Keeping your eyes on your thumbs, start to relax gently backward, exhaling in your maximum position (C). Again, don't worry if only an inch is possible to begin with. Breathing normally, hold your backward stretch for a count of five. Then inhale and slowly return to an upright position. Exhale, lower your arms, and relax. Repeat this movement once.

BENEFITS: An excellent stretch, this gently releases tension from the whole body and ensures wonderful flexibility of the spine. It tones the legs, especially the backs of the thighs, and firms the abdomen, midriff, waistline, and throat. It is great for the skin and hair because it increases circulation to these areas.

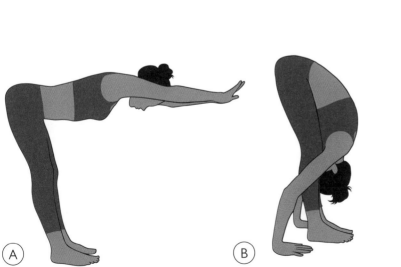

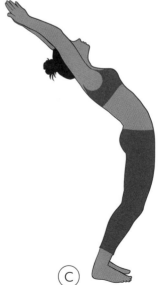

Rishi's posture

1. Stand straight with your feet 3 feet apart. Inhale and stretch your arms up in the air. As you exhale, move forward slowly and, with your legs straight and back flat, touch your left leg with your right hand (A). Eventually you will be able to slide your right hand under your left foot, but in the early stages just touch the leg where it feels comfortable, keeping both legs straight.

2. Slowly lift your left arm in the air and carefully turn your body so you are looking at your left hand (B). Breathing normally, hold for a count of five. Then slowly lower your arm and relax forward, clasping

your legs and gently pulling your upper body toward the legs. Breathe normally. Inhale, and then, as you exhale, grasp your right leg with your left hand and slowly lift your right arm in the air. Again, turn your body carefully to enable you to look up at your right hand (C). Breathing normally, hold for a count of five.

3. Relax forward, clasping both legs and drawing the body inward. Inhale and lift your head, then slowly return to an upright position, stretching your arms above your head. Now place your hands at your waistline with your thumbs in front and fingers behind, and with full lungs gently bend backward,

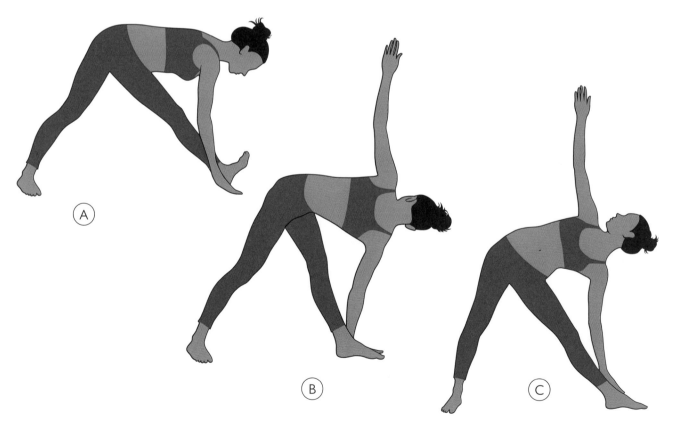

exhaling as you reach your maximum backward bend (D). Breathing normally, hold your maximum backward bend for a count of five. Then inhale as you return to an upright position. Exhale, relax, and repeat the entire movement.

BENEFITS: This is excellent for rebalancing the lower back and is great for people who suffer from tension in this region. I recommend it for tennis players and golfers, who can frequently suffer from aches and pain in the lower back. The movement also firms the midriff, waistline, bottom, and thighs and keeps the spine in an excellent condition, giving it great flexibility. A real gem of a movement.

The awkward posture

1. Stand straight with your feet about 1 foot apart and your toes facing forward, not outward.

2. Take a deep breath in and, as you exhale, keeping your back straight, gently lower your bottom to your heels (A). Don't worry if only halfway is possible in the beginning stages. Just do your best without straining.

3. Hold your maximum movement for a count of five. Then inhale and gradually return to an upright position, keeping your back straight (do not bend forward). Exhale, relax, and repeat this movement twice.

BENEFITS: This does wonders for your thighs—it really tones and firms them. It also greatly improves the flexibility of the knees and strengthens the arches of the feet, as well as the toes and ankles. In my opinion, this simple ten-minute sequence is worth its weight in gold. It will give you energy, improve your shape, and is excellent for helping with and preventing back problems.

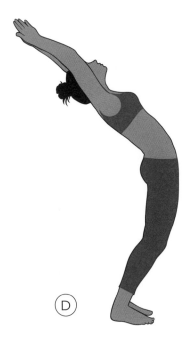

D

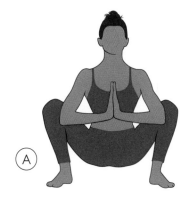

A

YOGA TONING: LOWER BODY

Yoga balances firm, tone, and strengthen virtually every muscle in the legs and bottom and are excellent for keeping our joints and lower back flexible. They help to strengthen the bones in the legs since the entire weight of the body is transferred to just one leg during these movements. The balances also teach us the power of focus and concentration as we learn to focus on a spot to enable us to do the movements. This takes our mind off our daily activities and gives it a rest, making us concentrate on the present moment. Although difficult to start with, most beginners are delighted that they are able to do these movements with ease in a relatively short time.

Tree pose

1. Standing straight, inhale and lift your right foot onto your left thigh. This sounds easy but can be quite difficult to start with. Don't worry or strain yourself. Even if you start by placing your foot on your ankle, calf, or knee in the beginning stages, you will assist your joints back to their natural flexibility. Yoga and perseverance will get you there!

2. Inhale and lift your arms in the air (A). Placing the palms of your hands together, stare at a spot on the floor or wall to help your balance. Breathing normally, hold this position for a count of five, increasing to ten as you progress. Exhale, lower your arms, replace your foot on the floor, and relax. Repeat to the other side, and then repeat the entire sequence.

> BENEFITS: This movement is excellent for toning and firming your inner and outer thighs and strengthening your legs. It also aids the flexibility in your ankles, knees, and hips. The balances take your thoughts off your day-to-day activities, so giving your mind a rest.

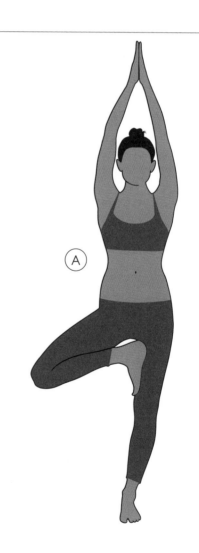

Standing stick balance

Standing straight with your feet together, inhale and lift your arms in the air, placing the palms of your hands together and crossing the thumbs. Inhale and place your right foot in front of the left. Exhale and, leaning forward, lift the left leg so that the entire body resembles a capital T (A). Stare at a spot to aid your balance. Breathing normally, stretch the body, fingers forward and the left leg back, and hold for a count of five, increasing to ten as you progress. Inhale and return to an upright position. Exhale and relax. Repeat on the other side, then repeat the entire sequence.

BENEFITS: This movement is excellent for toning and firming your inner and outer thighs and strengthening your legs. It also aids the flexibility in your ankles, knees, and hips. The balances take your thoughts off your day-to-day activities, so giving your mind a rest.

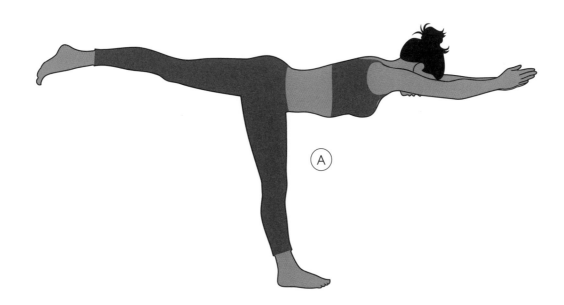

YOGA TONING: ABDOMINALS AND WAIST

Do not attempt any of these movements during pregnancy. These exercises are invaluable for keeping the abdomen firm, toned, uplifted, and youthful. The contraction massages your internal organs (your small intestine, colon, pancreas, gallbladder, and heart). The movement can help tremendously in stimulating peristalsis and relieving constipation, and gives relief to those who suffer from irritable bowel syndrome and abdominal bloating.

Boat pose

1. On a mat or blanket, sit straight with both legs straight out in front of you (A). Stretch out your arms parallel to the floor. Inhale and, as you exhale gently, lift your legs from the floor and balance on your bottom (B). Hold the position for a count of one to begin with, gradually increasing to ten as you progress, then gently lower your legs to the floor and relax. Repeat the movement twice. This can be hard work, but move carefully and build it up gently. Remember, never strain in the posture. Following the movement, lie on your back, draw your knees to your chest, and gently rock your back from side to side to relieve any tension in your lower back.

> BENEFITS: This is a powerful hamstring stretch. It tones the back of your thighs and is a help in getting rid of cellulite.

2. Once you are comfortable with step 1, repeat the instructions but try taking the pose further by fully stretching out your legs, so that your body forms a V shape (C). Exhale to the count of one to start with, increasing to ten as you progress. This is very powerful—do not strain!

3. Gently lower your legs to the floor, then relax. Repeat the movement twice. Following the movement, lie down and gently draw your knees to your chest and rock from side to side.

> BENEFITS: Again, this is a powerful toner for your abdomen, thighs, and lower back.

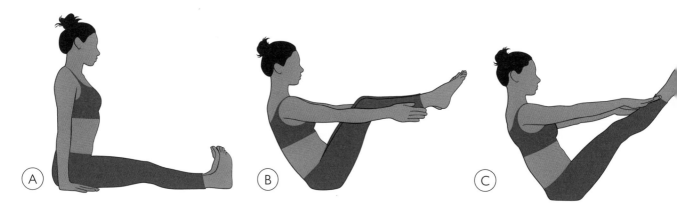

Slow motion firming

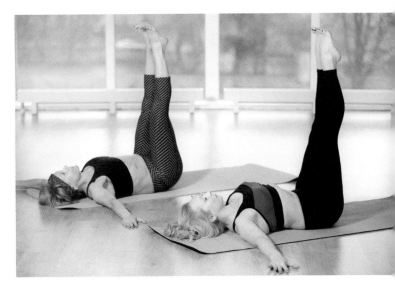

1. Sit up with your back straight and with both legs straight out in front of you and together. Reach out to touch your toes (A). Inhale and lift your arms in the air.

2. Exhale as you slowly move forward, keeping your back and legs straight—do not strain, just allow your body to flow easily and gently into your maximum position. You should eventually aim to clasp your feet and draw your chin to your knees (B).

3. Inhale as you slowly return to an upright position, then exhale as you gently lie flat. Place your arms flat on the floor behind your head. Inhale and gently bend your knees, lift your legs up, and straighten them so that they are at right angles to your body (see above picture).

4. Exhale as you slowly lower your legs to the floor. In the beginning stages, make this part of the movement relatively fast, then slow it down as your abdominals firm and strengthen. For people with weak backs, you may feel a small pull in your lower back to start with. If this occurs, immediately bend your knees and then continue to lower your legs with your knees bent.

As you progress, you will find that you will be able to go further before having to bend your knees. Inhale as you slowly come up into a sitting position, stretching your arms up in the air. If you find this difficult in the beginning stages, then use your elbows to help you push off. Exhale as you relax and stretch forward into a back stretch. Repeat this sequence twice, increasing to four times as your back and abdominals become stronger. Then lie down, draw your knees into your chest, and gently relax your back into the floor, rocking from side to side. Then lie flat, slow down your breathing, and relax.

BENEFITS: This beautiful sequence will deliver the results you want—a firm tummy and strong back—and it will really relax you, helping you to deep, restful sleep.

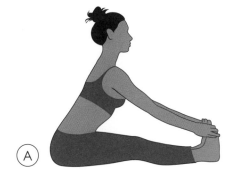

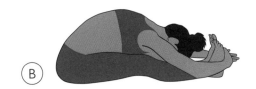

YOGA TONING: UPPER BODY

On the physical level, these exercises are amazing in how they tone your upper arms, neck, jaw, and throat, while releasing the tension in the back of your neck and shoulders. They also stimulate blood flow to the head and neck area, so benefiting your skin, hair, and brain cells. The tensions of the mind are frequently stored in the back of the neck (the proverbial pain in the neck) and lumbar spine. These powerful exercises carefully relax both these areas.

The chest expansion

1. Stand with your feet together and your back straight (A). Interlock your hands behind your back, gently pulling your shoulders back and straightening your arms.

2. Inhale and lift your arms up as high as possible behind your back, then exhale as you slowly bend forward into your maximum forward bend, keeping your back and legs straight (B). Breathing normally, relax and hold your maximum position for a count of five. Your aim is to be able to place your chin on the top of the shin, just under the knee. It will happen eventually, but remember not to strain!

3. Inhale and lift your head, then slowly return to an upright position and gently bend backward, pulling your arms back down and under your bottom. In your maximum position, exhale and hold for a count of five. Inhale and return to an upright position, hold your arms up behind your back for an extra count of two, then lower them and relax. Repeat the movement twice.

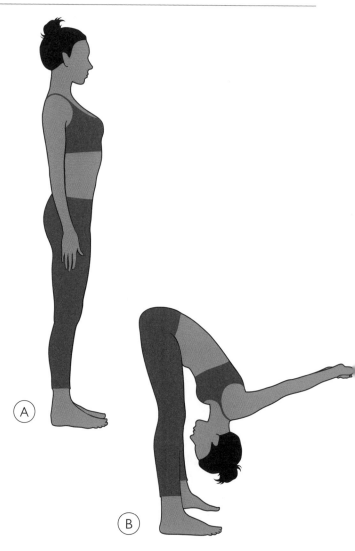

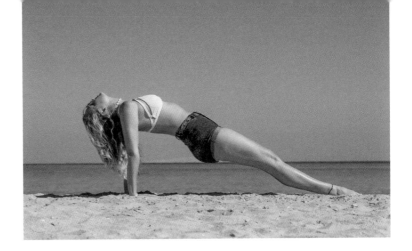

Planet pose

1. Sit straight with your hands comfortably on the floor behind you, about 1 foot behind your bottom, with your fingertips facing backward. Your legs should be straight out in front of you. Inhale and, as you exhale, keeping your body in a straight line, place your weight on your arms and gently lift your body from the floor (see above picture). Ensure that your legs are straight and your toes are on the floor. Hold for a count of one at first, increasing to ten as you become stronger. Slowly lower your bottom to the floor and relax. Repeat this movement once.

BENEFITS: This is so good for the strength of your hands, arms, wrists, and fingers. It gives great shape to your upper arms and shoulders, helps to correct drooping shoulders, and releases tension in the lower back.

Sideways body raise

If you have had a wrist or arm problem, follow the directions below but do not lift your bottom—just put a little weight on your hands to strengthen them gradually. Follow these instructions only when your arms are sufficiently strong.

1. Place both hands on the floor to the right-hand side of your body. Keep your knees bent and make sure that your hands and feet are on a nonslip surface. Inhale and, as you exhale, lift your body from the floor, ensuring that your weight is supported on both hands and both feet. Adjust your body so that your right shoulder is directly above your right wrist and that your arm is straight. Lift your bottom and make sure the left foot is on top of the right one and that the body is in a straight line. When, and only when, you feel strong enough, lift your left arm from the floor and stretch it toward the ceiling (A). Concentrate on a spot on the floor and hold your balance for a count of five, then relax. Gently lower your bottom to the floor and repeat on the other side. Repeat the whole movement once.

BENEFITS: An excellent arm toner and firmer that gives good shape to your upper arms and shoulders. This movement greatly strengthens the wrists, hands, elbows, and shoulders. An extra benefit is in the way it stretches the hands. For those who spend many hours at the computer, the wrists can become very stiff and painful and this movement can help tremendously.

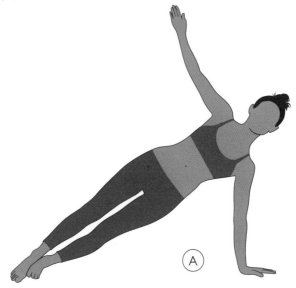

AEROBIC WORKOUTS

Aerobic, or cardio, exercise is so called because it gets your heart pumping and increases the flow of blood to your muscles and lungs. Aerobic exercise is known to improve fitness, burn calories, help with weight loss, and boost your overall physical and mental health.

Medical practitioners recommend that adults should do at least 150 minutes (2 hours and 30 minutes) a week of moderate-intensity aerobic physical activity, or 75 minutes (1 hour and 15 minutes) of vigorous-intensity aerobic activity each week. Vigorous-intensity activity means an activity that makes you breathe hard and fast—you're unlikely to be able to talk much without needing to pause for breath while you're doing it.

It's possible to meet your weekly target from just one single session of aerobic activity, but a lot of people find it more practical to break it into several smaller sessions spread out over a couple of days, or even do a little each day. Smaller chunks of exercise may fit in with your schedule and work commitments more easily and be more achievable than one long workout. One of the benefits of aerobic exercise is that there are a lot of options to choose from, so hopefully you should be able to find something that meets your needs and that you enjoy. You can mix it up, too, trying out different exercises when you fancy a change.

Types of aerobic exercise include running, swimming, hiking, jumping rope, dancing, kickboxing, brisk walking, in-line skating, water aerobics, tennis, working out on cardio machines, and cycling. To get you started, here are some simple aerobic workout ideas that you can perform at home, indoors or outdoors, to meet your fitness and exercise goals.

Warm up

Before you start doing an aerobic workout, you'll need to warm up. This will help reduce the risk of injuries and prepare your body by releasing the tension in different parts of your body. Ideally, aim to warm up for at least five minutes before you start exercising, or longer if you feel your body is stiff and needs it.

Start your warm-up by marching in place, then march back and forth, swinging your arms as you go. Then do the following:

• Ten shoulder rolls—continue marching in place with your arms loose by your sides and roll your shoulders forward ten times, then backward ten times.

• Ten head rolls—stand and rotate your head gently in a clockwise direction, then repeat in a counterclockwise direction.

• Ten upper body twists—stand with your feet shoulder-width apart, bend your arms in front of you, and have your hands clasped loosely in fists. Turn your body and hips to the right, hold for a few seconds, and return to the center. Repeat on the other side.

• Ten knee lifts—stand and, keeping your back straight, bring one knee up and touch it with the opposite hand. Repeat with the opposite side.

One of the benefits of aerobic exercise is that there are a lot of options to choose from.

• Ten knee bends—stand with your feet shoulder-width apart and your arms stretched out in front of you, parallel with your shoulders. Bend your knees slightly, lower yourself down a little, then stand back up and repeat.

• Ten simple squats—stand with your feet shoulder-width apart, with your knees facing forward, and let your arms hang down by your sides. Gently lower yourself down by bending your knees and pushing your bottom back, your chest over your knees. For extra balance, you can extend your arms forward as you bend.

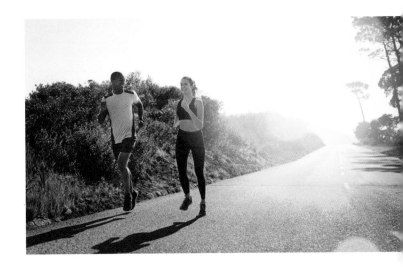

Main workout

Once you've warmed up your body sufficiently, you can start your aerobic workout. The following exercises can be performed in the order listed or mixed up for a bit of variety. Each exercise is beneficial to different parts of your body, while also giving you a good, thorough aerobic workout. Aim to repeat each exercise ten times before moving on to the next one, then try to do a few more each time as you build your fitness level. Even a short ten-minute aerobic workout will be beneficial.

Jump, squat, and turn: Stand with your feet slightly wider than hip-width apart. Jump on the spot, and on the second jump, turn to face the opposite way. Jump again and drop down into a squat by bending both your knees. If you feel comfortable, reach down and touch the floor with one hand. To vary things, try skipping the turn and just do the jump and squat.

Squat thrust: Stand with your feet hip-width apart and put your hands by your sides. Bend down, place both hands flat on the floor, and hop your feet so they land behind you in a high plank position with your legs straight, hips level, and your wrists in line with your shoulders. To complete the squat thrust, hop forward and stand up straight. If it's too much for you to hop back both feet together, try doing them one at a time.

You can continue your aerobic workout with these heart-pumping exercises.

JUMPING JACKS: Starting in a standing position, bend your knees slightly and jump, while extending your legs to each side and putting your arms straight up into the air. Jump again and move back to your original position. As you get fitter, try jumping a bit higher each time, with less time between jumps.

TOE TAPS: Put a small object that won't roll around (e.g., a small cushion) on the floor in front of your feet to act as a target. The aim is to tap the target with your toes while jumping from one foot to the other. Start with one foot resting lightly on the target, then quickly jump and swap so that your other foot is on the target. Repeat the move, alternating your feet and lightly tapping your toes on the target. The more you practice the quicker you'll get.

FAST FEET PUNCHES: Stand with your feet slightly wider than hip width, with your knees slightly bent. Close your fists, then bend your arms to bring your fists up to chin height. Take fast steps with your feet, and at the same time, move your arms out forward in a punching motion. If you find it tricky to do both movements at once, start by practicing them separately, then build them in together.

SQUAT JUMPS: Start these jumps from a squatting position, with your thighs parallel with the floor, your back straight, and your arms bent so that your fists are at chin height. Jump to turn 90 degrees, extending your arms down by your sides as you do so. You should land in a squat position. As you get better at this exercise, try to turn 180 degrees as you jump.

HOP AND TOUCH: Stand up and raise your right leg in front of you, keeping it as straight as possible. Hop on your left foot, then swing your opposite arm in front of your body and touch your right knee. Repeat with the other leg and try to keep hopping and moving as you go. As you get more flexible, aim to reach farther down your leg, until eventually you are able to touch your ankle.

MOUNTAIN CLIMBER: Start in a high plank position, with your palms flat on the floor and your hands shoulder-width apart. Your shoulders should be parallel with your hands and your legs extended. Move your right knee so that it comes up to your chest, while keeping your left leg and back straight. Move your leg back to the original position and repeat with your left leg.

SKIPPING: Skipping is perfect to add to your aerobic workout. Do 10–20 single skips with the rope. The fitter and more practiced you get, the faster you should be able to skip.

Cool down

Once you've finished your exercises, don't forget to cool down. In the same way that it's important to warm up before you exercise, it's also important to cool down properly; it will slow your heart rate and help you relax after your exercise session. Spend at least five minutes—longer if you feel you need it—cooling down.

As you get fitter, try jumping a bit higher each time, with less time between jumps.

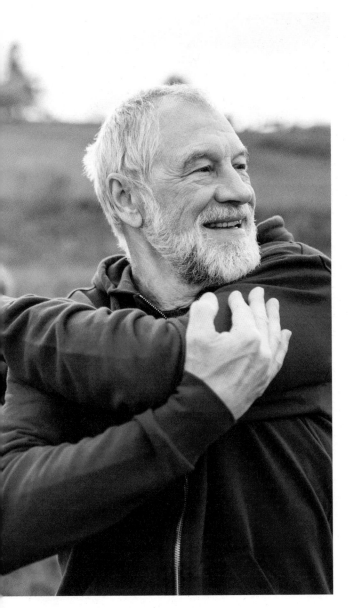

Here are some gentle stretches you can try.

UPPER BODY STRETCH: In a standing position, link your fingers together and turn your palms upward. Keeping your back straight, lift your hands up and backward as far as you comfortably can. Hold for a few seconds, then repeat.

CALF STRETCH: In a standing position, move your right leg forward, resting the foot on the floor, bend at the knee slightly, and lean forward a little. Keep your left leg straight and gently lower your left heel to the floor. Repeat the stretch with the other leg.

HAMSTRING STRETCH: Lie on your back and raise your left leg, keeping your right leg bent with the foot on the floor. Hold your left leg with both hands, below the knee, and gently pull your left leg toward you. Hold for a few seconds then repeat with the other leg.

THIGH STRETCH: Lie on the floor on your left-hand side, with your arm bent and supporting your head. Slowly bend your right leg upward and reach out to hold the top of your right foot. Aim to gently pull the heel toward your bottom to stretch your thigh. Keep your knees together and touching for this. Hold for a few seconds, then repeat with the other leg.

CHILD'S POSE: Sit on the floor on your heels with your knees open wide. Bend forward at your hips and gently lower yourself down, using your hands to walk your body along the floor until your forehead is resting on the ground. Extend your arms and place your palms on the ground. Hold for 30 seconds.

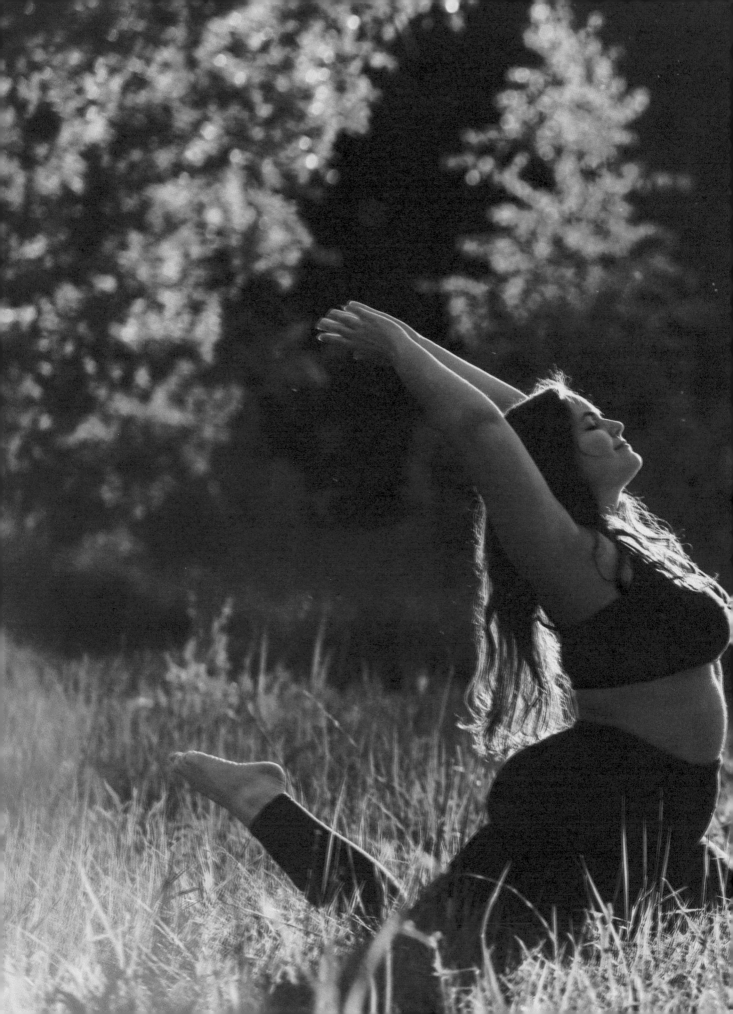

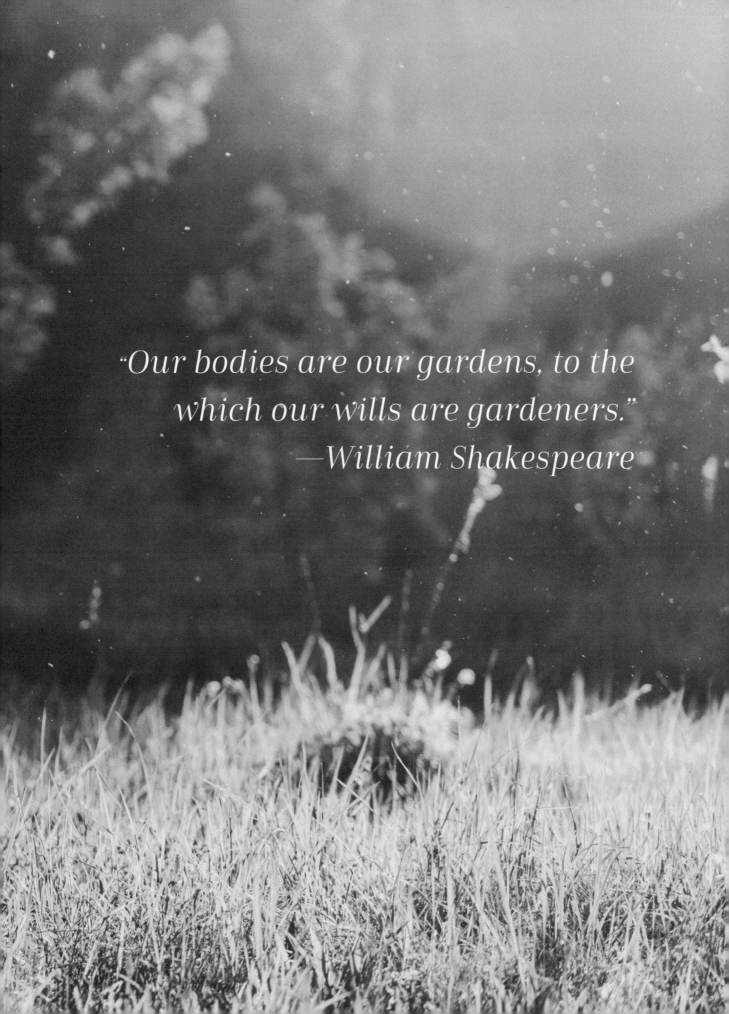

"Our bodies are our gardens, to the which our wills are gardeners."
—William Shakespeare

SLEEP AND REST FOR PHYSICAL WELLNESS

The amount of sleep needed, or taken, by individuals varies enormously. There's a standard belief that eight hours is the norm, but we all know of people who need much less. There have been a number of famous short sleepers, including Winston Churchill and Napoleon (both of whom catnapped during the day), and Voltaire, who needed only three hours.

It's important for couples to realize that these variations are real; a short sleeper married to a long sleeper can make their partner's life quite difficult if they insist on banging around at 6:00 A.M., or interpret the other's genuine needs as laziness. Short and long sleepers have been found by and large to have different personalities. Short sleepers tend to be hardworking, ambitious, and rather obsessive, as well as extrovert and efficient. Long sleepers worry more, are less self-assured, and value their sleep, which they may use as an escape. They are also often creative people—and creative people are said to dream more and to have more vivid and adventurous dreams than other people. Einstein was a long sleeper.

The ages of sleep

The amount of sleep we need also varies with age. The "average" 7.5 hours applies to adults between the ages of 16 and 50. Most small babies sleep about 16–18 hours a day, and toddlers still need a lot more sleep than adults. However, some older children may actually need less than adults, something that parents don't always recognize. With adolescence, the picture changes again: Some teenagers will sleep up to 15 hours a night. They are not necessarily being lazy and will grow out of it. However, parents should note that longer sleeping hours are also a symptom of depression, which can hit teenagers quite badly. At about the age of 16 we reach the "normal" adult pattern—that is, whatever is normal for us.

From the age of 40 in men and 50 in women, the pattern alters yet again. In some women menopause temporarily disrupts sleeping patterns. But in everyone, as they grow older, nighttime sleep becomes lighter and more broken, with fewer dreams. In addition, many older people take naps during the day, so they need less sleep at night. Including catnaps, the average sleep for a 70-year-old is about six hours. It's important to realize this, since many old people ask their doctors for help with their "insomnia" when in fact they are sleeping quite normally for their age.

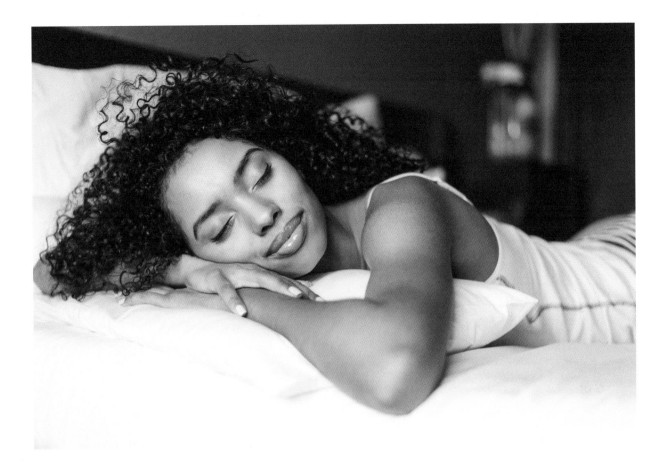

Your body clock

The functioning of our bodies is governed by an inner biological clock, known as the circadian rhythm (from the Latin *circa diem*, meaning "about a day"). This regulates the times when various organs become more or less active and when the production of various hormones peaks and tails off. The length of the circadian day is normally between 24 and 25 hours; some people have sleep problems because their body clocks are out of time with the norm, or disturbed by things such as shift work and jet lag.

The siesta, traditional in hot southern European countries such as Spain, is in decline as Mediterranean businesses come into line with the rest of Europe. Yet it could be much more natural than the worldwide norm. The circadian rhythm is set to bring on sleep twice a day, mainly at night, but also in the early afternoon, which is why many people feel sleepy after lunch.

The circadian rhythm also varies with age. Babies sleep regularly during the day, at first at around three-hour intervals, tailing off to a morning and an afternoon sleep; by the age of about two and a half they are sleeping only in the afternoon. In the elderly, the need for an afternoon nap usually returns.

It appears to be the circadian rhythm that is responsible for some people being "owls," finding it hard to wake in the morning but lively at night, while others are "larks," leaping out of bed first thing and drooping by ten in the evening. Interestingly, these differences seem to lessen as people age.

THE STAGES OF SLEEP

In sleep, the brain goes through four main stages, each characterized by different types of brain waves—the electrical impulses emitted by the brain.

Stage 1

This first stage, the lightest, is the transition from wakefulness to drowsiness. As we enter it our muscles relax, our blood pressure drops, and the heart rate and digestion slow down. The brain begins to produce hormones such as serotonin and melatonin, which are associated with sleep and sleepiness (whether they actually cause sleep is under debate). At the same time, there is an increase in alpha waves—brain waves of 7–14 cycles per second—which are typical of relaxed wakefulness; alpha waves also appear in people who are meditating or under hypnosis. This stage lasts between one and ten minutes in the normal sleeper; although we return to it at intervals during the night, it usually occupies only about 5 percent of our sleep.

Stage 2

This stage starts quite soon after falling asleep and occupies about 45 percent of human sleep. It contains a mixture of deeper, slower brain waves: theta brain waves (3.5–7.5 cycles per second) typical of drowsiness and light sleep, and slow delta waves (under 3.5 cycles per second), during which we are really unconscious.

Stage 3

Stage 3, which occupies only about 7 percent of sleep in young adults, is another transition phase to deeper sleep; as delta wave activity increases, we are taken fairly rapidly to stage 4.

Stage 4

Stage 4 is the deepest form of sleep, with delta brain waves predominating; it makes up about 13 percent of sleep in young adults. We stay in stage 4 for quite long periods before surfacing again to REM (see below) and stage 1 several times during the night.

REM sleep

Rapid eye movement (REM) sleep is so called because the sleeper's eyes move, indicating that they are dreaming. It occurs during stage 1 sleep and increases in quantity later in the night. It has been found that we also dream during deeper stages of sleep. It used to be thought that REM sleep was the part of sleep essential to us; it was believed that these periods were needed for brain rest, and that people deprived of them would develop psychosis. This last theory has been disproved, though deprivation of REM sleep does produce irritability and difficulties in concentration, and affects the ability to retain information learned the day before. People deprived of REM for more than three days have started having waking dreams, in the form of hallucinations. Others have been found to become less inhibited and conscientious.

Core sleep

In his book *Why We Sleep* (OUP, 1988), sleep neuroscientist Professor Jim Horne proposes that the really essential part of sleep consists of stages 3 and 4, which he calls collectively slow wave sleep (SWS).

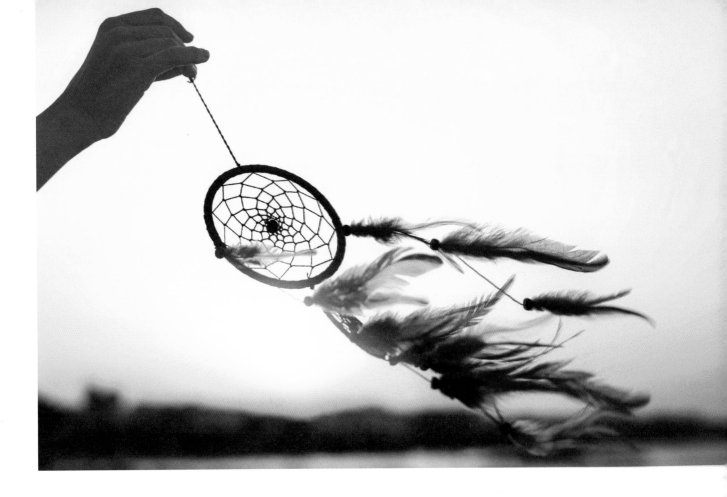

During these stages the brain is in what he calls an "off-line" state: It is the only time during which this hardworking organ is totally at rest. SWS occurs largely during the first three cycles, that is, during the first half of a night's sleep.

When people stay up all night and are therefore deprived of sleep, it has been found that they don't need to catch up with all the sleep they've lost. When they do finally sleep, they recover no extra light sleep and only a fraction of REM sleep. But they do recover all the lost deep sleep, which suggests that this is the sleep that is really essential.

In people who naturally need less sleep than the average, the same pattern is followed during the first few hours as in average sleepers. Although these people sleep for fewer hours, says Professor Horne, they are getting the essential slow wave sleep: "It is as though these short sleepers have somehow done away with what seems to be the flexible non-restorative sleep—the latter hours of sleep."

He defines "core sleep" as consisting of SWS and some REM sleep. His conclusion is that so long as we get our ration of core sleep, the brain will recover from its waking wear and tear. The rest he calls "optional sleep," which has no essential purpose but "fills the tedious hours of darkness until sunrise, maintaining sleep beyond the point where core sleep declines," and it may in fact not be necessary.

*Alpha waves **also** appear in people **who** are meditating or under hypnosis.*

WHAT IS INSOMNIA?

Insomnia is defined by sleep experts as a difficulty in initiating and maintaining sleep, which has continued for at least three weeks. Chronic insomnia can last for years, while intermittent insomnia can be triggered by particular anxieties or crises. People experience insomnia in different ways: for some it's the tossing and turning for what feels like hours before they drop off; others wake up at intervals and feel they never get a good night's sleep; and others wake early in the morning and can't get back to sleep again.

Measuring insomnia

Insomnia can't be measured by the number of hours you sleep, since people's needs vary so much. It's been found in sleep laboratories that some insomniacs actually sleep longer than "normal" sleepers: If you need ten hours and sleep only for eight, then you won't feel as refreshed as the good sleeper who needs seven.

Different types of insomnia have traditionally been related to different states of mind; it's often said that not being able to get off to sleep at night is a symptom of anxiety, while waking early is a sign of depression. In fact, it's not as simple as that. Some anxious and depressed people can actually sleep more, and some anxious people fall asleep normally, but wake in the early hours.

A number of sleep experts believe that anger and resentment are more frequent causes of insomnia than anxiety and depression. Others suggest that the overactive, churning mind may not be a cause of insomnia, but a result. In addition, there is often more than one factor involved, and as you can see from the checklist opposite, the causes are not always emotional.

Quality versus quantity

Insomnia is unpleasant. It is boring and uncomfortable in itself, and it can affect your daily activities, work, and relationships. However, it may not be quite as damaging as some fear. Sleep research laboratories have shown that people who normally sleep for seven or eight hours can adapt over time to as much as two hours less sleep daily without impairing their mental or physical ability. And when people have been totally deprived of sleep for between eight and eleven days, most of the body's organs, except for the brain, continue to function remarkably well. While the brain does need rest, Professor Horne stresses that "everything else from the neck down seems to cope very well, without sleep, provided you get regular rest and regular food."

Nevertheless, too little sleep does affect us, both because of genuine fatigue, but also because we believe that shortened sleep will cause us suffering. Our beliefs about how things should be have a major effect on how we react to them. So how much sleep do we really need? Professor Horne believes that around six hours is more than adequate for mental

Your attitude toward your sleep has a lot to do with the quality of the sleep you get.

health; any sleep after that comes into his category of "optional sleep." If his theory is correct, what the brain needs is core sleep. This should provide some reassurance: Core sleep predominates during the first sleep cycles, so even if you only sleep for a few hours, you will be getting a period of this important mixture of deep and REM sleep.

Conditions in sleep laboratories, of course, where the human guinea pigs are fed and rested and have chosen to lose sleep, are quite different from those of the person tossing and turning in bed at home—even if they end up getting the same amount of sleep. EEG readings that record brain activity show that most insomniacs actually sleep much more than they claim to: Quite often people who feel they have slept only an hour or two have actually slept for several. It appears that people's perception of their insomnia can cause as much stress as the insomnia itself. It may well be that worrying about insomnia can make you just as stressed, and tired as not sleeping. It will also contribute to keeping you awake.

So, if you are insomniac, there are three important things to remember. First, you may be getting more sleep than you think. Second, so long as you get some sleep and can relax your body, you will not come to long-term harm. Third, your attitude toward your sleep has a lot to do with the quality of the sleep you get. Essentially, the first step toward beating insomnia is not to worry about it.

TYPE OF PROBLEM: Taking a long time to get to sleep
Note: the first nine reasons in this list could also be contributing factors for the other three types of problems listed.
POSSIBLE CAUSES OR CONTRIBUTING FACTORS:
Needing less sleep than you think you do • Napping during the day • Jet lag, working night shifts, and other body clock disturbances • External disturbances such as noise • Habit
Dietary factors: Too much junk food • Stimulating foods and drinks • Eating heavy meals late at night
Digestive problems: Smoking, especially in the evenings • Lack of regular exercise
Emotional stress: Anxiety, depression, unhappiness, anger, guilt, etc. • Unsolved problems • Obsessive thinking
Psychiatric disturbances: Stress (at home or work) • Major life changes: moving, divorce, changing jobs, etc. • Certain medical conditions • Neurological problems

TYPE OF PROBLEM: Waking during the night
POSSIBLE CAUSES OR CONTRIBUTING FACTORS:
High degrees of anger and irritability • Heavy alcohol consumption • Withdrawal from alcohol or drugs (medical or otherwise) • Nightmares • Fear of nightmares (waking just before you are about to dream) • Not being adequately tired by the end of the day

TYPE OF PROBLEM: Waking early and not being able to get back to sleep
POSSIBLE CAUSES OR CONTRIBUTING FACTORS:
Severe depression • Sleeping pill dependency • Alcoholism

TYPE OF PROBLEM: Getting "enough" sleep but still feeling tired
POSSIBLE CAUSES OR CONTRIBUTING FACTORS:
Sleep apnea (a respiratory disorder) • Depression • Narcolepsy

BREAKING THE INSOMNIA HABIT

Most of us like to think we are independent, freethinking spirits. Yet a surprising amount of our behavior is totally conditioned, starting when we are very young. Much of our conditioning is helpful and life-supporting: It would be very inconvenient if every time you crossed a road you had to relearn the desirability of looking both ways. Unfortunately, the mechanical part of our brain absorbs other, less helpful lessons, such as associating bedtime with lying awake.

Self-talk

The best way to break unhelpful habits is to start exchanging them for helpful ones. The first thing is to recognize in what particular ways your habitual thinking or behavior is keeping you in that sleepless groove. How do you talk to yourself and others about sleep? If you label yourself "insomniac" and tell yourself every time you head for bed that it'll take you ages to get to sleep, you are simply reinforcing the programming that keeps you awake. You can change some of that thinking now, by telling yourself that you are now on the way to improving your sleep, and by no longer telling other people that you suffer from insomnia.

Start noticing your habitual thoughts about insomnia. In particular, look out for sentences starting with "I always . . ." or "I never . . ." or "I know . . ." For example: "I always take hours to get to sleep" or "I always wake up for hours in the middle of the night." These statements may not actually be true, although they feel true to you. As we've seen, most insomniacs overestimate how long they take to get to sleep or lie awake during the night. You could make a start by recognizing that your perception of the amount of sleep you get may be inaccurate.

Make a game of catching these kinds of thoughts. It may help you to write them down. Then try replacing your negative statements with positive ones; a good start might be: "I'm now learning how to sleep better." Make your positive statements ones you can believe. Telling yourself "I am going to sleep perfectly tonight" may not work, because at this point you probably won't believe it, and trying to convince yourself will just set up further tension. But you could try: "I will take tonight as it comes." You may be surprised by the results.

Starting to change your self-talk can be a way of opening up other possibilities. Once you realize that you don't have to be a victim of your own thinking and reactions, all kinds of barriers can begin to crumble.

Changing the pattern

A popular way of treating insomnia today is a behavioral psychology method called stimulus control, which consists of retraining yourself to sleep by learning to associate bed and bedtime with sleep, and sleep alone. This is the routine:

1. Don't watch television, listen to music, read, work, smoke, scroll through social media, surf the Internet, or eat in bed. Making love is permitted and can actually help you sleep.

2. Always get up at the same time, including weekends and vacation. If you find waking up difficult, place your alarm clock on the other side of the room so that you have to get up to turn it off. Put the light on straight away, as light can stimulate wakefulness.

3. Don't take naps during the day. You can overcome post-lunch sleepiness with some deep breathing or a quick walk around the block.

4. Don't go to bed until you are really sleepy.

5. If you don't fall asleep within ten minutes, get up and do something else in another room. Don't go back to bed until you are ready to fall asleep.

Further sleep-assisting habits you can develop:

1. Deal with anxieties during the day or early evening.

2. Avoid stimulating foods and drinks in the evening. These include coffee, tea, and alcohol. Smoking is also a stimulant; if you can't give it up immediately, at least cut down, especially in the evening.

3. Avoid stimulating activities late at night, including strenuous exercise, work, and arguments.

4. Establish a winding-down routine. Spend the last hour before bedtime preparing for sleep, by listening to some relaxation music or taking a warm bath.

5. Make sure your bedroom is both well aired and at a comfortable temperature.

Self-hypnosis and visualization

The imagination can have a direct effect on the body, for good or ill. When you imagine or remember a disaster, your pulse can start racing and your breathing can become more shallow, as the body's stress system starts revving up. It doesn't matter that the disaster isn't real—your body reacts as though it is. Similarly, when you imagine yourself healthy and happy, your body starts to feel as such.

In a relaxed, daydreaming state, you can mentally picture the outcome that you want, such as better sleep. In so doing, you are using an in-depth way of reprogramming your mental computer.

Visualization techniques may not be right for everyone, but even if you don't use specific techniques, you are using the power of thought and imagination throughout the day, both mentally and verbally. All the more reason to exchange depressing thoughts about your life and your sleep for positive ideas about what you really want.

For successful self-hypnosis, the first, essential step is to be able to relax deeply. If you are normally tense, you may need some help in learning to relax sufficiently. (See "Part Two: Mental Wellness," pages 118–191.)

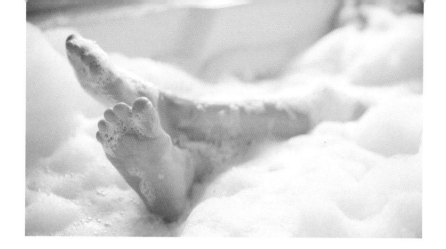

The churning mind

Probably the most common complaint among poor sleepers is difficulty in getting off to sleep. It's almost always related to a mind that won't switch itself off. Your thoughts go round and round, you toss and turn, and an hour later you're tired, twitchy, and wide awake.

The churning mind may be caused by anxiety about something specific—an exam, a job interview, a work project, a partner's illness, or the state of your finances. Possibly even more often it is caused by resentment or anger, brooding over unpleasant events, sometimes from the recent past, sometimes from way back. You relive the scenes, inventing scenarios in which you find just the right words to put down that person who insulted you yesterday, or even years ago. Or you may be feeling depressed and lonely, wishing your life were different, blaming yourself or others because it isn't, and replaying past regrets, missed opportunities, or lost happiness.

A great deal of nighttime churning is connected with unfinished business, something that computer in your head can't stand. It chugs away looking for solutions and won't shut up. Or it allows you to get to sleep and then wakes you up with a bad dream to remind you of a problem, or to tell you, "Hey, we really must do some worrying about this!"

Regularly waking with nightmares or bad dreams can make you anxious about going to bed in the first place: Usually these, too, concern unfinished business. Night terrors—suddenly waking from nondreaming sleep with a sense of fear and doom—are often the result of past traumas. Recurring dreams may also stem from traumatic past events—car crashes, an abusive partner, or an assault—which the conscious mind has tried to forget. But the unconscious mind is still trying to cope with these traumas in the only way it knows how. In such cases it is important to seek professional help from a counselor, psychotherapist, or hypnotherapist who can work with you to heal your fears, so that they no longer fester and cause you misery.

Some people aren't particularly worried about anything, but just have very active minds. Many of them accept this, often creative people who come up with creative ideas as they lie awake. But if your thoughts are unpleasant, sad, or anxious, they are crying out to be dealt with, and bed is not the place.

Establish a winding-down routine before you go to bed.

Who's in the driver's seat?

Rushing around all day and going to bed with a mind that's exhausted but awake is all too common these days. Modern life doesn't encourage natural rhythms. We start work at the same time all year round, whether it's dark or light. Commuter travel is uncomfortable and frustrating, office atmospheres are often unhealthy as well as fraught, and lunch may be a hastily devoured sandwich or burger. For many people, "relaxation" takes place in the artificial surroundings and noise of bars and clubs.

Small wonder that those who rush around can't sleep. The whole physical and nervous system becomes jangled and out of gear. There is no breathing space to look at problems—or even just to breathe! Body and mind are poorly nourished. And underlying this frantic rush, an anxious little voice is often sending anxious little messages that we don't want to hear: "Am I good enough?" "Is this all there is to life?" "Why am I unhappy?" If your life is anything like this, and it has resulted in insomnia, ask yourself what you are truly getting out of it. OK, so modern life is like that. But does that mean yours has to be? What or who is driving you to eat badly, maybe drink too much, or work until all hours so that by bedtime your brain is buzzing?

Much of our busy-busy behavior is due to conditioning by other people, and our beliefs about how life should be lived may not be aligned with what we really need. The work ethic says we shouldn't waste a moment; societal standards say we must have a "good time" and be successful. We must also be seen to be successful through buying more and more goodies for ourselves and our families, and to keep the merry-go-round turning we have to work even harder. Yet when you were a child, was this what you wanted from life? Who programmed your computer?

Our beliefs come from a number of different sources, which is why they often conflict. Some psychotherapists point out that we all have multiple personalities, often referred to as sub-personalities or "voices." For example, most people have an inner critic sitting in judgment on their every action; at the same time there's an inner child, made to feel small by the critic's remarks. And many of us have an inner saboteur, doing its best to get us to make a mess of things. But there are other parts of us that often don't get addressed—for example, a wise self, a peaceful self, and a creative child who wants to play.

So, try listening to the thoughts and voices underlying your daily rush. Who's driving you on? Are you responding to other people's programming—perhaps a critical father demanding that you prove your worth, or a perfectionist mother setting you impossibly high standards? Do you have to believe those voices from the past? What does the real you need and want from life, and are you getting it?

A HEALTHY BEDROOM

Ideally, your bedroom should be associated with sleep, and not with other activities; it should be warm and welcoming, with a peaceful and healthy atmosphere. Yet some bedrooms can actually damage your health.

Colors

Colors have an influence not only on our visual sense but on our nervous system; they radiate at different wavelengths, some of which are stimulating, and some calming. Calming colors for bedrooms are soft blues, greens, pastel pinks, and peaches; neutral colors such as beige and cream are also appropriate. Avoid vivid colors, particularly in a child's bedroom—they might seem cheerful but can be overstimulating.

The bed

Your bed should obviously be comfortable, ideally with a firm but not overhard mattress. People's tastes in mattresses vary, and if you're happy with a squashy one, that's fine. But soft mattresses are not good for your back in the long run.

It's best to sleep with a single pillow, which keeps your neck at a natural angle. A stiff neck is often greatly improved when two or three pillows are replaced with a single one. (It's been suggested, incidentally, that if you sleep badly in strange houses, taking a familiar pillow with you will provide the link with home that will allow sleep to come.) Some people find hop- or herb-filled pillows help them to sleep; you can find these at herbalists and some health-food stores. Make sure you like the smell before buying.

Fresh, clean air

Fresh air is important, provided it doesn't make the room too cold. If you don't like sleeping with an open window, consider getting an ionizer. Ionizers replace negative ions in the atmosphere. Negative ions are electrically charged molecules that are found in abundance in mountain air and around waterfalls, and keep the air healthy and clean.

Crystals and natural materials

Crystals are very popular as aids to healing, meditation, and clearing the atmosphere. If the idea appeals to you, rose quartz and amethyst are both considered suitable stones for sleep; keep one by your bedside. When you buy a crystal, it should be thoroughly cleansed before you use it, since crystals absorb energies from the atmosphere around them. Soak it for several hours in a bowl of salt water, rinse it under the cold faucet, don't wipe it with a cloth, but place it to dry on a sunny windowsill.

Over the last few years complaints of headaches, skin rashes, nausea, lethargy, depression, stress, and fatigue have been related to "sick building syndrome." The health of workers in modern buildings has been affected by factors such as artificial lighting, static electricity from synthetic furniture and fabrics, low-frequency electromagnetic radiation from electronic machinery, and airborne particles. Air-conditioning and windows that can't be opened further deplete the atmosphere of negative ions.

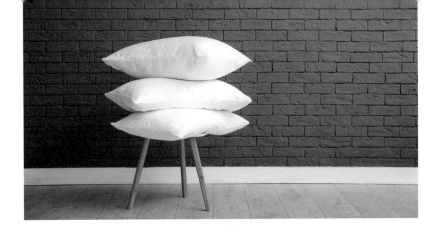

We don't hear too much about "sick bedrooms," but some of these factors can also affect your home, particularly if you are sensitive to them. It is increasingly likely that there will be a computer, smartphone, or tablet in the bedroom. An increasing number of synthetic fabrics are used in furnishings, bed linen, and nightwear, while harmful gas can be given off by insulation materials, lacquers, glues, and vinyls. There is also increasing evidence that radiation from electric pylons can affect the health of people living near them.

Ideally, use natural fabrics for your bedroom furnishings, linen, and nightwear, and don't have a TV set in there. Although individual items of electrical and electronic equipment are said to give off safe levels of radiation, we are increasingly exposed to radiation of all kinds, and the accumulation from various sources can ultimately get to us. It's also best not to use an electric blanket; if you do, unplug it before going to bed.

Keep the air in your bedroom fresh and clean for a restful night.

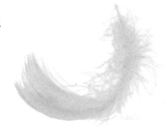

Looking after your body

Anxiety, depression, and obsessive thinking all have a strong physical component, since they trigger the production of stress hormones that create further anxiety, depression, and obsessive thinking. Breaking the cycle by looking after your body will have a positive feedback effect on your emotions. Stress hormones are actually produced to gear us up for action. If you start exercising regularly, you will get rid of these hormones healthily.

Evening exercise

A word of caution. Avoid exercising late at night, as it overstimulates the body. One man who sought help for insomnia was found to be running several miles every night. The simple answer was to schedule his exercise earlier in the day. While a gentle walk around the block to unwind last thing is fine, the best times for strenuous exercise are the afternoon and early evening.

LEARNING TO RELAX

The onset of normal sleep is a drowsy, relaxed state of peaceful letting go. We should be able to drift into this naturally, yet in this busy, stressed age, many people have simply lost the art of relaxation and have to relearn it.

Meditation

Watching TV, socializing, and other off-duty activities all have their place, but they are not really relaxing. True relaxation involves switching off the active left brain, and also the part of the nervous system that gears us up for action. It reverses the process of building tension by bringing into play the parasympathetic nervous system, which counteracts the effects of stress and helps to strengthen the immune system. Regular relaxation can actually alter body chemistry, and deep states of relaxation can help the brain to produce endorphins—hormones that have been called "the body's own morphine," which can lift the mood and relieve pain.

Meditation has many similar effects. Though relaxation is aimed chiefly at the body, and meditation at the mind and spirit, both slow down and rebalance the body–mind system. Many people who meditate regularly find they need less sleep than before, because during their meditation periods they are giving their systems deep rest. Both meditation and relaxation require us—and also enable us—to let go of worry and tension and focus on the present moment. Some people are quite scared of letting go; they feel they must hang on and stay in control. This is partly because many of us have been brought up with the idea that "doing nothing" is a waste of precious time, and partly because of a not-always-conscious fear that something terrible will happen if we let go.

Letting go is a normal part of life's rhythm; hanging on to control builds physical tensions that go to bed with you. A tense mind is less able to solve problems than a relaxed one: If you learn to relax you will find that it will not make you less efficient, but better able to cope, and give you more control over your waking and sleeping patterns.

Most people in these tense days could benefit from regular relaxation or meditation. Build it into your day: give yourself a space to practice for 20 minutes at least once a day.

Relaxation techniques

Although there are some excellent books on relaxation, if you are under severe tension there is nothing to beat personal tuition, in a group or class where you can get individual attention. If you want to make a start on your own, choose a time and a place where you will be peaceful and undisturbed. Tell yourself that you are going to devote the next 20 minutes to completely letting go. Sit comfortably with your back supported and your feet flat on the floor, your hands loose in your lap and your eyes closed. Or lie down, with your head and knees supported by cushions. There are several relaxation techniques favored by experts. Here are two.

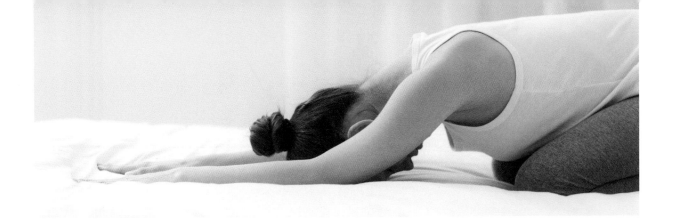

• Progressive relaxation consists of consciously alternately tensing and relaxing all the muscles in your body, from head to toe, in turn. If there are any tense spots left, let them go. Then enjoy the sense of relaxation until your 20 minutes are up. Come out of your relaxation position slowly.

• Stretching the whole body, then letting go, is another method. Then simply sense that waves of relaxation are flowing through your body as you

breathe in, while more and more tension is leaving you with every out-breath.

Relaxation can be aided by using mental imagery, such as imagining floating on a cloud. Podcasts also help you learn to relax on your own—don't, however, become dependent on one product. What you are aiming for is the ability to relax whenever you want to—not just at special times.

Guided meditation: calming the mind

For this meditation, choose something that will serve as your meditation object. It can be a flower, a candle, or an object that symbolizes calmness for you. It is best not to select anything that is overly complex or emotionally charged for you.

• Place the object on the ground in front of your meditation place. Let your body settle into a posture of calm alertness. Lower your eyelids.

• Take a few moments to soften your body, noticing the points where it connects with the ground, cushion, or chair. Take a few slightly fuller breaths to establish your attention in the moment. Now open your eyes and let your gaze rest gently on the meditation object in front of you.

• Take a few moments to familiarize yourself with the object, noticing its textures, color, and shape.

• Let your eyes rest gently on the object, not wandering the room to notice anything else. Whatever other sensations or thoughts appear, give them minimal attention, bringing a dedicated focus to your meditation object.

• Now close your eyes and see if you can bring an image of that object to life. See if you are able to hold a visual impression of your object in your mind, sensing the same detail of textures, color, and shape. Initially you may be able to do this only for a few moments. If the image begins

to blur or fade in your mind, don't struggle to maintain it, simply open your eyes to visually connect with the object once more.

• You may need to shift your attention from the inner impression to the visual object a number of times before you find yourself able to sustain the impression in your mind for longer periods of time.

• As your attention deepens, you will find a greater ease in accessing the visual imprint of the object. The image will become increasingly clear in its detail and vividness.

• Let your attention rest within it, fully connected with it. Sense the calmness that emerges with the deepening attention, filling your whole consciousness.

• If your attention becomes distracted, know that you can simply open your eyes and renew your connection visually with the object in front of you. Then close your eyes once more, recalling that image and resting within it.

• When you are ready, open your eyes and move out of your meditation posture.

FOOD AND SLEEP

It's impossible to get a truly healthy balance in life without including nutrition. Food and drink have a direct chemical influence on our body, nervous system, and mood. Overindulgence in junk food, coffee, or alcohol—all of which often accompany a stressed lifestyle—affects our well-being, simultaneously overstimulating the adrenal glands and nervous system and depleting the body of essential vitamins and minerals.

We get many contradictory messages these days about what's good for us and what isn't. And of course individual needs differ: While more and more people are becoming vegetarian, for instance, there are others whose systems really seem to need meat. If you're in any doubt, consult a naturopath or nutritionist about your own needs. Meanwhile, here are some general guidelines for everyone who wants to sleep better.

Foods and drinks to go for

Choose plenty of fresh fruits and salads, dried fruits, green and root vegetables, live yogurt, whole grains (brown rice, oats, and whole-grain bread), pulses (lentils and dried beans), fish and free-range chicken rather than red meats, and a moderate amount of fats, eggs, cheese, and other dairy products. Among these foods, the more stimulating are raw vegetables, salads, and fruits, so naturopaths recommend these at breakfast and lunch times. Root vegetables are believed to be more sedative than those growing aboveground; also sedative are the unrefined carbohydrates—potatoes and whole-grain bread, pasta, and rice—so these are best eaten with the evening meal.

Many foods, when combined with carbohydrates, lead to the production of an amino acid called tryptophan, the main building block of serotonin, a neurochemical that is produced as a precursor to sleep. These include milk, eggs, meat, nuts, fish, hard cheeses, bananas, and pulses. Drink herbal teas, spring water, and pure fruit juices, or some of the noncaffeinated drinks you can buy in health-food stores, such as dandelion coffee (made from the dried root rather than powder) or cereal drinks.

Foods and drinks to avoid

Steer clear of refined carbohydrates (white flour and sugar), which fill you up and overwork the digestive system without giving your body any real fuel.

Avoid processed foods. We have been made aware of the dangers of chemical additives, especially to the allergy-prone, but many processed foods still contain additives to which some people have an adverse reaction without always realizing it. In particular, tartrazine (E102, a yellow food coloring) and monosodium glutamate can upset people's sleeping patterns, especially if eaten in the evening. High-fat foods also put a strain on the digestive system when eaten in the evening, and caffeine doesn't only affect you late at night; it can contribute to nervousness and depression at any time. Excess salt raises the blood pressure and puts the body into overdrive.

You're giving your body—especially your hardworking liver—a nice rest!

A word about alcohol

It's true that a small amount of alcohol is a relaxant and can blur the edges of anxiety. But there are both disadvantages and risks in the alcoholic nightcap.

Alcohol is a drug; it's possible for one glass to turn into two, or more, and before you know it you have developed a dependency. And even if it helps you to get off to sleep initially, alcohol can actually cause insomnia. To digest it, your liver and kidneys have to work extra hard, and your body has to provide extra adrenaline—which is, of course, a stimulant. It has been found that after alcohol intake, sleep is more disturbed with more awakenings; alcohol also reduces REM sleep.

So, ideally, stick to no more than a glass or two of wine, two or three days a week; you'll feel better for it all around. If you feel deprived on nonalcohol days, boost your morale by telling yourself you're giving your body—especially your hardworking liver—a nice rest!

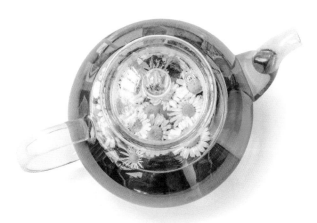

Smoking

Nicotine is also a stimulant, which can exacerbate sleeplessness, particularly as you grow older. Non-insomniac smokers have been found to take longer to go to sleep than nonsmokers and wake up more often during the night. In a trial at Pennsylvania State University, when eight heavy smokers gave up abruptly, the time they took to get to sleep dropped from an average of 52 minutes to 18 on the first two nights, and this pattern continued in four of them who continued without smoking for two weeks.

Initially, giving up smoking may cause a short-term increase in tension, and if you are under a lot of stress at the moment this may not be the best time to stop. But cutting down in the evenings, and avoiding smoking during the last hour before going to bed is beneficial. One way of cutting down is to tell yourself, every time you reach for a cigarette, that you'll have it later. But if you make a real commitment to stop, this could improve your sleep quite rapidly.

You can get many forms of help and support from a number of natural therapies, which will help to calm your nervous system and support you during the withdrawal phase. These include acupuncture, homeopathy, herbalism, hypnotherapy, kinesiology, and relaxation.

HEALTHY BEDTIME HABITS

The hour or two leading up to bedtime should be a time of slowly winding down, letting go of the day and its busyness. If you need to have a family discussion (or even an argument), get it out of the way early, and leave matters as resolved as they can be. The same goes for anything else that might be worrying you. Early in the evening, write any worries down, along with any decisions you have made about dealing with it, and then say goodbye to it for today. You have done all you can.

Keep your bedtime as regular as possible; while you are retraining your body–mind system, late nights are not a good idea. Although it's not been proven scientifically that the hours before midnight are best for sleep, some natural practitioners believe that they are. Around 10:00 P.M. our body clocks begin to slow down and gear themselves up for sleep.

Try to observe your own natural rhythm, and don't stay up beyond the time you naturally feel sleepy, even if that means forgoing the end of an interesting TV program. Some experts recommend that you don't watch television during the hours before bedtime, since the flickering image can stimulate the nervous system. However, I think this must depend on both the person and the program. A cheering or funny program may help you go to bed in a good mood. But don't fall asleep while you're watching it: You'll have to wake up again in order to go to bed, which is very confusing to your body clock and makes it hard to get to sleep again. The same goes for reading in bed. While the stimulus-control program described on page 75 says the bedroom is only for sleep, some people do find reading in bed a good way to switch their mind away from the worries of the day. This too must be your own choice. But don't waver between systems: If you've chosen to adopt the stimulus-control program, stick to it for the whole three weeks.

Bedtime drinks

A hot bedtime drink can be soothing and comforting—but bear in mind that it will reach your bladder during the night. This might seem obvious, but I've come across more than one elderly person complaining of having to get up to go to the bathroom, without connecting it with their late-night cup of tea! As we get older, our kidneys become more active during the night, so the amount an elderly person can comfortably drink before bed will be less than in their younger days. If your bladder is a problem, try having your bedtime drink no later than an hour before bedtime.

The tradition of having a hot milky drink at bedtime is probably based on the fact that milk contains tryptophan, which is a muscle relaxant and is soothing to the nervous system. A cup of hot milk accompanied by a couple of dolomite tablets (containing calcium and magnesium) can help you get off to sleep, and can also help those who suffer with restless legs. Not all milky drinks are good for sleep,

Around 10:00 P.M. our body clocks begin to slow down and gear themselves up for sleep.

however: Chocolate, for instance, has a high caffeine content. The best is plain hot milk, with maybe a teaspoon of honey, or a malted milk. A sprinkling of grated nutmeg on top is also sleep-inducing. If your sleeplessness is related to indigestion, you could try a drink made from slippery elm.

Some people find milk hard to digest, and as it is a food in its own right, dietary purists would not recommend it last thing at night. This also applies to late-night snacks, of course. Some people recommend eating a snack of foods containing tryptophan before bedtime—a bowl of cereal, a banana, or a lettuce sandwich for instance. As discussed previously, this is the time when the body should be gearing up for sleep, not digesting food—and food eaten last thing

is more likely to end up as stored fat. However, this is a choice you must make for yourself: If a late-night snack suits you and helps you sleep, that may be the most important factor for your sleep pattern.

Some people find cider vinegar and honey helps them to sleep; the mixture contains a good supply of trace elements, including calcium. Take a teaspoonful of each in a small cup of boiling water.

A very pleasant late-night drink is Norfolk Punch, a nonalcoholic blend of herbs and spices found in health-food stores and recommended as a relaxant. Some people find that it loses its efficacy if drunk every night—have it as a treat after a particularly fraught day.

Chamomile for relaxation and sleep

• Chamomile is a small, perennial herb with daisylike white flowers and feathery leaves. In herbalism, chamomile may be taken freely, except during early pregnancy.

• As a sedative, make a double-strength tea, using 2 teaspoons of flowers or 1 tea bag. Use a covered vessel, so the steam does not escape. Linden flowers, chamomile, and four cloves make an effective drink before bed, relaxing the body and the mind and bringing satisfying sleep.

• For times of severe stress, make a mixture of 3 parts chamomile to 2 parts sage and 1 part basil (a pinch of ginger powder is optional). Take twice a day to reduce tension and conserve your resources.

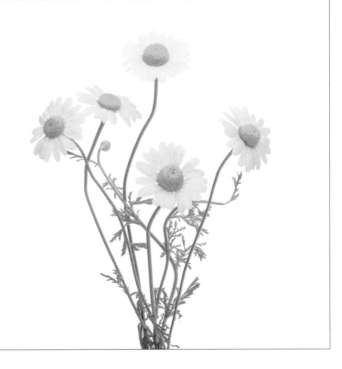

THE BENEFITS OF BATH TIME

Wash off any remaining stresses of the day by having a bath before bed, and make it sleep-inducing with the help of herbal or aromatherapy preparations. Enjoy your bath as a relaxing treatment; make it warm but not too hot, and give yourself time to soak in the oils or herbs so that you get the full, soothing benefit.

Suitable aromatherapy oils include lavender (used regularly, it has the advantage of boosting your immune system), chamomile and orange blossom (both rather expensive), meadowsweet, geranium, and hops. Use no more than 4–6 drops of oil or oils altogether, using the smaller amount if your skin is very sensitive. Agitate the water so that the oil spreads evenly and reaches your whole body. Allow yourself time to soak, relax, and absorb the oil both through your skin and by inhaling the vapor.

Herbs can also be used in the bath by making an extra strong infusion, which is then strained and poured into your bath water. Lime flowers are good, and so are hops: pour a cup of boiling water over three crushed heads and steep, covered, for ten minutes. You can also use lavender or a mixture of herbs: Fill a muslin bag with the heads and tie it to the faucet so that the hot water runs through it. Before getting into the bath, add a strained infusion of the same herbs.

Herbal baths are also soothing for babies. Herbalist Michael McIntyre says: "Chamomile herb is a very suitable way to get your baby to sleep. You can give your baby a chamomile bath. Make a strong tea using an ounce to two pints of water, strain it, and add it to the water in the baby bath." And herbalist Barbara Griggs quotes the French herbalist Maurice Mességué, who "recalls being put in a bath of Lime Flowers and Leaves as a child when he couldn't sleep—with magical results . . ."

Caution: If you are pregnant, consult a medical practitioner before using aromatherapy oils or herbs.

Mustard foot bath

Mustard is an annual plant cultivated as a spice all over the world. It has been used for centuries as a pungent condiment and healing herb, by the Greeks, Ayurvedics, and folk practitioners. Mustard's strong taste develops only after the seeds are crushed and come into contact with water or saliva. Large amounts of mustard can cause irritation and inflammation. Avoid contact with the mucus membranes and with sensitive skin.

For a warming mustard foot bath, put ¼ cup mustard seeds in a small cloth bag or a large tea strainer. Steep in hot water for five minutes. Soak the feet in the water until it cools.

Melissa mind and body soother

For frazzled nerves, irritability, and exhaustion, dilute 3 drops of Melissa essential oil, 2 drops of chamomile oil, and 2 drops of bergamot oil in 1 teaspoon of sweet almond oil and add to your bath water.

Allow yourself time to soak, relax, and absorb the oil.

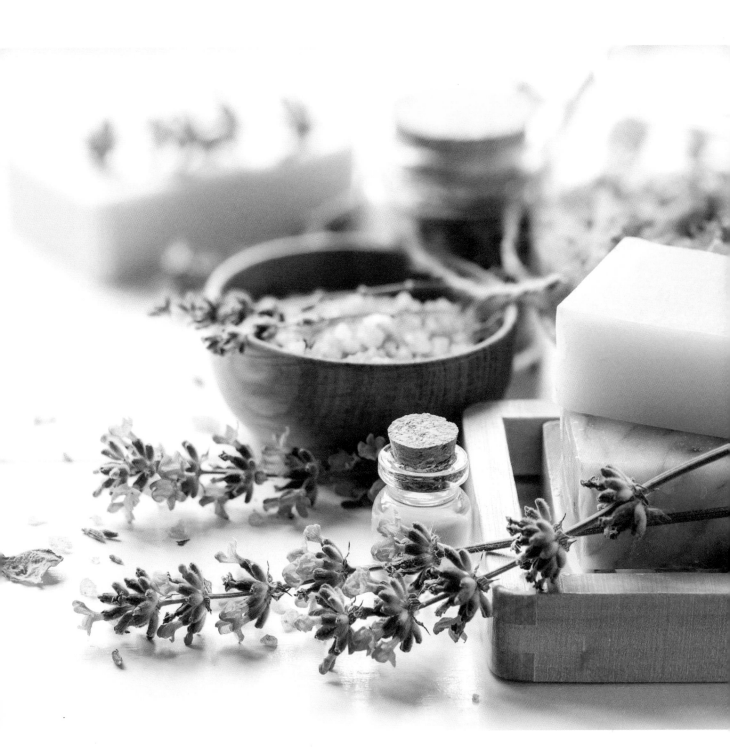

DEALING WITH NIGHT THOUGHTS

If your body is relaxed but your mind still active, either before going to sleep or after waking up in the early hours, you can train yourself not to focus on anxiety and worry by concentrating on something else.

Methods to aid sleep

One method is to play mental games, which will keep your mind occupied (and possibly rather bored) until you drop off. Try things like counting backward from 100, or listing the names of your friends, or countries, or flowers in alphabetical order. You could consider learning a verse or two of a poem before turning in, and reciting it to yourself mentally in bed. Or just pick a harmonious line of poetry and repeat it to yourself over and over.

Listening to the radio has been the resort of many insomniacs, but it has the disadvantage that if there's a really interesting program, you may stay awake to hear it to the end.

If worrying thoughts come into your head, let them go, with the knowledge that you will deal with them at the proper time. As you breathe in, think of peace, tranquility, and calmness entering your system: Breathe the worry away.

Another way of dealing with negative or anxious thoughts is not to fight them, but to listen to them in a detached manner, as if they were a rather boring radio program, without trying to find solutions.

You could also use visualization to help activate the alpha waves that precede sleep: You could take yourself on an imaginary or remembered walk in the country or by the sea. Or through a film you have

---

Flower essences for night thoughts

The scent of these essences may help to dissipate night thoughts:

WORRYING THOUGHTS AND MENTAL ARGUMENTS might respond to white chestnut.

INDECISION can be treated with Scleranthus.

STRESS, STRAIN, FRUSTRATION, AND INABILITY TO RELAX might respond to vervain or rock water, vine, elm, beech, or impatiens.

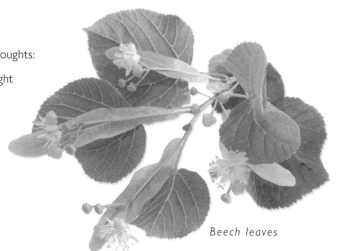

Beech leaves

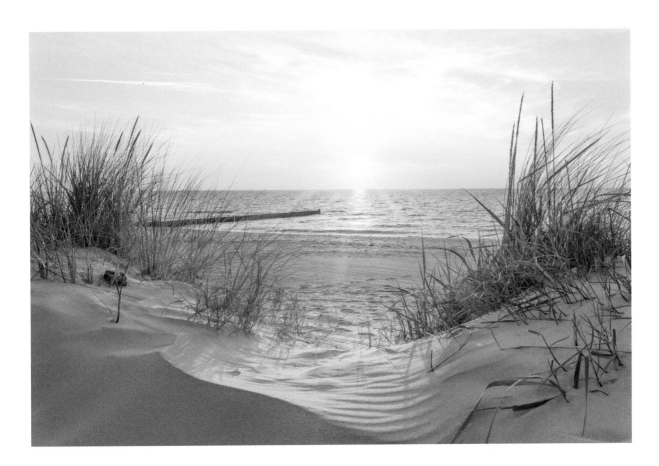

really enjoyed. The more pleasant your thoughts, the more likely you are to relax and go off to sleep.

Remember the strength of your mind energy: Negative thoughts press down on you, while happy ones lift depression away from you, as do thoughts that are not focused on yourself. I discovered accidentally one wakeful night that praying for other people sent me off in no time. Obviously, the purpose of prayer is not to send you to sleep, nor do I assume that everyone believes in prayer. But if you find your mind returning to your own problems, it may help you to switch your attention to a friend or friends who would benefit from a healing or positive thought from you. If they are ill, don't focus on their illness, but visualize them well and happy, or imagine a stream of healing white or gold light going from your heart to surround them. If you don't visualize clearly, this is not important: Simply send them well-wishing thoughts.

If someone pops into your mind who has hurt, insulted, irritated, or angered you, send them a healing thought, too—they probably need it. And if you're one of those people who lies awake worrying about the environment, try sending healing thoughts to the planet, to animals, trees, and nature—this will do both you and the environment much more good than if you lie there worrying about it.

One final technique to help with night thoughts could be the use of self-massage to calm the body and mind (see pages 110–117).

YOU ARE WHAT YOU EAT

Food is required for life. From the simplest of animals—a single-celled amoeba—to the most complex, all require a variety of essential nutrients to stay alive and to function healthily. Over the years, a number of diets, both fad and scientifically led, have been suggested to promote a healthy lifestyle, reduce obesity, and improve well-being. Countless diets and nutrition regimes have come and gone, including, among others, the Paleolithic (Paleo) diet, with its focus on wild foods; the low-carbohydrate Atkins diet; and the nutrition-based, low-carb diet promoted by Dr. Broda Barnes. To feel empowered to make your own decisions about your diet, it is key to understand why your body needs nutrients and how it uses them.

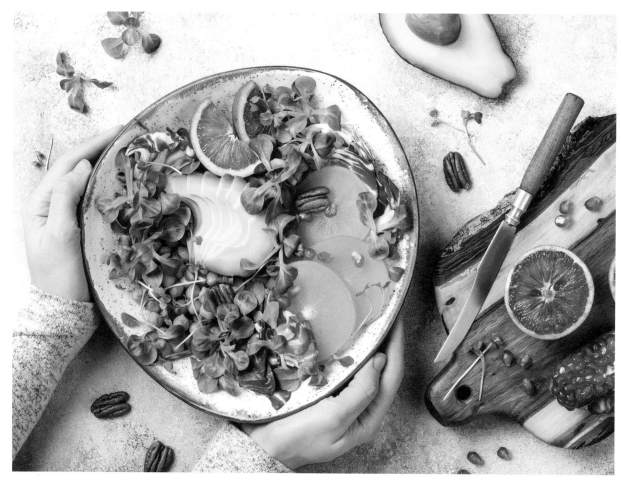

It is key to understand why your body needs nutrients.

The digestive system

Your digestive system starts in your mouth and continues through the esophagus, stomach, and intestines—ending, of course, in the rectum. Along the way, other organs play an essential role, including the liver and gallbladder, which respectively make and supply bile, which helps break down fats. Your digestive system's job is to break down the food you eat into its basic parts, called nutrients. The body uses nutrients to supply energy to all the body's cells, so they can do their work, or to make materials that the body needs. Before the nutrients in food can be used, they must be broken down into smaller, simpler molecules, which the body can easily transport and use.

After food has been pulped by the teeth, tongue, and saliva, it travels to the stomach along the tube known as the esophagus. The stomach's muscly walls and digestive enzymes get to work, turning food into a souplike mush named chyme. Enzymes are chemicals that bring about change, with different enzymes targeting different food groups. After chyme trickles into the intestines, tiny, fronded cells called enterocytes soak up its nutrients and water, passing them into the bloodstream. Indigestible material, some water, and bacteria are expelled as feces. Indigestible material includes cellulose fibers from plants, which help to move material through your digestive system and prevent constipation.

Nutrients

Your body needs two types of nutrients: macronutrients, which are needed in large quantities; and micronutrients, which are needed in much smaller quantities. The macronutrients are carbohydrates (found in foods such as bread and pasta), proteins (found in foods such as meat and eggs), and fats (found in foods such as fish and nuts). The digestive system breaks carbohydrates down into glucose, a sugar used by cells to produce energy. Proteins are broken down into amino acids, which the body uses for making cells and tissues. Fats are broken down into fatty acids and glycerol, which are used for tasks such as absorbing vitamins and making chemical messengers called hormones.

The micronutrients are vitamins and minerals, which the body needs to stay healthy. For example, vitamin C (found in foods such as oranges and broccoli) helps the body grow and to repair blood vessels, skin, muscles, and bones. The mineral calcium (found in foods such as dairy products and canned salmon) is needed for strong teeth and bones.

Nutrient-rich blood from the intestines travels to the liver, which sorts material into nutrients the body needs immediately (which are passed to the heart for pumping around the body), nutrients that need to be saved for later use, and toxins such as alcohol. The liver converts toxins into more harmless waste products and passes them to the urinary system, but the liver can be scarred by excessive and continual toxin intake. With the help of insulin made by the pancreas, excess glucose is converted into fatty acids and sent for storage in fat cells and other body tissues.

A HEALTHY DIET

Getting the macronutrients

A healthy diet needs to include all the macronutrients: carbohydrates, proteins, and fats.

• Carbohydrates: There are different types of carbohydrates, including fibers, starches, and sugars. Healthier carbohydrates contain more fibers and starches but less sugar. Good sources of carbohydrates include whole grains (such as brown rice), legumes, vegetables, and fruit. Less healthy sources are refined carbohydrates, including white bread, sodas, and cookies, in which the carbohydrates have been stripped of fiber. Refined carbohydrates can lead to a rapid rise in blood sugar.

• Proteins: Healthy sources of protein include poultry, fish, tofu, beans, and nuts. Less healthy options include processed meats (which may contain excess salt or chemicals), along with red meat and full-fat dairy, which are high in saturated fat (see below).

• Fats: Fats are either saturated or unsaturated. Saturated fats (including trans fats) are solid at room temperature. These can increase the level of a fatty substance called cholesterol in the blood, which in turn increases your risk of heart disease. Unsaturated fats—which are mostly found in plants and are liquid at room temperature—do not increase cholesterol levels. Sources of unsaturated fats include plant oils and spreads, nuts, seeds, and fish. Foods high in saturated fat include red meat, full-fat dairy products, and many baked goods.

Getting the micronutrients

Your body needs to intake around 30 vitamins and minerals. A balanced diet that includes vegetables, fruits, legumes, whole grains, lean proteins, nuts, and plant oils will certainly contain the tiny quantities of micronutrients that the body needs. However, it may be useful to know which foods contain high quantities of key vitamins and minerals.

Vitamin A: Necessary for maintenance of the eyes, found in carrots, sweet potatoes, and spinach.

Vitamin B6: Used for making red blood cells and maintaining the immune system, B6 can be found in chicken, whole grains, bananas, and potatoes (with their skins on).

Vitamin C: This vitamin helps to maintain the skin. Good sources include oranges, grapefruits, kiwis, broccoli, tomatoes, and sweet peppers.

Vitamin D: Benefiting the immune system and bone growth, this vitamin can be found in fish oil and skim milk. Sunlight is also a key source of vitamin D.

Vitamin E: Needed by the immune system, found in peanut butter, almonds, and sunflower seeds and oil.

Vitamin K: This vitamin helps the blood to clot after injury. Sources include leafy greens, soybeans, and pumpkins.

Calcium: Needed for strong bones and teeth, calcium is found in dairy products, leafy greens, and broccoli.

Iron: Needed in very small quantities, iron helps to transport oxygen around the body. Oysters, spinach, and white beans are rich in iron.

Magnesium: This mineral helps to regulate blood pressure. It is found in whole-grain wheat, black beans, nuts, and seeds.

Phosphorus: Needed for bone maintenance, phosphorus is found in salmon and turkey.

Potassium: Essential to nerves and muscles, potassium is found in lentils and bananas.

Zinc: For growth and for wound healing, zinc is in crabs, oysters, dark turkey meat, and chickpeas.

Creating balance

The best way to ensure that your body receives all its nutritional needs is to ensure that your diet contains whole grains, lean proteins, vegetables, fruits, and healthy oils. As a guide, imagine that the food you eat during one week is laid out on a (large) plate:

Processed foods

We are often told to avoid processed foods, including cured meats, packaged pastries, and ready-made sauces and meals. The fact is that all these foods contain some materials that can be damaging in large quantities. These include saturated fats (see page 92), refined carbohydrates (see page 92), and salt. Adults are advised to eat no more than 1 teaspoon of salt per day. Excessive salt can raise blood pressure, which increases the risk of stroke and heart disease.

The healthy eating plate

Vegetables and fruit
Around half of each meal can be vegetables and fruits. Aim to eat more vegetables than fruits, which contain natural sugars. Try to build a multicolored plate containing a wide variety of produce.

Whole grains
can form about a quarter of your diet, while refined grains (such as white rice and white pasta) should be eaten less frequently.

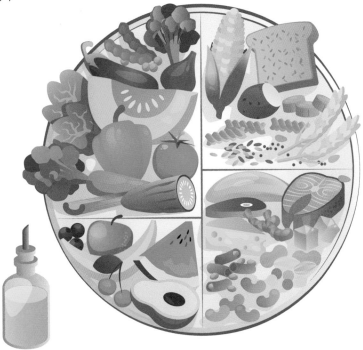

Healthy oils
Try to use healthy plant oils for cooking and as dressings.

Healthy protein
A range of healthy protein, including plant-based sources, can cover around a quarter of your plate.

DRINKS FOR WELLNESS

Drinking enough

Physicians tell us we should drink 6–8 glasses of fluid per day. To be more exact, an adult woman needs to drink about 64 ounces per day, while an adult man needs about 84 ounces. In hot weather, or when you are exercising, remember to drink plenty more. If you feel thirsty or notice that your urine is dark yellow, you are already a little dehydrated. Water, juices, smoothies, skim milk, tea, and coffee can all count toward that total, although caffeinated drinks should be limited.

Wonderful water

The healthiest drink of all is water. Around 60 percent of the human body is water. Water has myriad roles in the body, including: allowing cells to grow and survive; transporting oxygen and nutrients in the bloodstream; flushing out waste through urination; regulating body temperature through sweating; making saliva; and lubricating joints. Although most drinks contain water, pure water is the healthiest choice as it contains no fats and sugars. If you find pure water a dull drink, open a bottle of sparkling water and add a squeeze of lemon or a splash of unsweetened fruit juice. However, avoid store-bought flavored water, which can contain large quantities of sugar.

Fruit juices and smoothies

Just like the fruits and vegetables they are made from, juices and smoothies contain a wide variety of vitamins and minerals, making them a healthy choice as well as a delicious one. However, when fruits and vegetables are juiced or blended, they release their sugars, making them "free sugars." Free sugars can damage your teeth, so limit these drinks to one small glass per day.

Milk choices

Cow's milk contains calcium, which helps to maintain healthy bones, as well as protein, vitamins, and minerals. It does not contain free sugars that contribute to tooth decay. However, cow's milk is high in saturated fat, so adults should choose skim milk and limit their overall cow's milk consumption. Alternatives to cow's milk that are high in calcium, protein, healthy fats, and minerals include: soy, hemp (which is not psychoactive in this form), oat, potato, and quinoa milks, as well as fortified rice, almond, and coconut milks (check the label for the nutritional content).

Caffeinated drinks

Coffee, tea, hot chocolate, colas, and energy drinks contain caffeine, which is a stimulant. Low doses of caffeine make you feel alert, but higher doses can make some people irritable and unable to sleep. Caffeine is a diuretic, which means it increases water loss from the body through urination—which means it can lead to dehydration if drunk excessively. If excessive caffeine is drunk over a long period, it depletes the body of nutrients and unbalances

Pure water is the healthiest choice as it contains no fats and sugars.

hormones. Caffeine is also addictive; its withdrawal symptoms include headaches and indigestion. However, caffeine is harmless—and pleasurable— if drunk in moderation. The average adult can safely drink up to 400mg of caffeine a day, which is equal to around 4 cups of coffee, or 5 cups of tea, or 44 hot chocolates, or 10 colas, or 2 energy drinks. Of course, uncaffeinated fruit or herbal teas are a healthy choice, as long as they do not contain added sugar.

Caution: Pregnant women should consult with their health-care provider about limiting caffeine to 200mg per day.

Drinks to limit

Try to limit drinks that are high in sugar, which can damage teeth and contribute to weight gain. Sugary drinks include sodas, smoothies, flavored milks, milkshakes, sports drinks, and energy drinks. Keep in mind that energy drinks also contain high quantities of caffeine, so they should be factored into your caffeine calculations. Drinking alcohol is linked with health problems such as high blood pressure and breast cancer, as well as behavioral disinhibition. Adult women are advised to drink no more than one alcoholic drink per day, while men should have no more than two. For help with reducing your alcohol intake, start with a visit to your primary care doctor, who can evaluate your health, offer treatment referrals, and help you craft a plan of action.

Caution: Pregnant women should not drink alcohol at all.

Breakfast juice

For a morning pick-me-up high in vitamins A and C, this zingy recipe makes one small glass:

1 mandarin orange
½ carrot
¼ pineapple
¼-inch piece of fresh root ginger

Peel the ingredients, cut into chunks, then put in a juicer or blender and blend until smooth.

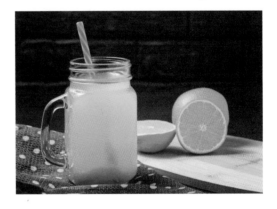

ARE NUTRITIONAL SUPPLEMENTS BENEFICIAL?

Should you take supplements?

Vitamins, minerals, and other elements work together within the body to ensure that all bodily processes can be carried out. When even one element is missing, the body becomes unbalanced and unable to work at its optimum level. The best source of all micronutrients is food. Supplements are not a replacement for food, and most cannot be ingested without food. They cannot be taken in place of a good diet, but their beneficial effects will be optimized if combined with a balanced intake of nutritious foods. People suffering from chronic conditions or who smoke or drink regularly may need to take supplements to ensure optimum health.

Micronutrients work in conjunction with one another, and taking large doses of any one supplement can upset the balance within the body. A good vitamin and mineral supplement will ensure that you are getting the correct amounts of each, according to the relationships between them. Extra supplements should be taken only on the advice of a registered nutritionist or medical practitioner. Where supplements are taken to discourage the course of illness—for example vitamin C for colds or flu—it is safe to take larger doses than usual. Read the package for further information.

Registered nutritionists have achieved great success with using supplements to treat conditions such as rheumatism and arthritis, high blood pressure, fatigue, constipation and other digestive disorders, the healing and recuperation processes following injury or surgery, skin problems, and many psychological and behavioral problems.

Neuralgia, osteoporosis, PMS, postnatal illness, pregnancy problems, reduced immunities, stress, and viruses may also respond to treatment with supplements.

When to take supplements

The best time for taking most supplements is after a meal, on a full stomach, although some vitamins and minerals work best on an empty stomach. Read the label on any supplement to find out the ideal time to take it.

Time-release formulas need to be taken with food, as their nutrients are released slowly over a number of hours. If there is not enough food to slow their passage through the body, they can pass the sites where they are normally absorbed before they have had a chance to release their nutrients. Take supplements evenly throughout the day for best effect.

When to see a practitioner

Most supplements can be taken safely without input from a registered nutritionist, but if you suffer from chronic health problems or a specific ailment, it is best to seek expert advice. Amino acids and other elements should be taken only with the advice of a professional. A nutritionist will make sure that you are taking a balanced combination of nutrients that will work together to make you healthy. Remember that everyone's needs are different, based on overall health, diet, whether or not you smoke or drink, are pregnant, and other influences. It is sensible to ensure that you receive advice that is tailored specifically to your individual needs.

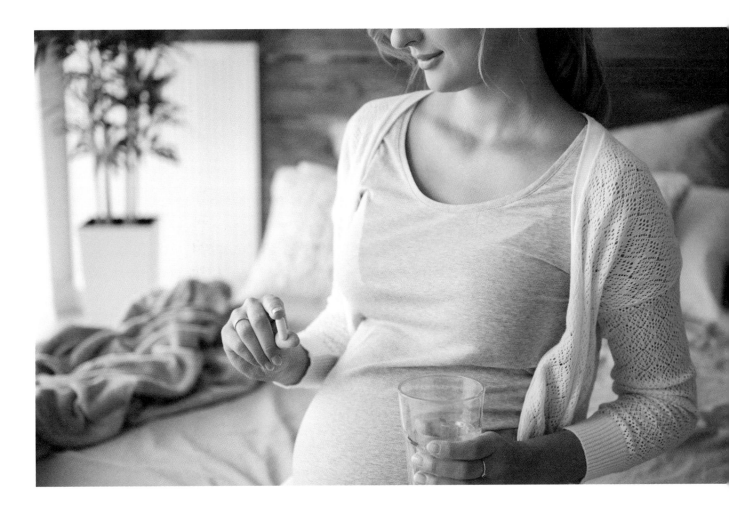

Always take care to consult with a registered nutritionist or a dietician, as the term "nutritionist" is not legally protected in many states and countries. Any person can call themselves a nutritionist, even if they are wholly self-taught.

Children

Children will of course need far lower doses of nutrients than adults, and a healthy, organic diet should offer a large proportion of their nutritional needs. A good vitamin and mineral supplement will provide anything extra that is required, but if you feel your child needs further supplements, see a practitioner. If you are buying products yourself, read the label to ensure that the product is safe for children, and follow the advice carefully.

Pregnancy

A growing baby puts heavy demands on your body, and it is more important than ever to ensure that you have a good diet. Research has now proved that women need extra folic acid and iron during pregnancy, and a good multivitamin and mineral supplement is often suggested. Consult with your health-care provider about which supplements are recommended during pregnancy. Do not take vitamin A supplements while pregnant.

FORMS OF NUTRITIONAL SUPPLEMENTS

Which supplement?

Most supplements come in a variety of forms. They are also prepared with different quantities of the active ingredients, so read the label carefully to ensure that you are getting the correct quantity for your needs.

• Powders: Many supplements come in powder form, which will usually provide you with extra potency, with no binders or additives. This is useful for people with allergies, or those who find it difficult to swallow a tablet. Powders are particularly useful for children—sprinkle a little in their breakfast juice, or stir it into some yogurt or dessert.

• Capsules: These are convenient to take and easy to keep. Fat-soluble vitamins are normally taken in capsule form, but many contain vitamin and mineral powders that allow a higher potency. Garlic and evening primrose oil are commonly available as capsules, and these can be broken apart and applied externally as necessary.

• Tablets: Many supplements come in tablet form, and these are the most practical for many people because they can be stored easily and will keep for a long time. Check the label to see what is added to your tablets in the form of binders or fillers, which preserve or bulk out the active ingredient.

• Liquids: Liquids are appropriate for people who have difficulty swallowing tablets or capsules. Many children's formulas come in liquid form for easy administration. Liquids can be mixed with food or stirred into drinks. They can also be applied externally.

Reading the label

Supplements work in different ways, and you will need to understand some of the key words that appear on the labels in order to choose which are most suitable for you.

"Chelated" is a term that appears on mineral supplements, and it means that the mineral is combined with amino acids to make assimilation more efficient. Most nutritionists recommend taking chelated minerals because they are 2–5 times more effective than other forms.

Time-release formulas are created via a process that allows them to be released into the body over an 8–10-hour period. These are particularly useful for water-soluble vitamins (the B vitamins and vitamin C), any excess of which is excreted within 2–3 hours of taking the supplement. Time-release formulas are reputed to provide stable levels of the relevant supplement during the day and night.

RDA and supplements

Governments provide guidelines for how much of each vitamin or mineral we need in our diets. These specify the recommended daily allowance (RDA) or recommended daily intake (RDI), and they apply to healthy individuals with a good, balanced diet. These levels are an "adequate" intake for the average person. In other words, they are not therapeutic levels and they do not take into account the varying needs of the population. People with illnesses, a stressful lifestyle, or who are on medication, or eat a highly refined diet, may need much more than the RDA. RDAs are given in mg (milligrams) or mcg (micrograms).

The therapeutic dosage for different vitamins and minerals may be many times the RDA. For example, the RDA for vitamin C is 60mg, while the therapeutic dose is 2,000mg. The RDA for vitamin E is 10mg, while the therapeutic dose is 400mg. The RDA for zinc is 15mg, but the therapeutic dose is 30–60mg.

Antioxidants and superfoods

Much of the cell damage that occurs in disease is caused by highly destructive chemical groups known as free radicals. These are the products of oxidation, a process that occurs naturally in our bodies as we breathe. Today, because of the other elements in the air, there are more free radicals than ever. In small quantities, free radicals can fight bacteria and viruses; in larger quantities, they encourage the aging process and cause damage to our cells.

Many nutritionists believe that free radicals can be combated by antioxidants—the ACE vitamins (vitamin A in the form of beta carotene, vitamin C, and vitamin E), the minerals selenium and zinc, and to a lesser extent manganese and copper. Antioxidants protect other substances from oxidation. Trials have shown that additional antioxidant vitamins—such as 2,000mg of vitamin C and 400mg of vitamin E daily— can reduce the incidence of heart attacks, strokes, cataracts, and other diseases, and slow down the process of aging.

Many "superfoods" are high in antioxidants, including blueberries, goji berries, pomegranate, and broccoli. Although not all physicians agree on the power of antioxidants, they do agree that these vitamin-rich, high-fiber foods are a good addition to a balanced diet. Other foods that are high in antioxidants, such as green tea and chocolate, are also high in fat or caffeine. These can be consumed as part of a healthy diet, but not to excess.

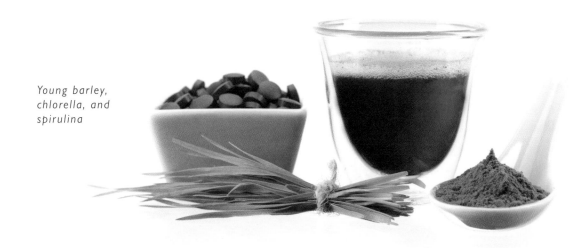

Young barley, chlorella, and spirulina

BODY IMAGE

Body image is how we think and feel about how our body looks, how other people view our body, and whether others find our body sexually attractive. Our body image depends on our feelings about our weight, shape, height, face, skin, hair, and age. Yet those feelings do not come into being like a rabbit pulled from a magician's hat. Our feelings about how we look depend on the society in which we live and our own experiences of growing up and making our way in that society.

Positive vs. negative body image

A positive body image makes us feel attractive, even powerful. Yet few of us are blessed with a continuously positive view of our own body, particularly as we age. Even a mildly negative body image causes loss of confidence and anxiety from time to time, if only when we are on the beach or in the changing room. If anxiety about how other people view our body prevents us from working out at the gym, from baring our swimsuit-clad body at the swimming pool, or from heading out for a jog in sweats, then it is directly impacting our physical wellness.

When negative body image becomes overwhelming, it can lead to crash dieting or even to long-term eating disorders such as anorexia nervosa.

Many patients with eating disorders are suffering from body image disturbance, a condition characterized by an altered and distressing perception of one's body. Body dysmorphic disorder is characterized by obsession with a perceived flaw in the face, body, skin, or hair. Thoughts about the flaw are intrusive, occupying hours of every day and severely affecting quality of life. Some sufferers seek cosmetic surgery, but this rarely alleviates the disorder as the perception of the flaw is not based on reality. If you or a loved one is suffering from an eating disorder or mental health issue related to your body, you are far from alone. Make an appointment with your primary care doctor, who can offer referrals for support and treatment.

Society and the body

Everywhere we look, advertising presents us with flawless faces and glossy skin. Knowing that most advertising images have been digitally enhanced does not prevent us from absorbing their unrealistic standard of beauty. Feeling the eyes of the world on them, social media influencers and movie stars feel perhaps greater pressure than the rest of us to meet this standard. We read that many celebrities have changed their appearance with the help of medical procedures, yet we still judge our thinner lips and laughter lines against their faces. When a female celebrity dares to be seen in public with a post-baby tummy or a naturally aged face, the body shaming is quick and merciless, reinforcing the message that our society values physical perfection above honesty or even kindness.

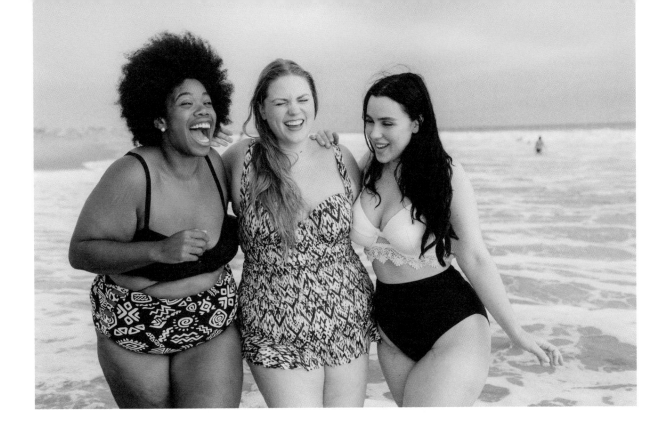

A positive body image makes us feel attractive, even powerful.

Judgment of women's—and, of course, men's—bodies is nothing new. Neither is the effect on our minds and bodies. In the seventeenth century, women painted their faces with lead-based makeup to cover the ubiquitous effects of smallpox and aging. Women of the nineteenth century wore breathtakingly tight corsets to give themselves unnaturally tiny waists. In the 1920s, women wore brassieres to flatten their chests in search of the then-fashionable androgynous look. Yet, today, the Information Age—and in particular the advent of social media—has handed us an endless and inescapable mirror on ourselves that is affecting our body image with perhaps greater intensity than ever before.

In a survey by Sheryl Monteath and Marita McCabe, published in *The Journal of Social Psychology*, 44 percent of women expressed negative feelings about their body. Girls are developing a negative body image at younger ages than ever before. The National Eating Disorders Association reports that 81 percent of ten-year-olds already express a fear of being fat. And men are suffering no less from unrealistic ideas about the masculine body, based on bulked-up action heroes in movies and video games. The National Association for Males with Eating Disorders estimates that 25 to 40 percent of people with eating disorders are male.

BODY POSITIVITY

The body positivity movement urges us to celebrate our body, whatever its shape, age, skin tone, or physical ability. The movement encourages us to unshackle ourselves from the tyranny of body image, which is founded on cultural standards that change with time and place. Body positivity enables us to focus on the health of our body, not its physical appearance.

Forget body image

Society's insistence on body image teaches us to place our own body in a hierarchy, based on desirability. Consciously or subconsciously, we judge our own body as less attractive than that body but—thank goodness!—more attractive than that one. Not only does this self-imposed ranking dent our confidence and distract from true worth, but it discourages us from valuing our body for the miracle it truly is: trillions of dividing cells, dozens of busy organs, and billions of firing neurons that allow us to learn, laugh, and love.

By forgetting societal constructs about shape and muscle mass, we can focus on eating and exercising to be healthy rather than to change how we look. We can forget about crash diets to squeeze into a smaller dress, or lunge reps to develop a perfect rear. Instead, we can eat a healthy diet, containing all the nutrients the body needs to function well. We can develop a well-rounded exercise program that offers aerobic activity to strengthen the heart, and muscle-building activity so we can stay fit into old age.

Focus on what matters

Being truly body positive does not mean forgetting that body mass—at both ends of the scale—can impact on physical wellness. Instead it means focusing on how diet and physical activity make us feel, rather than on how they make us look. Focusing on body image and worrying about hard-to-lose pounds can have a negative effect on our desire to exercise and stay active—where exercise does not have the desired effect on appearance, it comes to feel pointless and depressing.

When exercising, we need to forget about excess pounds or wobbling thighs and focus on the invisible benefits of exercise. Exercise releases brain chemicals that boost mood. In the long term, it reduces the risk

of anxiety and depression. Regular exercise helps the cardiovascular system work more effectively, which improves our energy levels. It helps us sleep better, provided we do not exercise immediately before bed, and combats countless health conditions and diseases, including strokes, high blood pressure, arthritis, type 2 diabetes, and many types of cancer. Exercising regularly into old age can reduce the risk of falls and even dementia. Physicians also tell us that regular exercise can boost our sex life, enhancing arousal in women and reducing the risk of erectile dysfunction in men.

Finally, we can use exercise as a way to spend time with friends or to make new ones, whether

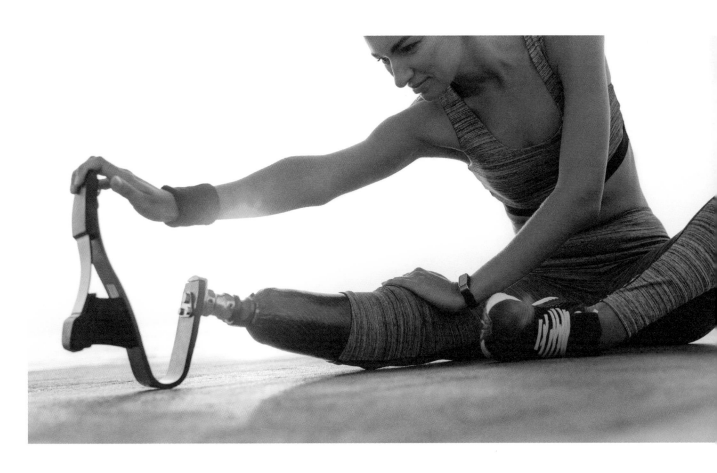

they be workout buddies or fellow Sunday strollers. Exercising with a friend is the ideal way to make it a lasting habit. A good friend likes us for who we are rather than what we look like. They can bolster us through times when anxiety about body image stands in the way of exercise, such as when we are joining a gym for the first time. If you cannot find a like-minded friend, join a local class—and remind yourself that you will never be the only person worried about how they look.

We can use exercise as a way to spend time with friends or to make new ones.

SELF-CARE FOR YOUR BODY: MASSAGE

Massage is probably one of the most popular forms of health activity today. It is used in relaxation groups and workshops, in leisure centers, and as a form of natural therapy for injury and the wear and tear of daily life. Whether performed by a trained professional or a gifted amateur, it offers the experience of touch, movement, and energy, qualities that are associated with the well-being of the whole person, and the act of giving massage has deep significance for both the giver and the receiver.

By treating symptoms, or suppressing them, we are doing nothing to treat the root cause of a problem. Eczema sufferers apply ointments and creams to the surface of the skin; they may take anti-inflammatories or antihistamines to ease the itching, but the cause of the eczema is still there—the body's reaction has just been masked by drugs. They have not been cured; their illness has merely been controlled.

Origins of massage

The physical and psychological benefits of massage have been recognized and valued since ancient times. Working within their limited concepts of body function, early physicians were able to use massage very effectively in the treatment of fatigue, illness, and injury. In the fifth century BC, Hippocrates described anatripsis—literally, "rubbing up"—as having a more favorable effect than rubbing down on the limbs, although the understanding of the blood's circulation was at that time incomplete.

Aesthetically, the ancient Greeks associated physical fitness with the unfolding of mental and spiritual faculties, and set up massage schools in their beautifully built centers of health known as gymnasiums. In the Far East, performing musicians and actors have always learned massage practices as aids to their artistic development; exponents of kathakali, an early dance form originating in southern India, are treated with deep massage from the feet of their teachers. In some societies, massage has even been used socially as an act of hospitality; in Hawaii, for example, passive movements called lomilomi are traditionally bestowed on honored guests.

In Europe, massage remained an important element of health care throughout the duration of the Roman Empire and is widely referred to in the literature of the era. The development of massage in the West seems to have been interrupted by the disintegration of the Roman civilization, although the unbroken tradition continued in the East. It is not until the sixteenth century, at a time when relatively sophisticated surgical techniques were being developed in France, that we hear of massage reemerging in Europe in connection with healing.

In the late nineteenth century, the demand for therapeutic massage led to the formation of societies of therapists. These societies aimed to promote the science of massage, organizing training and "safeguarding the interests of the public and the profession." The desirable characteristics of a practitioner were held to be "good health, intelligence, and a high moral tone." At the time they succeeded in their aims, but later developments were to undo much of their work.

Eclipse and revival

In the twentieth century, the great strides made by conventional medicine have tended to eclipse traditional therapies, even though—or perhaps because—they have been practiced for centuries. Dazzled by the achievements of science and technology, most people in the developed world all but ignored the therapeutic value of human touch until a few decades ago. Yet massage and its sister therapies are enjoying a renaissance. This can be partly explained by a return to "natural" values in reaction to the highly stressful conditions of modern life, but there is also a growing resistance to the dehumanizing aspects of modern health care.

Today many people yearn for an approach to health care that is based not on drugs and technology but on the healing value of physical contact. There is nothing mystical or romantic about this idea. The human body is a physical object that responds to physical influences, and a grasp of human anatomy is central to any understanding of the role of massage. This book is partly a celebration of our wonderful anatomy—an appeal to the imagination, because anatomy is imagination. You can learn little about the body unless you can imagine, for example, your heart's powerful beating, the delicacy and strength of your muscles, and the balance of the bony arrangements that support you. An appreciation of the body's engineering is as vital to good massage as any psychological insight.

Massage is now firmly established as an effective therapy, yet despite growing awareness of its value, the idea of massage often meets with some resistance. Massage has been abused socially, leading to doubts about its morality, and there is still much confusion about its role in healing. Should it be seen as an alternative to conventional medicine, or a complementary therapy? How safe is it? Does it have any real physiological effects, or is it primarily psychological in value? These questions, and no doubt many more, will be examined in the pages that follow.

MASSAGE STYLES

There are many interpretations of massage, and each emphasizes the benefits of a particular technique or style. There are two main categories: Oriental and Western. Oriental styles tend to be stimulating, and use direct, focused pressures. Western styles are more concerned with soothing and calming the patient. The rationale for massage is quite different in each culture. Although formal anatomy is accepted in the East, practitioners there use unconventional theories to explain the interactions between the body and its "owner." So whereas a Western therapist may speak of the liver as an organ of the body, the Eastern therapist refers to the energy that organizes the liver, and will use massage to adjust that sense of energy, rather than treat the organ in isolation.

Massage for illness

Traditional health-care systems throughout the world recognize that massage can play an important role in treating illness. In India, for example, it is not uncommon to see children massaging the legs of their hospitalized parents. For many years, massage has been ignored by orthodox Western medicine, but, increasingly, medical practitioners have come to recognize the potential of massage therapy, especially in connection with those diseases in which personal stress is acknowledged to be an important factor. In many such cases, orthodox treatments have achieved limited success, while holistic therapies involving massage have been of help.

We recognize illness as having two distinct aspects: "acute," which is an active or regenerative stage, and "chronic," in which degenerative processes feature. The stimulating and supportive influence of massage has much to offer in both cases, helping to alleviate acute conditions and reduce the emotional and psychological disturbance associated with chronic conditions.

Massage is valuable during illness because of its recognition that being ill involves being disordered neurologically. The term "being ill" is another way of expressing that the body is under the dominance of the sympathetic nerves: the part of the autonomic nervous system that governs the system's response to irregularity. Sympathetic nerve activity is also associated with fear and distress, and this is why even the simplest manifestation of disease tends to be associated with emotional upset.

Extreme cases of this are sometimes described as psychosomatic conditions, in which the fear generated and the condition provoking it fuel each other in a relentless, self-perpetuating cycle. Massage can interrupt this cycle and relieve the distress of illness by modifying sympathetic nerve activity and encouraging the activity of the parasympathetic nerves, which have a relaxing effect. This increases the patient's tolerance of pain, which is a good indicator of recovery, enabling the patient to make a swifter return to full health.

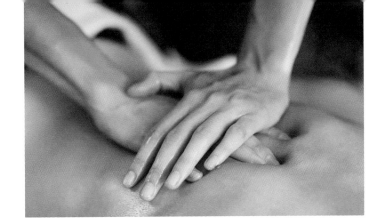

Massage for injury

The influence of massage on the circulation is very helpful in alleviating pain after accidents and injuries. In the case of serious injury, the pain can be greater during the recovery stage than immediately after the accident, and is often associated with the return of functioning. Vigorously massaging the opposite limb to the injured one, or the lower limbs in cases of upper-body injury, alleviates pressure without compromising the healing processes.

An injury harms the tissue, interrupting normal functioning. It is accompanied by pain, swelling, and inflammation. Pain draws conscious awareness to the site of the injury so that irritating movement is discouraged. The increased circulation to the injured tissue is responsible for the swelling, which also helps immobilize the damaged area. Inflammation involves a rise in local temperature that helps destroy debris within the injury. Appropriate massage treatment helps modify these responses so that injuries are easier to bear and quicker to heal.

The blood that is attracted to an injury is thicker than usual because of the increase in white cell activity. The lymphatic system is also mobilized to supply a watery disinfectant that protects the body from any external contamination. It is unwise to reduce the resulting swelling artificially since it contains healing ingredients. Raising the injured part higher than the heart usually makes the congested state much more tolerable; meanwhile, the gentle strokes of massage, above and below the injury, are helpful in maintaining an effective drainage.

The inflammatory response is necessary to help dispose of disintegrating body tissue. It is an uncomfortable experience, however, and the most obvious, effective way to minimize this discomfort is through the use of cooling hydrotherapy. The heat from the inflammation is transferred to a cool compress and the effect on the nerves and the blood vessels is very soothing.

Massage types

WESTERN MASSAGE	INNOVATIVE	PHYSIOTHERAPY	EASTERN
Swedish Massage (Europe)	Bowen Technique (Bowen)	Vacuum Suction (Effleurage)	Ayurveda (India)
Esalen (California)	Polarity (Randolph Stone)	Gyrator (Kneading)	Tuina (China)
Aromatherapy (Anglo-French)	Rolfing (Ida Rolf)	Ultrasound (Petrissage)	Lomilomi (Hawaii)
Holistic Massage	Reflexology (Bailey)	Vibrator (Percussion)	Shiatsu (Japan)

BENEFITS OF MASSAGE FOR PHYSICAL WELLNESS

The benefits of massage are extensive. It can be used to help preserve health and treat illness. It can work in conjunction with orthodox and complementary therapies, and is in itself an enjoyable and healthy activity. As the popularity of massage increases, more opportunities are being identified for its use—from easing the discomforts of childbirth to providing emotional and physical support to a wide range of individuals.

In India, massage is considered to be indispensable, and beneficial literally from the cradle to the grave. In Japan, people are regularly roused by the shiatsu practitioner who calls from house to house asking, "Shiatsu today?" The whole family may then each enjoy ten minutes of refreshing treatment. Throughout the world, massage is employed in preparation for surgery, and it is also used for postoperative therapy. In the United States it is an important element of stress-management programs, and it has been found that the act of giving simple massage reduces stress even in the givers.

Physiological benefits

The benefits of massage as injury therapy have always been appreciated in sports, but in recent years its use has developed and expanded. Massage is now an intrinsic part of an enlightened attitude that embraces the care as well as the repair of athletes. Its importance as a means of combating the stresses of competitive sports has made it a major component of training and fitness regimes.

The value of massage as therapy for a variety of subclinical conditions has been demonstrated by its application to long-distance air travel. Although in some respects less arduous than in the past, modern air journeys are nevertheless capable of producing symptoms such as dehydration, indigestion, stiffness, and disorientation. Massage can help with all these, and one airline company offers in-flight therapy, in which passengers receive facial, foot, or hand massage. They are also advised on simple de-stressing movements. Another airline has developed a seat with built-in massage technology that intermittently stimulates passive posture throughout the flight. Passengers have reported that these treatments reduce the impact of jet lag, especially when combined with rest and further massage soon after landing.

It has been found that the act of giving simple massage reduces stress even in the givers.

Psychological benefits

It is one of the many joys of massage that its therapeutic benefits are not exclusive to professional treatment. Even at a spontaneous level, massage provides an opportunity for us to offer help to both family and friends.

It seems almost instinctive to squeeze the shoulders of a tired or anxious friend or smooth the brow of a startled child. Most people know how it feels to be under strain, and this may be our guide when giving untutored massage. For those who find it natural to extend a helping hand, it is not difficult to convert a tentative approach into a lasting, beneficial exchange for both receiver and giver. A little experience, coupled with a little knowledge about how massage works, can transform the instinctive touch into a precious gift.

Massage has been found to be a useful extension of communication between partners or colleagues when verbal and familiar patterns of relating become exhausted. Massage can create emotional space, reducing the intensity of conflict, and provide cooling-off time without repressing the real issues. The powerful nonverbal communication of massage enables friends to address the physical burden of each other's problems without necessarily involving direct or unwanted confrontation.

Ultimate benefit

Enjoying and appreciating the benefits of massage requires a physical receptivity and a willingness to be benefited by our bodies. Throughout history, certain religious codes of conduct have demanded restraint and control at all times, and these precepts have become ingrained in our culture. Consequently, some people find their access to the pleasure of massage blocked by their own physical inhibitions. Fortunately, nature has arranged that the benefits of massage, once they have been experienced, become inviting, magnetic, and irresistible.

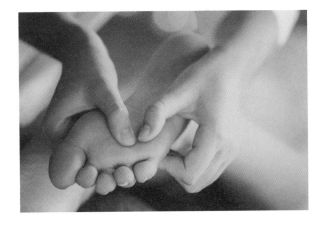

MASSAGE SELF-TREATMENTS

While massage is generally most beneficial when given by another person, it can also be used as a safe and effective self-treatment. Practitioners often teach self-applied movements to use at home to extend the effects of a professional massage. There may also be occasions when treatment is required urgently, and such emergencies nearly always occur when helpful friends or therapists are unavailable. When the immediate need is to contain a problem or deal with acute pain, self-treatments can be extremely valuable.

Aside from any physical benefit, the feeling that you are able to respond physically to a problem can be very reassuring as you await the attention of an expert therapist. It is very comforting to have techniques readily available that are helpful in managing pain, refreshing, and emotionally sustaining. Self-massage has a variety of applications. Chronic conditions and problems associated with wear and tear often respond well to self-treatment. Self-massage is also known to be beneficial for respiratory distress and exhaustion, and can provide stress relief in the workplace. In parts of China, for example, it is a recognized part of the daily routine of many workers. The most obvious practitioners of self-massage are massage therapists, who enjoy its benefits through the rhythmic strokes and movements they apply to their patients.

A softer option

While self-treatment is primarily a maintenance therapy, it also has a role in the prevention of problems. By including self-massage as part of a fitness program, it is possible to avoid the buildup of conditions that may precede an emergency.

Learning self-massage can be an important step toward accepting treatment from someone else. If given massage feels too pressurizing or threatening for those who are reclaiming their bodies from self-harm or another type of trauma, tentative self-massage can encourage recognition of positive sensory experiences. This is particularly true of reservations about abdominal massage.

It is understandable that we should feel physically protective of the abdomen since, considering its importance, it is a relatively unprotected area of the body. It is quite possible that, because of the ideal position of our hands relative to the abdomen and the sensitivity of its muscles, self-massage of the abdomen may initially be more effective than given massage. The realization of its benefits may then allow a deeper, therapeutic treatment to be received from an experienced massage practitioner later.

Self-massage in practice

Given reasonable privacy, self-treatment can be applied wherever and whenever possible. There are some simple movements that can be done anywhere, such as squeezing the fists or wriggling toes within shoes; both of these are useful for relieving fatigue. It is also possible to apply self-help therapy at antisocial times, such as in the middle of the night. The below self-massage may help with insomnia, and other techniques such as self-applied neck massage (see page 112) can also help deal with broken sleep.

Self-treatment is rarely contraindicated, even when given massage may be inadvisable. This is because you have total control over the level of pressure—an important feature of appropriate massage. There is also less chance that the treatment may irritate underlying conditions, because the feedback is immediate and the movements can be finely adjusted. Self-massage can even assist in reclaiming self-control after the incapacitation of illness or injury.

Self-massage for insomnia

If you are unable to fall asleep, then tossing and turning and furiously rubbing your head will only succeed in increasing the blood supply to your brain. Instead, try this hydrotherapy massage, which harmlessly reduces blood flow to the head and helps the brain to naturally switch off.

1. Go to the sink and turn on the cold water. Place each wrist under the flow of water for one minute. Your wrists should feel cooled but not chilled.

2. Use a towel to mop the water from your hands rather than fully drying them. Then go back to bed.

3. Lie on your side so you can insert your hands beneath your underarms. Breathe deeply and assume a sleepy attitude by pretending to be fast asleep.

4. Almost immediately, you will be aware of increasing warmth in your hands. While this is happening, the blood supply to your brain is reduced.

The first time you use this hydrotherapy, you will imagine that you must be dreaming, by which time . . .

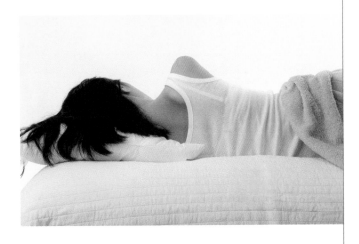

SELF-MASSAGE FOR YOUR NECK

The neck is a vulnerable structure. The heels of shoes cause the head to tilt backward and shorten the neck; most of us hear better from one ear and twist the neck around to the clearer side; violent movements may tear at the neck's delicate nerves and blood vessels. This in turn may lead to referred pain in the head and arms. Compensatory tensions build up around the bones, often heard as crackling during neck exercises.

This self-massage encourages a relaxed centeredness of the neck. It is also worth trying for sinus congestion, with the addition of a hot cloth over the cheeks and a cold cloth around the feet.

1. Roll a small towel to a diameter of roughly 3 inches. Lie down and place the towel directly beneath your neck, taking up the normal neck curvature. Relax your jaw.

2. Draw your feet up closer to your hips (A). Without deliberately moving, your head will have rocked slightly backward.

3. Keeping your head in contact with the floor, roll the head to the left and right against the towel a few times, then come to rest on the right side. Breathe deeply for a few seconds.

4. Roll again two or three times and rest on the left side, breathing as before. If one side of the neck feels tighter, roll the head back toward the stiffness for a few seconds, then slowly roll as far as possible in the opposite direction.

5. Return to center, reach up, and hold the ends of the towel (B). After a deep inward breath, exhale, while at the same time rolling your supported head comfortably forward, chin toward your chest. Repeat once more.

6. Lower your head slowly and replace your arms by your sides. Relax completely with your mouth slightly open. To recover without strain, roll your whole body over and push yourself upright from the side.

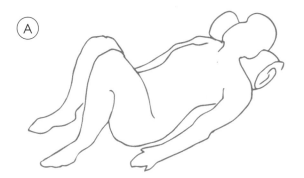

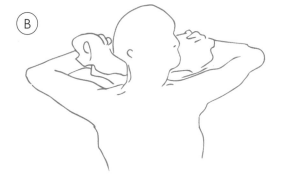

Self-massage encourages a relaxed centeredness of the neck.

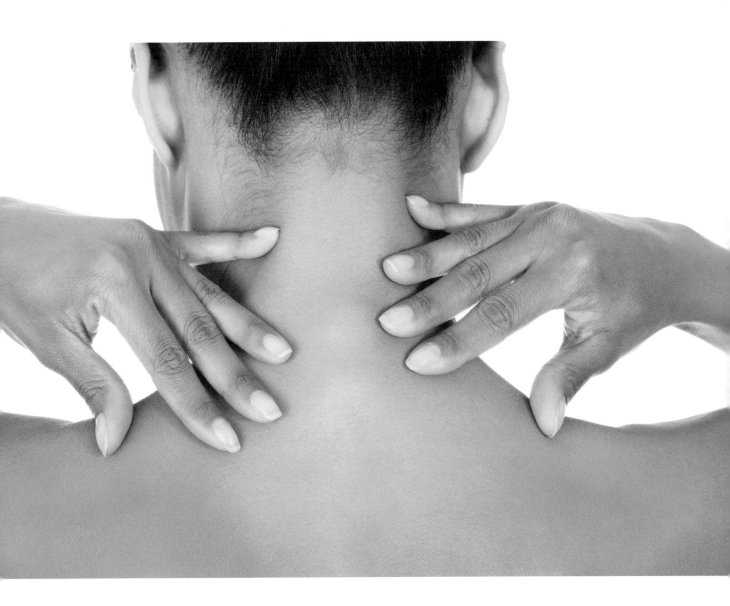

ABDOMINAL SELF-MASSAGE

Massage for abdominal pain

The usual cause of abdominal pain is indigestion. Excessive consumption of any food tends to overwhelm the system, and when someone is exhausted or nervously upset, food that has been eaten is hardly processed at all. The pain associated with the symptoms is connected to the slow but steady cramping of the muscles of digestion, which normally squeeze food gently through the system. Since this process is itself a massage system for food, self-massage is a very appropriate treatment.

1. Lie down with a pillow under your knees (A). Take a few deep breaths. Investigate your abdomen with gently probing fingers. If you feel a tightening over a painful area, begin a smooth, continuous, reinforced effleurage, clockwise, massaging with lighter pressure over the uncomfortable part.

2. If this helps, use the knuckles or fingertips to give little bounces over the painful part, pressing enough to stretch the skin. You may detect some movement within the abdomen. Alternate this pressure with effleurage.

3. Where there has been focused tension in the abdomen, the remaining area will have gone slack. Do a quicker, upward effleurage with one or both hands to encourage toning (B).

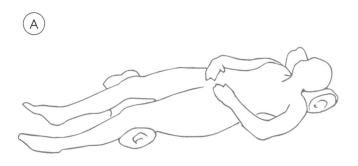

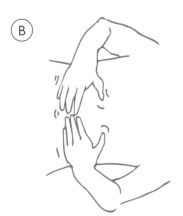

Massage for constipation

The internal body massage responsible for moving food through the digestive tract is called peristalsis. The action of peristalsis is continuous to the very end of the digestive process in the large intestine or colon, but action of the sympathetic nervous system can disrupt the activity of the colon and cause constipation. Self-massage can help relieve the problem by converting the sympathetic nervous activity to parasympathetic activity. The position adopted for this massage is well known outside English-speaking countries.

1. If needed, practice squatting by holding on to a stable chair or door handle and lowering your hips as far as you can go (A). Try to keep your feet flat.

2. When you have made your hips supple, squat on the toilet seat in the same way. If you can't manage this without fear of falling, sit down and raise your feet on a box so that your knees are higher than your hips.

3. Retract and slowly release your abdomen a few times. Make a fist and press gently but deeply around the edge of the abdomen, especially on the left side. Relax and breathe deeply and avoid bearing down.

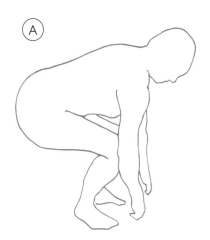

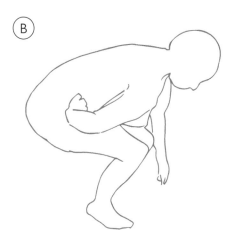

SELF-MASSAGE FOR YOUR EYES AND FEET

Massage for tired eyes

Although it may not seem possible to overuse the eyes, the monotonous gazing and fixed focusing associated with modern living can become strenuous. The strain affects the eyes' external muscles, causing them to sting and ache. Eyesight is also known to be affected by stressful events. This self-massage, known as palming, has both physical and mental benefits. It deeply relaxes the eyes and eases tension in the neck muscles, which is important for the circulation to the eyes. If you are becoming concerned about your eyes, do these movements twice a day along with a neck massage.

1. Wearing loose-necked clothing, sit close to a table. Shrug your shoulders, rolling them forward and backward six times.

2. Rub your hands together vigorously for a few seconds to generate some friction and make the palms feel warm.

3. Place both your palms (not your fingers) over your closed eyes so that no light can leak through the gaps.

4. Rest your elbows on the table and take a few deep breaths. You will begin to feel your neck muscles relaxing.

5. Let your arms slide apart a little and slowly sink your head into your hands, taking more weight on your elbows (A). Spend a few moments visualizing a vivid, colorful scene from nature, with changing perspectives.

6. After approximately one minute, let the imagery fade and breathe deeply six times. Lightly make contact with the eyeballs by extending your thumb and fingers and flattening your palms over your eye sockets (B).

7. Lower your hands to your cheeks and make smooth effleurages from between the eyebrows to the temples (C), six times.

8. Relax your arms. Widen your eyes for a moment and breathe deeply to conclude the self-massage treatment.

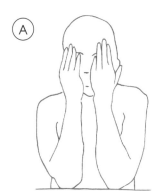

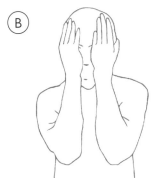

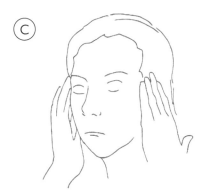

Massage for feet

From an early age our feet are confined by shoes in a way that would be unacceptable to any other part of the body. This may result in irreversible compensations such as fallen arches and toe deviations; freely moving feet are known to provide significant help in preventing heart disease and assisting postoperative circulation. This self-massage can be helpful with headaches, as well as foot discomfort. The water massages are useful when you are suffering from low energy or just getting back on your feet after an illness.

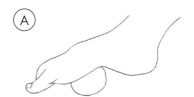

1. Fill a basin with ankle-deep cool water. Take off your shoes and socks and paddle for two minutes, lifting each foot clear of the water with every paddle action.

2. Mop your feet dry. Place a ball under one instep and roll the foot backward and forward for one minute (A). Repeat with the other foot.

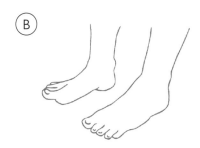

3. Walk your feet slowly forward, one foot length at a time, using creeping movements of your toes. Then creep backward.

4. Press your left toes onto the floor while drawing your right toes firmly upward, keeping the foot flat (B). Hold for three seconds, then repeat on the other side.

5. While keeping the toes on the ground, bounce the heel of each foot up and down 20 times.

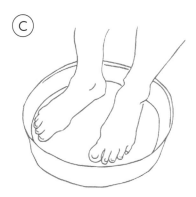

6. Keeping the heels on the ground, bounce the rest of the foot up and down 20 times. Paddle again for one minute (C), then wrap the feet in a towel without drying, and rest with your legs elevated.

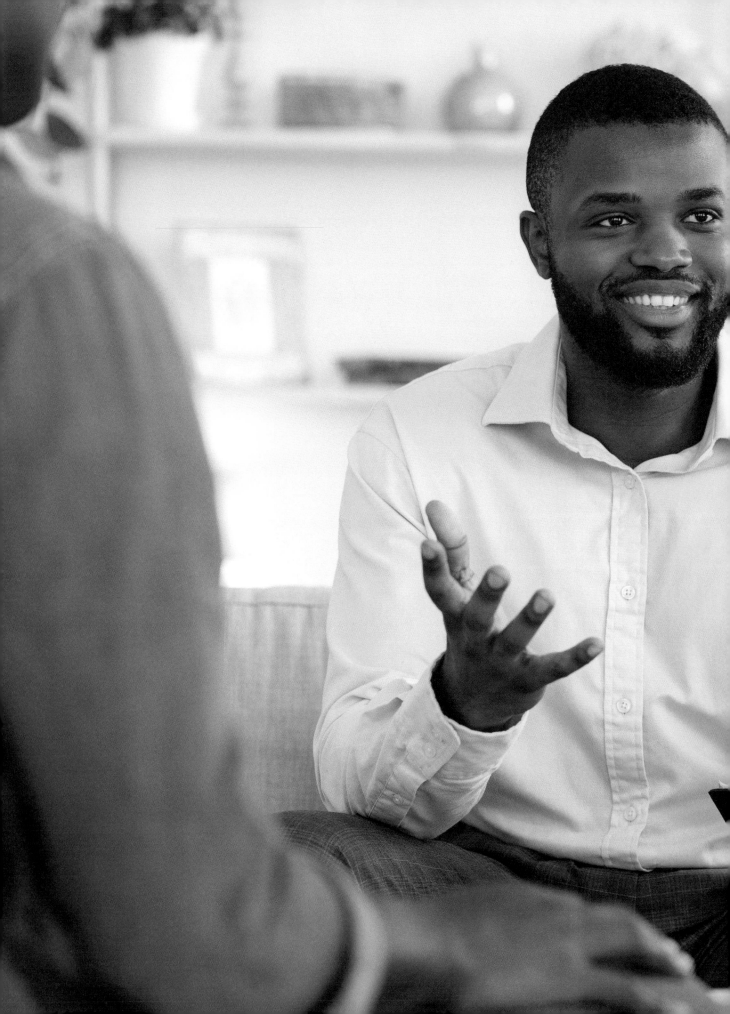

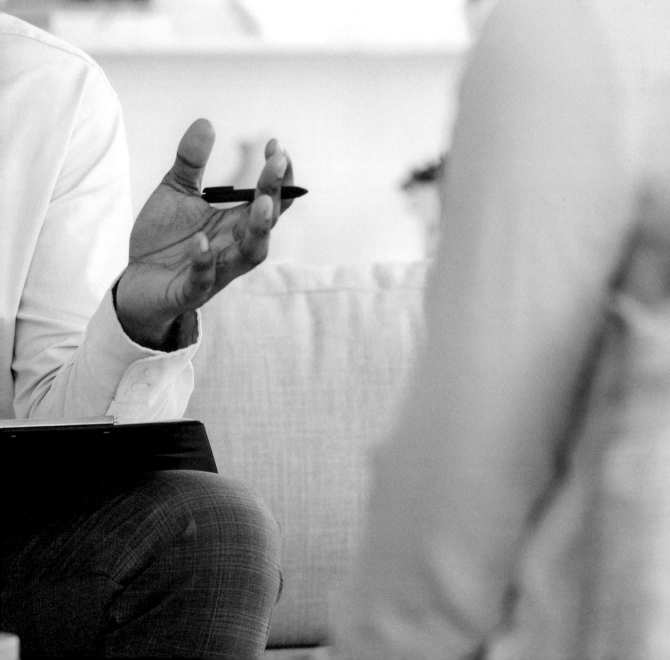

PART TWO

Mental Wellness

THE IMPORTANCE OF MENTAL WELLNESS

Mental health and wellness includes your emotional, psychological, and social well-being, affecting how you think, feel, and act. If you have a healthy and balanced state of mental wellness, you're better equipped to handle stress, make decisions, socialize with other people, and deal with your day-to-day home and work commitments with ease.

Issues with mental health are common, affecting an estimated one in five adults. Yet in the past there's been a stigma associated with mental health that's led people to hide their illness and suffer in silence. Mental health and wellness are talked about more openly now, although there's still room for improvement, and awareness about the importance of looking after your mental health is growing.

Looking after your mental wellness should be part of everyone's self-care regime. It may seem like your mental health is separate from your physical health, but when one is out of balance, it can affect the other. In fact, some physical health problems are directly linked to mental health conditions. Stress, for example, can raise the risk of heart disease, so managing stress could have a positive impact on your physical heart health.

There are plenty more benefits to be gained from looking after your mental wellness needs. For example, you may experience improvements in your mood, a reduction in feelings of anxiety, an ability to think more clearly, and find that your self-esteem and confidence are boosted, your relationships improve for the better, and you feel more at peace and content with yourself.

Self-care for mental wellness

There are many aspects involved in self-care for mental wellness, in particular looking after your physical and mental health. For example:

EXERCISING REGULARLY—find something you enjoy doing, from yoga or tai chi to running, tennis, or going to the gym.

EAT A HEALTHY, BALANCED, AND NUTRITIONALLY RICH DIET—include lots of fresh produce to get a good range of vitamins and minerals; regular meals help balance blood sugar levels.

MAKE SURE YOU GET ENOUGH SLEEP—sleep is essential for both physical and mental wellness and to help you cope with life's demands.

DRINK PLENTY OF WATER—you need it to stay properly hydrated.

SET YOURSELF GOALS AND PRIORITIES—decide what you can and can't do and learn to say "no" to demands that are too much.

BE GRATEFUL—practice gratitude and learn to be grateful for everything in your life, however big or small.

DEVELOP AND NURTURE FRIENDSHIPS—social connections are important for everyone.

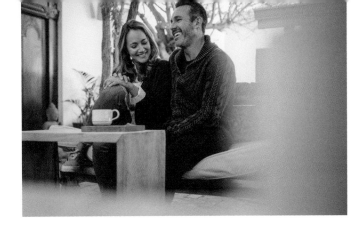

How to spot the signs of potential mental health issues

If you're struggling mentally or you suspect that someone else is, there are some warning signs that you can look out for. It's not unusual to initially be unaware that your issues could be related to mental health, as this can be hard to spot in yourself; or it's possible that a person may have an inkling, yet try and hide their condition from other people for fear of shame or embarrassment.

Common signs of potential mental health issues include:

• A change in social behavior—not attending social situations, and being on your own more.

• A change in eating habits—overeating, undereating, or eating more erratically.

• Low energy levels and sleeping more than usual.

• Sudden onset of insomnia and not sleeping properly.

• Mood swings and sudden anxiety.

• Falling out and picking fights with friends and family.

• Not keeping in contact with people—not replying to texts, phone calls, or messages when you usually do.

• Feeling in a constant state of despair or hopelessness.

• Being confused, forgetful, on edge, upset, or scared.

• Not coping with everyday tasks—anything from not looking after pets or being able to cope with the demands of work, to not washing or caring for yourself properly.

• Harming yourself or other people.

• Suddenly drinking or smoking more than usual or taking drugs.

• Believing things that aren't true.

• Feeling suicidal.

These signs and symptoms don't affect everyone in the same way and can also be associated with other health conditions. If you feel like you're struggling with your mental health, or you know someone else who might be, seek help from a medical practitioner. There are lots of treatments available, including talking therapies and medication, and it's much better to get treatment than to hide how you really feel, especially since symptoms may get worse without intervention.

It's also good to open up and talk to friends or family about how you're feeling. The chances are they may have been through a similar experience themselves, and talking about it with them can make things seem more manageable.

MENTAL HEALTH AND ITS EFFECTS

Mental health issues can have a huge impact on your life, your ability to perform simple daily tasks, your work, family, and social life. The longer you ignore your mental health and any potential symptoms you may be experiencing, the worse things can get. There are a variety of different mental health problems, some of which have similar symptoms.

Anxiety

It's normal to feel anxious from time to time, but if you suffer from anxiety, it's a regular occurrence. Anxiety can be mild, moderate, or severe, where it seriously disrupts your life. Feelings of anxiety can be paralyzing, stopping you from doing your usual activities like shopping, socializing, or things you enjoy. There's likely to be a cycle of fear, whereby you live in fear of fear, and the anxiety can be overwhelming.

Depression

Depression is more than just feeling down every now and again. It's a persistent low mood that lasts for weeks or months and has a direct impact on your life. Depression can be mild or severe and cause physical symptoms such as exhaustion, a change in appetite, and insomnia, as well as make you feel worthless, unmotivated, and hopeless.

Panic attacks

Panic attacks are sudden attacks of extreme fear and anxiety that cause intense and scary physical and mental symptoms. They typically come on suddenly and often for no apparent reason, causing symptoms such as a racing heartbeat, feeling faint, chest pain, nausea, trembling, dizziness, and hot flashes.

Phobias

Phobias are extreme fears that are triggered by certain circumstances or objects. For example, an extreme fear of snakes, of driving, or of being in social situations. Fears become phobias when they are completely out of proportion to the actual danger faced, if they last a long time, or if they significantly impact your daily life.

Obsessive-compulsive disorder

Obsessive-compulsive disorder (OCD) is a form of anxiety disorder. It's characterized by having obsessions—unwanted thoughts, worries, doubts, or urges that keep coming to mind and won't go away; and compulsions—repetitive actions that you keep needing to do to try and reduce the anxiety of the obsession.

Learning to accept help

Acknowledging you're not feeling well and admitting and accepting help, whether from a friend or family member in the first instance, followed by medical expertise if required, is one of the most important steps you can take. It gives you the opportunity to gain the support you need and puts you on the path toward getting better. The exact treatment you'll need depends on your individual symptoms and mental health diagnosis, so you'll need to accept

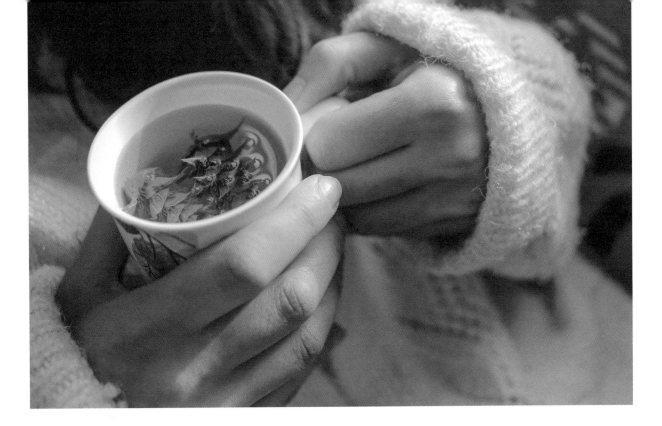

Learn to focus on the good things in your life that make you feel brighter.

guidance as to what is deemed best for you. One part of your treatment may involve learning to develop coping skills and strategies to help you deal with difficult symptoms, so they don't overwhelm you to the same extent in the future. Mental health issues don't necessarily go away instantly, and it can take time to get symptoms under control, but with the right help, you can learn to successfully manage your symptoms and live a happier life.

Self-help for mild mental health issues

In cases of mild mental health issues, where you're not at the stage of needing conventional treatments or forms of therapy, but you could do with a boost and extra support of some kind, there are self-help methods you can adopt to help deal with mild symptoms.

For example, your diet and nutrition can have an impact on your health, and making small changes to eating habits could have a beneficial effect. Exercising is important, too, and there are some forms of exercise, such as yoga, that combine a focus on both the body and the mind, making them ideal for mental wellness.

Natural remedies such as the use of herbs may offer an alternative treatment for mild symptoms that don't require conventional medication, and there are some remedies that you can have a go at making yourself at home, such as herbal teas. Other more unusual approaches include the use of crystals, which work on a vibrational level and may offer an extra way to help soothe your soul.

In the rest of this section, you'll discover lots of different ways to take care of your mental wellness, nurturing your body and mind and learning to focus on the good things in your life that make you feel brighter.

STRESS

Stress describes the feelings you have when the demands made on you, or that you feel are being made, are more than you are able to fully cope with. Stress can affect all ages and is a normal reaction to pressure. It can be caused by external stressors, such as pressure from work, life experiences, family, or finances; or internal stressors, such as thoughts and feelings of inadequacy, uncertainty, or low self-esteem.

Sometimes the effect of stress can be positive; for example, if it acts as encouragement or motivation to get on with the task in hand. This is because stress is a physical response, causing your body to move into the fight-or-flight mode. As it does so, the body releases a mix of hormones and chemicals, such as adrenaline, cortisol, and norepinephrine, that prepare your body for action. That is what causes physical symptoms such as a pounding heart, a rush of energy, and fast breathing, which can prove to be exhilarating and motivational for some.

However, stress is healthy and positive only when it is short-lived. Stress becomes a problem when you experience too much of it, causing it to become overwhelming and resulting in both physical and mental exhaustion. Too much cortisol can also affect your immune system, making it less efficient.

Stress can cause emotional and behavioral changes. You may be plagued by feelings of anxiety, fear, anger, depression, and frustration, and lack concentration, sleep, and the ability to make decisions. In turn, a buildup of all these feelings can produce physical symptoms, such as heart palpitations, headaches, and aches and pains.

Stress can be a highly unpleasant experience, and an important part of tackling stress is to accept you have a problem. As well as identifying the root causes and making lifestyle changes, exploring ways to release your stress, relax your mind, and rebalance your body are some of the key ways of combating it.

Nutrition

Eating a good, balanced diet will make your body stronger and able to cope more efficiently with stress. B vitamins are often depleted by stress, so ensure that you are getting enough in your diet, or take a good supplement. There is some evidence that bee and flower pollen can boost immunity and energize the body. However, do not eat them if you are allergic to honey or bee stings.

An amino acid called L-tyrosine appears to energize, and studies show that people taking this

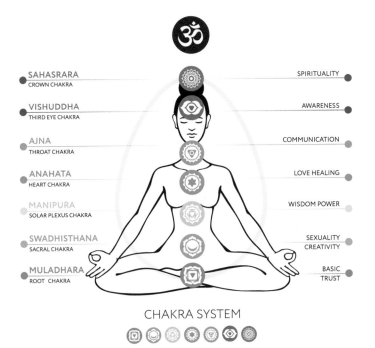

The chakra system is key to placing crystals in the healing practice.

SAHASRARA
CROWN CHAKRA

VISHUDDHA
THIRD EYE CHAKRA

AJNA
THROAT CHAKRA

ANAHATA
HEART CHAKRA

MANIPURA
SOLAR PLEXUS CHAKRA

SWADHISTHANA
SACRAL CHAKRA

MULADHARA
ROOT CHAKRA

SPIRITUALITY

AWARENESS

COMMUNICATION

LOVE HEALING

WISDOM POWER

SEXUALITY
CREATIVITY

BASIC
TRUST

CHAKRA SYSTEM

supplement react better to stressful situations, staying more alert and less anxious, and have fewer complaints about physical discomforts. Vitamin C, found in oranges, blackcurrants, and bell peppers, is a great stress reliever and boosts immunity, making you fitter and healthier.

Pumpkin seeds, which contain high quantities of zinc, iron, and calcium, as well as B vitamins and proteins, which are necessary for brain function, will help you to deal with the effects of stress. Oats are vital for a healthy nervous system. In periods of stress, start the day with oatmeal, which will help to keep you calm, and prevent depression and general debility.

Herbal remedies

Herbs that encourage relaxation and act as a tonic to the nervous system include lemon balm, lavender, chamomile, passionflower, and oats. These can be drunk as an infusion when in a stressful situation. Ginseng is an "adaptogenic" herb, which means that it lifts you when you are tired and relaxes you when you are stressed. It also works on the immune system and energizes. Some therapists recommend a daily dose at stressful times. It is not suitable for use during pregnancy or by those with high blood pressure.

Crystals

Crystals can work on an emotional level, so may be useful to help you cope with mental wellness concerns.

AMETHYST—has a gentle, calming energy, so is ideal to wear or keep close to you during times of stress.

HEMATITE—a stone of grounding, this crystal will help you to maintain balance and soak up negative energies around you.

TIGER'S EYE—the energies of this warm and earthy stone will help you keep focused and reduce the chance of you being diverted off course by other distractions.

AMAZONITE—a stone that could help transform negative thoughts associated with stress into positive ones.

ANXIETY

It's normal to feel anxious from time to time, but some people are plagued with constant anxiety, worries, and fears. Feelings of anxiety can range in severity from mild to severe. When anxiety is constant, it can take over and affect your home, work, and social life. The symptoms may start off as psychological, but constant anxiety can lead to physical symptoms such as restlessness, insomnia, dizziness, palpitations, irritability, fatigue, and difficulty concentrating. You may experience trouble sleeping or have nightmares, and you may find it hard to switch off painful or traumatic memories and thoughts.

Anxiety is likely to be caused by a combination of factors, including brain chemistry, genetics, and environmental factors. Severe anxiety may prevent you from doing daily activities and the things you enjoy, from going shopping and attending social events, to getting in an elevator or even leaving your home. Without treatment, anxiety disorders will worsen. See your doctor if you're experiencing signs of anxiety, especially if anxiety is seriously affecting your life, as sometimes it can be caused by an underlying health condition.

Nutrition

If you're feeling anxious, it's important to practice self-care and look after your body. In general, eating a healthy, balanced diet rich in fresh fruits and vegetables containing plenty of vitamins, minerals, and antioxidants will play a part in nurturing your body. Make sure you include plenty of complex carbohydrates, too, as they may help to increase the natural levels of serotonin in your brain, which can have a calming effect. Good examples of such foods include whole-grain bread, whole-grain cereals, oats, and quinoa.

Magnesium is associated with easing anxiety and promoting calm, so try and include foods rich in magnesium in your diet. There are plenty to choose from, including leafy greens such as spinach and Swiss chard, nuts, seeds, and whole grains. Foods containing zinc could be beneficial, too, examples being cashew nuts, liver, egg yolks, beef, and oysters.

Avoid drinking caffeine and alcohol if you're feeling anxious, as they can both affect your sleep. Caffeine can also make you feel jittery, which is the last thing you need with anxiety. Instead, switch to calming herbal teas and drink plenty of water to keep hydrated.

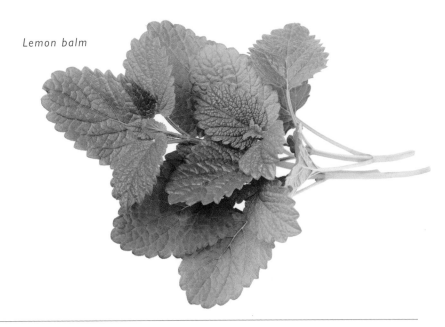

Lemon balm

Herbal remedies

Lemon balm and chamomile both have calming properties and can be helpful to ease mild feelings of anxiety. You can make your own herbal tea and drink a cup when you're feeling anxious. To make lemon balm or chamomile tea, infuse 1 tablespoon of the herb in one mug of boiling water for 10–15 minutes, then strain, warm through and drink it, adding a teaspoon of honey if desired.

The herb passionflower contains naturally occurring phytochemicals and the alkaloid harmine, which can have a calming effect on the mind. Popular passionflower remedies include tea, tinctures, sprays, or ready-made tablets. To brew passionflower tea, infuse 1 tablespoon of the herb in a mug of boiling water and let it steep for 10–15 minutes. Strain, warm through, and enjoy.

Another useful herb to have on hand if you're experiencing anxiety is valerian, which has natural sedative properties and is effective in dealing with anxiety-related insomnia and promoting natural sleep. Try drinking a cup of valerian tea before bed, or take ready-made capsules or a tincture for convenience.

Note: If you are on any medication for anxiety or other health conditions, always check with a medical practitioner first, as some herbs can react with this.

Crystals

GREEN CALCITE—a comforting crystal that could help to restore balance in your mind and help you let go of negativity and worries. Keep a piece in your pocket—a smooth tumble stone would be ideal—and hold it in your hand if you feel anxious.

BLACK TOURMALINE—place black tourmaline on the root chakra to help ground you and release tension. If your crystal has a point, place it with the point facing away from you, to draw off negative thoughts.

AMETHYST—wear an amethyst crystal pendant on a necklace to help calm your body and mind. It may help with decision-making if you're feeling anxious about making the right choices.

DEPRESSION

Everyone feels down or unhappy from time to time, but depression is much more than that. Depression is a health condition where you feel constantly and intensely low for weeks or months at a time. There are physical and mental symptoms, such as anxiety, stress, feeling hopeless, being tearful, and losing interest in everything, and they can range from mild to severe. Other symptoms may include insomnia, waking up in the night, irritability, worry, low self-esteem, changes in appetite, fatigue, aches and pains, lack of energy, withdrawing from social activities, and loss of libido. Severe depression can also be associated with suicidal thoughts.

Depression can be caused by stressful life events, such as changing jobs, losing a job, financial worries, bereavement, or trauma. As discussed, there's often a stigma associated with mental health, and depression is one of the conditions where people may be afraid or embarrassed to admit how they're feeling and ask for help. But symptoms won't go away on their own, and could worsen, so it's essential to see a medical practitioner for diagnosis and treatment.

Nutrition

If you're feeling depressed, it's easy to fall into bad habits and eat unhealthily, overeat, or skip meals completely, but a good balanced diet is really helpful. Your mood can be affected by what you eat and drink, so steer clear of processed and refined foods such as fried foods, junk foods, lots of sugar, and fat. Instead, try to eat foods rich in essential vitamins and minerals.

Avoid skipping breakfast, and instead eat oatmeal. Oats are rich in saponins, alkaloids, B vitamins, and flavonoids and will keep you fuller for longer and your blood sugar levels stable. Other breakfast cereals and whole-grain breads that are fortified with folic acid help with increasing blood levels of the B vitamin folate. Depression can be associated with low levels of folate, so it's important to get this B vitamin into your diet. Other good sources include cabbage, broccoli, beet, spinach, kale, asparagus, and black-eyed beans.

If you experience a craving for carbohydrates, eat complex carbohydrates such as whole-grain foods instead of simple carbs (such as cakes or cookies). It's possible that a craving for carbohydrates may be linked to the chemical serotonin, which is known as a mood-boosting brain chemical. Lean meats and low-fat milk will give you a good dose of vitamin B6, which the body needs to convert the amino acid tryptophan into serotonin. Include protein-rich foods such as turkey, tuna, and chicken in your daily diet.

Avoid drinking caffeine and alcohol if you're feeling depressed, as they can both affect your sleep, plus caffeine can make you feel jittery. Instead, switch to calming herbal teas and drink plenty of water to keep hydrated.

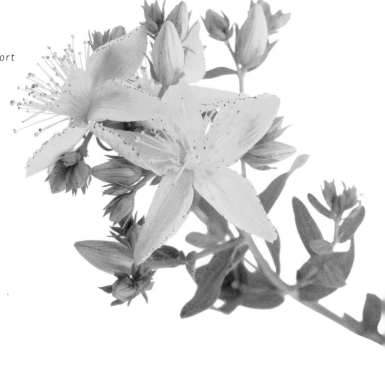

St. John's wort

Herbal remedies

The herb vervain has natural sedative properties and may help with easing feelings of depression. If you have access to fresh or dried vervain, you can make your own herbal tea by adding 1–3 teaspoons of the herb to a mug of boiling water. Let it infuse for 10–15 minutes, then strain, warm through, and drink. For ongoing depression, aim to drink a cup up to three times a day. Ready-made herbal remedies are available, too—look for vervain capsules or tinctures and take according to the guidelines.

The herb St. John's wort has a natural sedative and pain-reducing effect and may be beneficial for mild symptoms of depression. It can be found in health-food stores in the form of tablets, capsules, and tinctures that should be taken as recommended on the packaging.

Sage may also be helpful for depression. Sage tea can be drunk, but isn't to everyone's taste. Instead, try adding fresh or dried sage leaves into meals as you cook for a tasty and nutritious dish.

Note: Do not take herbal remedies (especially St. John's wort) if you're taking prescribed medication, as the herbs can cause unwanted interactions. Speak to your medical practitioner or pharmacist for advice.

Crystals

MOSS AGATE—Hold moss agate to access the stabilizing energies of this crystal. It can help remove negativity and fear, boost self-esteem, and generally help you see things from a different perspective.

AMETRINE—Place on the solar plexus chakra to help bring mental clarity and release physical, emotional, and mental blockages. It's also useful for easing headaches, tension, and stress associated with depression.

TURQUOISE—Place on the throat, solar plexus, or third eye chakras to relieve mental and physical exhaustion and instill a sense of inner calm.

SUNSTONE—Hold sunstone to help lift a dark mood. The positive energies of this crystal could help increase self-worth and enable you to see light at the end of the tunnel.

OBSESSIONS AND COMPULSIONS

Obsessions and compulsions often go hand-in-hand. Obsessions are unwanted thoughts that keep popping up in your mind, causing anxiety and stress, whereas compulsions refer to the need to keep repeating certain behaviors to relieve the obsession. Common types of obsessive and compulsive behaviors include the need to clean surfaces several times in case of bacteria, switch off all the electric sockets before you go to bed "just in case," or obsessively check that your doors and windows are locked before you go out. The compulsive actions provide only short-term relief and can be a cycle that becomes difficult to break free from or stop. It can take a considerable amount of time each day dealing with compulsions, impacting on your daily life and responsibilities, such as going to work or looking after your family. You may experience worry and distress and feel you have to act on every compulsion, even if you'd rather not.

Obsessions and compulsions can affect anyone of any age, and they can vary in severity from mild and moderate to severe. They can be distressing and have a significant impact on your daily life. OCD is a known and recognized medical condition and help is available, so don't suffer alone, and please see a medical practitioner for diagnosis and treatment.

Nutrition

It's worth ensuring you have omega-3 in your diet. Fish such as salmon, sardines, trout, mackerel, and herring are rich in omega-3 fatty acids, such as alpha-linolenic acid (ALA), eicosapentaenoic acid (EPA), and docosahexaenoic acid (DHA), which play a part in healthy brain and cognitive function.

Sometimes a zinc and magnesium deficiency is found in people with obsessive-compulsive behaviors, so eating foods that naturally include zinc and magnesium is worth trying. Good options for zinc include pumpkin seeds, beef, oysters, cashew nuts, spinach, and mushrooms; magnesium-rich foods include spinach, chard, almonds, avocado, dark chocolate, bananas, and pumpkin seeds.

It's important to eat regular meals, too, as when your blood sugar drops it can affect your mood. Complex carbohydrates such as whole grains, fruits, and vegetables will help keep your blood sugar levels stable. Try to avoid drinks containing caffeine, such as tea, coffee, soda, and energy drinks, as they can increase anxiety.

Avoid drinks containing caffeine, such as tea, coffee, soda, and energy drinks, as they can increase anxiety.

Herbal remedies

Hypericum, the key ingredient in St. John's wort, is believed to affect serotonin in the brain and may be beneficial to take as disruptions to serotonin have been linked to obsessive-compulsive disorder. Similarly, milk thistle may be beneficial, too. Both are available as supplements; follow the dosage guidelines.

The herb borage has been linked to reducing obsessive and compulsive anxiety symptoms. You could try brewing a cup of borage tea daily, or purchase a ready-made borage oil to take as a tincture.

It's also possible that the Indian herb ashwagandha might be useful to try. It has been linked with increasing serotonin in the brain and lowering cortisol levels, which may help with obsessive-compulsive behaviors.

The Bach flower remedy white chestnut may help to encourage peace of mind if you have obsessive thoughts. Put a few drops on your tongue when needed, or add to a glass of water and sip it.

Crystals

CHAROITE—a stone associated with transformation, which can help overcome obsessive and compulsive behaviors. Place the crystal on the heart and crown chakras to provide balance.

CHRYSOPRASE—the calming nature of chrysoprase can help deal with impulsive actions and thoughts. It encourages positivity and can also help with getting a good night's sleep. Place or wear on the solar plexus. Alternatively, hold the stone in your hand, carry it with you in your pocket, or pop it under your pillow at night.

PERIDOT—a cleansing crystal. As such, it can help cleanse the burden and guilt of obsessions and compulsions. It helps to release negative behaviors and encourages motivation and growth to move forward from old patterns. Use it in conjunction with the heart and solar plexus chakras.

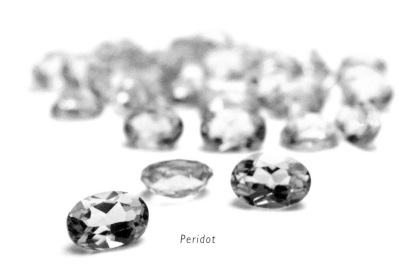

Peridot

PALPITATIONS AND PANIC ATTACKS

Palpitations is the name given to the feeling that your heart is beating faster, missing a beat, or fluttering, often suddenly and for a few seconds or minutes at a time. You may feel it in your chest, as well as in your neck or throat. It can be scary, especially the first time it happens, but in many cases it's not serious. Palpitations can commonly be triggered by stress and anxiety, by drinking too much caffeine or alcohol, or as a result of being pregnant or perimenopausal. If you are concerned, have regular palpitations, or experience shortness of breath, dizziness, fainting, or bad chest pain, seek medical help.

A panic attack is a sudden and intense feeling of fear that occurs, often without warning, and causes symptoms such as a rapid heart rate, sweating, trembling, shortness of breath, a tight feeling in your throat, hot sweats, nausea, chest pain, dizziness, numbness, and a sense of impending doom. The symptoms are so sudden and debilitating that they can be mistaken for a heart attack, but as intense as they are, your heart should be fine. Experiencing a panic attack can be scary, and if you have them frequently, seek help from a medical practitioner. Learning breathing techniques may help you cope with the attacks.

Hyperventilation occurs when you breathe very fast and exhale more than you inhale, and is common in association with panic attacks. As you breathe faster, your levels of carbon dioxide rapidly decrease, leading to a narrowing of the blood vessels that supply your brain. This can result in symptoms such as feeling faint or light-headed, tingling sensations in your fingers, sweating, feeling sick, or passing out. It can be scary, especially when it happens for the first time and you don't know why; trying to calm yourself and slowing your breathing can help. Sometimes it can be caused by a lung infection, lung disorder, heart attack, asthma, or other medical condition, so seek advice from a medical practitioner to check the cause.

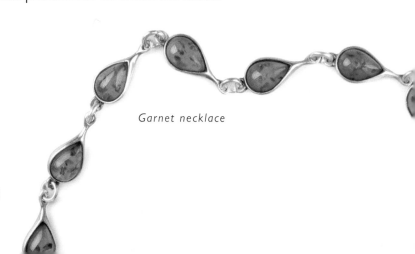

Garnet necklace

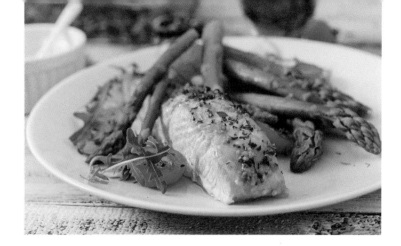

Nutrition

The minerals magnesium and potassium play a role in helping to keep your heart stable, so it's worth ensuring you're eating magnesium- and potassium-rich foods if you experience palpitations or dizziness. These include spinach, edamame beans, cannellini beans, salmon, avocado, squash, and potatoes.

Oily fish such as mackerel, herring, sardines, tuna, and salmon are good for heart health, too, and may help to reduce the occurrence of palpitations, so include one or two portions (approximately 3.5 ounces of fish) in your diet every week.

Remember to eat regular, balanced meals as this will help your blood sugar levels to remain stable and reduce the risk of sudden dips that may make you feel dizzy or faint.

Herbal remedies

Traditionally, the herbal remedy hawthorn was used to treat irregular heartbeats and palpitations, so you could try sourcing hawthorn supplements or tea bags.

The herb lavender is renowned for having calming properties, so try adding a few sprigs of dried lavender, or a few drops of lavender essential oil, to a bath at night to promote calm. You could also make your own lavender spray to spritz on your wrists if you experience sudden feelings of panic. Combine 2 tablespoons of dried lavender flowers, 30 drops of lavender essential oil, and 2 tablespoons of witch hazel together. Add them to an amber glass spray bottle and top up with water. You can spray the mist on your clothes to help ward off feelings of panic, or spritz it on your wrists, neck, or hair when needed.

If you're prone to panic attacks, keep a bottle of Dr. Bach's Rescue Remedy, or another similar emergency flower remedy, in your purse. This flower remedy is designed for times of sudden panic or shock and works on a vibrational level to gently calm and soothe the soul.

Crystals

GARNET—if you keep having palpitations, wear garnet on a necklace, so that it's close to your heart chakra.

CHRYSOPRASE—place chrysoprase on the heart chakra to encourage the flow of qi energy and release any blockages.

LEPIDOLITE—hold lepidolite and breathe slowly, to calm nerves and anxiety and instill a sense of peace.

KUNZITE—place a piece of kunzite on the solar plexus chakra, to help relieve emotional stress and feelings of panic.

RHODONITE—the calming energies of rhodonite make it a good first-aid crystal. Hold it in your hand to encourage calm breathing and release of panic and emotional stress.

PYRITE—hold pyrite in your hand, or place on the throat chakra, to help get your breathing under control.

PHOBIAS

Phobias are overwhelming irrational fears of objects, events, situations, animals, or people that cause significant distress. They are a form of anxiety and can develop if you have an unrealistic sense of danger or fear about something. Phobias don't have a single cause, but can be triggered by traumatic incidents, genetics (some people are more prone to anxiety than others), and learned responses.

Phobias can be mild or severe, and symptoms include sweating, shaking, palpitations, feeling dizzy, nausea, shortness of breath, and an upset stomach. Simple phobias tend to start during childhood, and you may grow out of them as you get older. Complex phobias, on the other hand, are more likely to start during adulthood, and can be far more debilitating, impacting your daily life. Examples of complex phobias include agoraphobia (fear of open spaces and public places) or social phobia (fear or anxiety about social situations).

Sometimes simple phobias can be tackled by desensitization, or gradual exposure to the animal, place, object, or situation that causes anxiety and fear. Other treatments for phobias include therapies such as counseling, psychotherapy, and cognitive behavioral therapy.

Nutrition

If you tend to experience dizziness in association with your phobia, it's beneficial to ensure that you're eating a healthy balanced diet and not skipping meals or going a long time without food. Skipping meals can cause your blood sugar levels to fall, which in turn can lead to hunger and dizziness.

Herbal remedies

If a phobia is making you feel anxious and jittery, use the herb chamomile to help promote a feeling of relaxation. You can make your own tea by steeping fresh or dried chamomile flowers in boiling water, use ready-made chamomile tea bags, or take chamomile supplements. The compounds found in hops can also have a calming and sedating effect, so it may be useful to try taking hops extract, too; look for this in your local health-food store.

The herb passionflower contains naturally occurring phytochemicals and the alkaloid harmine, which can have a calming effect on the mind. Popular passionflower remedies include tea, tinctures, sprays, and tablets. To brew passionflower tea, infuse 1 tablespoon of the herb in a mug of boiling water and let it steep for 10–15 minutes. Strain, warm through, and enjoy.

Another useful herb to have on hand if you're experiencing fear is valerian, as it has natural sedative properties. Try drinking a cup of valerian tea,

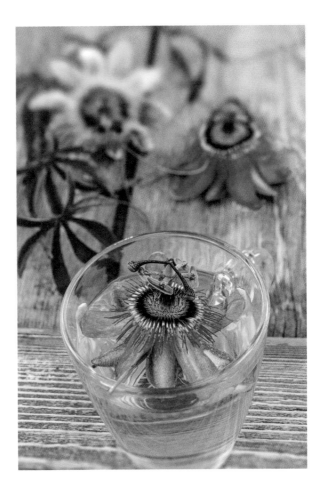

Passionflower tea

especially before having to face any situations where your phobia may arise, or take ready-made capsules or a tincture for convenience.

The flower remedy mimulus is designed to be taken if you feel frightened or anxious, so is a useful remedy to have on hand if you experience phobias. Take a few drops directly on your tongue, or add to a glass of water and sip slowly. The rock rose flower remedy may help if you're learning to face your fears, while aspen could promote feelings of security.

Crystals

AQUAMARINE—hold or wear aquamarine to boost your sense of courage. Its calming energies may help you focus and look closer at the cause of your phobias. Place on the throat chakra to encourage confidence in speaking up about your true feelings and sharing details of phobias with a therapist.

RUTILATED QUARTZ—wear or place on the solar plexus chakra to help deal with negative energy and facilitate transition. It can help balance the energy field when confronting emotional issues, which can be at the root of phobias.

CITRINE—this warming, energizing, and cheery crystal is a good all-purpose crystal for balancing and boosting energy, and can be helpful to use when you're coping with, or feeling drained by, emotional phobias. Wear a citrine necklace or place a stone on the throat chakra.

CHRYSOCOLLA—keep a piece of chrysocolla under your pillow. The crystal has a soothing and calming energy and could help bring a feeling of tranquility to a troubled mind.

Wear a citrine necklace or place a stone on the throat chakra.

MENTAL CLARITY

When you're grounded, you feel stable, calm, and at ease in the present moment. You're not fazed by what's going on around you, however stressful or chaotic it can be, and you feel positive and able to cope with whatever happens. When you're grounded, you feel in complete control of yourself physically, emotionally, and mentally and you're not easily influenced or affected by the views and opinions of others. Even when you come into contact with stressful situations or difficult people, you cope with it easily and carry on with your objectives.

When life is busy, though, it's easy to become distracted and dislodged from a secure, grounded feeling. It's also common for your grounded state to be knocked off-balance if you're involved in healing and spiritual work, or as a result of being around lots of negative energies. Regrounding will help you get back in control and feel better.

If you have mental clarity, you're blessed with a clear and focused state of mind that isn't clouded by worries, indecision, brain fog, or endless "what if?" questions. You're sure of who you are and what you think. In contrast, if you don't have mental clarity, you're likely to be your own worst inner critic, letting yourself get distracted from goals or intentions and talking yourself out of doing things. Mental clarity helps gives you focus and direction—it's easier to get things done and prioritize tasks, and it can help you push through worries and doubts. Mental clarity can also help you feel happy, at ease, and content with your life and the hand it has dealt you.

Nutrition

Eating a healthy diet, including fruits and vegetables in a variety of different colors, should provide you with the key nutrients needed for balanced cognitive function. Omega-3 fatty acids that are found in foods such as fish help to support brain function, too.

Turmeric, a spice that contains a compound called curcumin, has been found to have antioxidant and anti-inflammatory effects that may also have benefits for brain health. Turmeric is often one of the key ingredients in curry powders, so you could try eating more curry or adding turmeric to soups and other dishes.

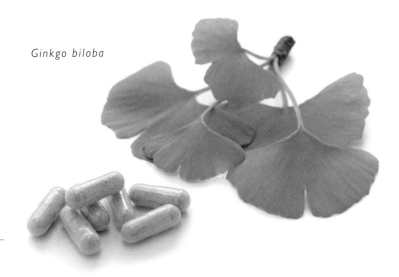

Ginkgo biloba

Herbal remedies

There are various herbal remedies that are associated with boosting cognitive function and mental clarity. Ginkgo biloba comes from the leaves of the ginkgo tree, which is native to China. It's thought that ginkgo can help improve the flow of oxygen to the brain, so it may help to improve mental clarity. It's best taken in tablet or capsule form and should be available in health-food stores. Check with a pharmacist or medical practitioner first if you're taking any prescribed medication, as interactions may occur.

The herb lemon balm can help calm feelings of anxiety and may make you feel more grounded. Brew up a refreshing cup of lemon balm tea (see page 127) and sip when needed. For an extra boost, add a few freshly chopped sage leaves, as this herb may be beneficial for cognitive function.

Crystals

HEMATITE—Place on the root chakra to ground and stabilize you. The energies of hematite will help restore harmony to your body, mind, and spirit.

OBSIDIAN—Place on the root chakra to help stabilize the chakras and enable you to become physically, emotionally, and mentally grounded.

SMOKY QUARTZ—Hold smoky quartz or use on the root chakra to bring back harmony and promote positivity.

AMAZONITE—The energies of amazonite are soothing and comforting and ideal for washing away negative thoughts, doubts, and worries. Place on the heart or throat chakra to help clear unwanted thoughts from your head and provide a more balanced outlook.

AMETRINE—Wear ametrine as a pendant on a necklace. The energies of ametrine promote clarity of mind, aid concentration and clear thought, and help you persevere with plans.

When you're grounded, you feel in complete control of yourself.

"Hope is important because it can make the present moment less difficult to bear. If we believe that tomorrow will be better, we can bear a hardship today." —Thich Nhat Hanh

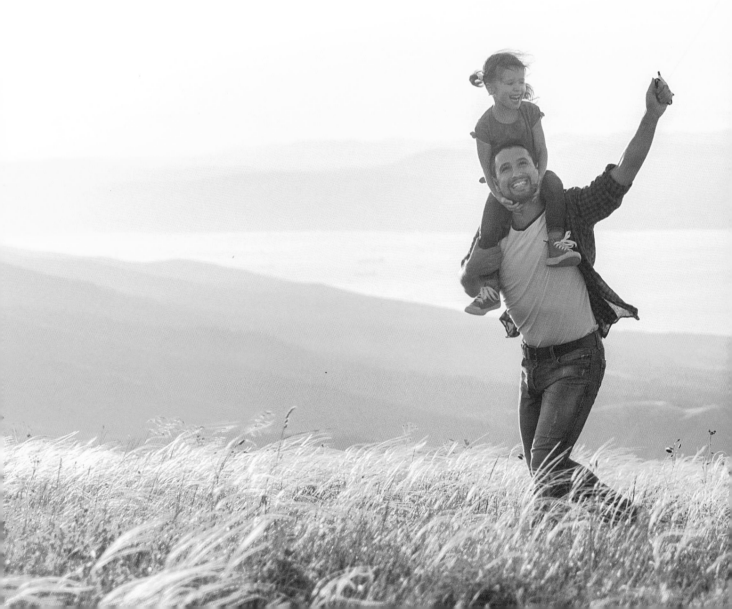

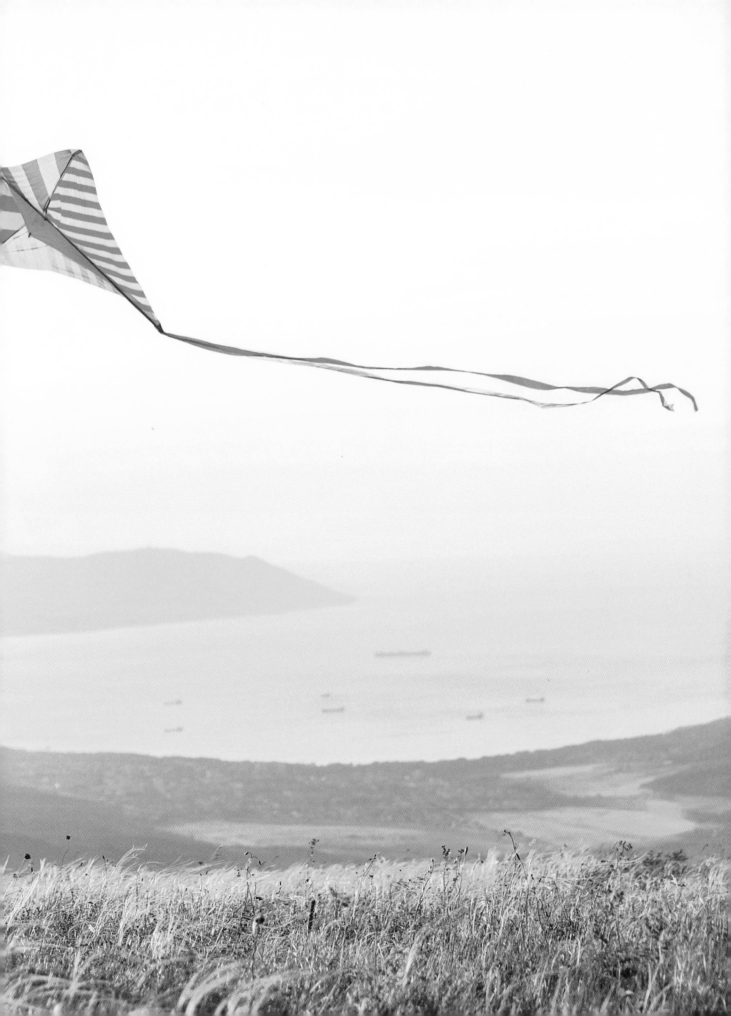

THE BENEFITS OF MIND AND BODY EXERCISES

Exercising can involve both your body and mind. Physical exercise means moving more—not necessarily going to the gym or running a marathon—but any form of additional movement or activity. Mental workouts, such as doing crosswords or solving puzzles, give your brain a valuable workout, too. Exercising your body and mind can have beneficial effects on your mental wellness. Here's an insight into some of the key benefits you could unlock.

Endorphin boost

Physical exercise is a mood booster. It activates endorphins, the so-called feel-good chemicals that are produced by the brain, helping to lift your mood and make you feel better and happier in yourself. You may find that you have more energy, too. In fact, regular moderate exercise can help ease the symptoms of mild depression and anxiety.

Reduced stress

Both physical and mental exercises can help reduce stress and anxiety. Getting involved in an activity gives you something else to focus on and, hopefully, get absorbed in doing, taking your mind off any thoughts or worries you may have. If you're doing physical exercise, the exercise reduces the levels of hormones such as cortisol in your body, which helps decrease your stress levels.

Improved sleep

Exercising can help you get a better night's sleep. It uses up physical and mental energy, which can help you feel calmer and more relaxed. If you're plagued by insomnia or continuous thoughts that you can't get out of your mind at night, you may find that exercising helps you feel better and more tired by the evening, giving you more of a chance of falling asleep.

Boosted self-esteem

Being active and taking part in different activities, either on your own or with other people, can have a beneficial effect on how you feel about yourself. It can boost your self-esteem and make you feel good about your achievements, and having goals can help keep you motivated to continue and achieve more.

A boost for your brain

Doing activities that require you to think can benefit your mental alertness and cognitive function. They get your brain working, perhaps in ways that it hasn't in a while, and help you focus. Physical exercise can have a benefit on your brain, too, as exercise can lift your energy and mood and help you feel more positive.

Connecting with other people

Getting involved in activities or exercise with other people helps you connect and enjoy a shared experience. This has a positive impact on your mental well-being, helping you make new friends and meet new people. Being connected socially can reduce the impact of isolation and help you feel a part of your local community.

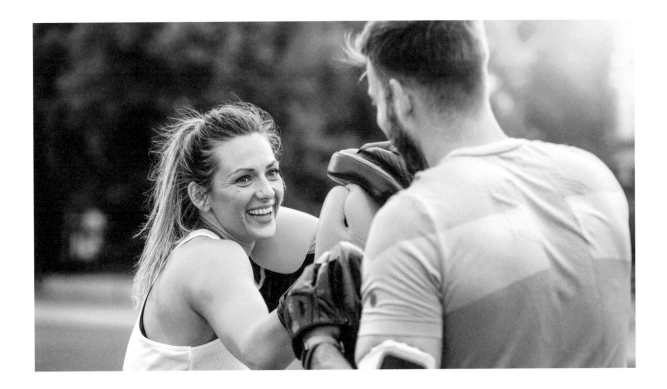

Distraction

If you are experiencing mental health issues, then being active provides the practical benefit of distraction. It helps take your mind away from negative thoughts and feelings, even if only for a short time, and it can be a good coping strategy.

Health prevention

Taking part in regular body and mind activities has been shown to reduce the risks of developing mental health conditions, such as depression, as well as numerous other health conditions, such as heart disease and high blood pressure.

Mind and body exercises combined

Some forms of physical exercise, typically those that originated in Eastern traditions such as yoga and tai chi, combine a focus on both the body and the mind and can be particularly beneficial for promoting mental wellness.

There are various different forms of yoga, some ranging from slow and gentle, to other, more challenging forms. For beginners, hatha yoga is a good starting point as it involves physical poses, called *asana*s, as well as controlled breathing and meditation, which can both help calm and center the mind. Although the movements of yoga are slow and controlled, they still work your muscles effectively, improve balance, increase your heart rate, and stimulate the release of feel-good brain chemicals. Learning the breathing methods and forms of meditation can be useful for dealing with issues such as stress and anxiety, and the general ambience of a gentle yoga session tends to be relaxing.

Like yoga, tai chi involves slow physical movements, slow breathing, and a meditative approach. The physical movements can improve strength and balance, while the meditative side of it is gentle and relaxing for the mind.

No wonder these have both become popular forms of exercise for today's busy modern life.

WALKING, GARDENING, AND BEING IN NATURE

One positive thing you can do for your mental wellness is to go outside. The simple act of being outdoors in the fresh air, breathing it in and moving around, has been shown to lower stress and blood pressure, improve your heart rate, and lift your mood.

It's interesting to note that the colors green and blue have been linked to feelings of relaxation, and they appear frequently in the natural world. Green is the color of grass, leaves, trees, and bushes, while blue (can be!) the color of the sky and the ocean.

Walking

When you walk or indulge in any form of physical activity, brain chemicals called endorphins are released. Often referred to as "happy chemicals," endorphins can relieve discomfort in your body and boost your mood. Being outdoors is good for the creation of vitamin D, too, which happens when sunlight interacts with your skin, plus walking can help to balance the natural circadian rhythms in your body, helping you get a better night's sleep.

When you walk, you could try out this simple meditation, which helps you connect with and observe the natural world around you in a calm and relaxed manner.

Walk at a natural, normal pace, and with each step you take notice the movement of your feet, legs, and body and the sensations you feel.

Next, pay attention to the sounds you can hear. Perhaps there's birdsong, traffic, noise from other people, or the sound of dogs barking. Don't worry about whether they're pleasant or unpleasant sounds, just listen and observe.

Slowly move your awareness to what you can see. Look at the surroundings you're walking in, the colors, designs, and textures. Don't be critical of it, just observe and acknowledge it.

Next, bring your awareness to the aromas in the air around you. What can you smell? Notice and be aware of the scent in the air, be it car fumes, fresh grass, the smell of rain, or your own perfume.

As you continue to walk, focus your awareness on everything around you, both in your near vicinity and the wider world. Acknowledge its existence and your part in it, but leave judgments out of the picture.

Finally, bring your awareness back to your body and the sensations you feel as you walk, be it your feet touching the ground with each step, the sensation of your shoes on your feet, or how your clothing feels against your legs as you move.

Gardening

If you have a garden, puttering around outside can be good for your health. Whether you're actively growing fruit and vegetables, pruning trees, mowing the lawn, or potting up flowers and cuttings, the simple of act of being outside and interacting with nature can have a beneficial effect. Even planting some window boxes or pots to put out on a balcony can be therapeutic.

If you enjoy gardening but don't have your own space, look for local allotments or join a community garden scheme, where you share access to a plot.

If you enjoy walking around gardens, take the opportunity to visit public gardens or garden open days when you can, to explore and be inspired.

Being in nature

The Japanese traditionally practice *shinrin-yoku*, or "forest bathing," a simple relaxation process which is great for physical and mental well-being. It involves being quiet and calm among the trees while observing nature and breathing deeply. There's a lot to be said for this approach, which can bring about a sense of calm and serenity, while also helping you to de-stress and take a step back from your hectic life.

Anyone can have a go at the concept of forest bathing. Find yourself a wooded area and enjoy a quiet time among the trees. It's beneficial to turn off your phone so you won't be disturbed, and to walk slowly through the woods so that you can fully absorb the atmosphere. Take time to stop, stand, or sit and take a few deep breaths as you look at the colors of nature. Carefully take in the landscape around you and use your senses to pick up the aroma of the trees, the feel of the breeze ruffling through leaves, and all the tiny details you can see and hear.

Urban nature

You don't have to live in the countryside to find nature—there are urban nature spots in cities, too, and they're just as beneficial. Look for parks, canals, roof gardens, and even small courtyards that are planted with flowers or trees, and take time to visit them. A simple stroll through a city park can be just as beneficial as being in the quiet countryside, and can help boost your physical and mental health. Part of the reason for this effect is believed to be the sense of connection with the natural world triggering a sense of happiness. Look for and observe birds, squirrels, and other wildlife. You can even spot signs of nature in unexpected places in cities, such as seeing urban foxes in car parks.

SWIMMING, CYCLING, AND DANCING

Any form of physical activity can be beneficial for both your physical and mental health, boosting your well-being and lifting your mood. From gentle activities to more vigorous exercise, there are choices and options for everyone.

Swimming

Swimming is a gentle form of exercise that helps build muscle strength, but it's also beneficial for your mental health. Like any exercise, swimming releases endorphins, which can increase your sense of happiness and positivity, but it may also boost your brain health by increasing the flow of blood to the brain. Many people find swimming useful for relieving stress and reducing anxiety, as being in water can help relax your body and soothe your mind. Look for leisure centers and swimming pools near you; becoming a member may make it cheaper to swim regularly. Some centers have regular lane swimming sessions, which can also be a good opportunity to socialize and meet people.

Open-water swimming has also grown in popularity in recent years. It's not for everyone, as the water is a natural temperature and can be a lot colder than you're used to in a swimming pool. If you're going to try open-water swimming, it's crucial you're a confident swimmer, that where you go is safe and free from strong currents and waterfalls, and that you watch out for sharp and slippery rocks and weeds that could entangle your legs. It's a good idea to join a local open-water swimming group, as they will be able to recommend the best places to swim outdoors in your area and often organize group swims.

Cycling

Cycling is a good form of aerobic exercise and can be as gentle or as invigorating as you like—and it's not only physically beneficial but mentally, too. Riding a bike takes you outside, enabling you to breathe in fresh air and get a healthy dose of vitamin D. Cycling increases endorphin levels in your body, leaving you feeling energized and positive. It can be a great form of stress relief and a good distraction, as it keeps your mind from dwelling on worries and gives you something else to focus on.

If you haven't ridden for a while, the chances are you'll pick up the skills again quickly. And if you're not keen on cycling on roads with automobile traffic, look for quieter backroads or specially designated bike paths, which can be safer.

Cycling doesn't have to be a solitary activity—you can ride socially, too. A bike ride with friends or family can be made into a day out (take a picnic lunch or stop at a café for a break), or you could join a local cycling club and take part in group rides.

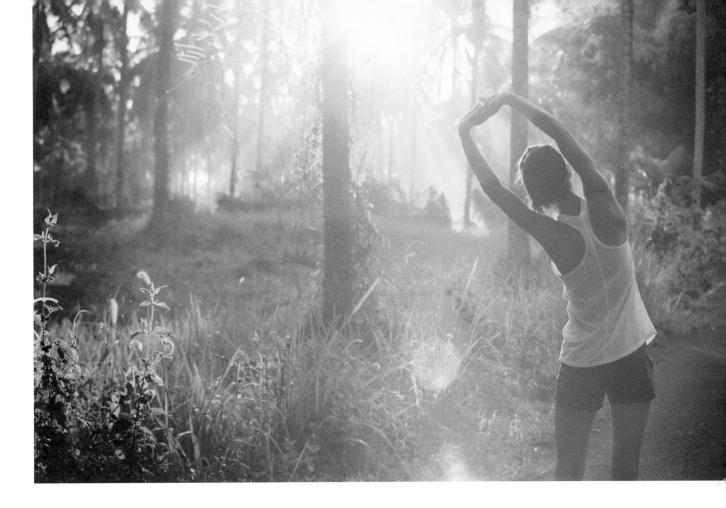

Exercise doesn't have to be aerobic every time—a good, gentle stretch is really beneficial, too.

Dancing

Dancing is a great way of exercising in a fun and enjoyable manner. At a basic level you could dance around at home as you do the housework, dance along to an exercise DVD, or enjoy a boogie at a weekend disco.

But if you want to explore the benefits of dancing more regularly, attending organized dance classes can be beneficial. There are a range of different dance classes available, from ballroom, ballet, tap, and salsa, to street dance, swing, Bollywood, jive, and jazz.

If you're unsure what type of dance would be best for you, see if you can go along to a few classes and have a trial session. That way you can try out the different methods and see which suits your fitness level, interests, and ability the best.

One of the best aspects of a dance class is that it often doesn't feel like exercise. You can get so absorbed in the rhythm of the music and be enjoying yourself so much that the time will fly.

MEDITATION

Meditation is a technique used to calm and quieten the mind. It's been practiced for thousands of years all over the world and is noted for its positive benefits on mental health and wellness.

Why meditate?

It's not unusual to long to be happy and free from the struggles and conflicts that scar our lives. Many people search for ways to find a heart of wisdom and a mind of calm, and yearn to be a conscious participant in creating a world that is imbued with peace and understanding. Throughout our lives we do all that we can to bring an end to feelings of alienation, estrangement, and suffering, and to forge relationships of intimacy and warmth. Meditation is intended to transform us, to show us the way to free ourselves from the grip of fear, division, and confusion. The practice of meditation illuminates our life, inwardly and outwardly, showing us the path to freedom and wakefulness.

A healing path

Meditation is not a means of fleeing from life, nor is it a quick-fix solution to all of the difficulties and challenges we may meet. But it is a path that teaches us to be increasingly present, honest, and awake in each moment of our lives. It is a direct means of healing the estrangement and division that too often separate us from others and ourselves.

Depth of wisdom, compassion, and peace are not sought in transcendent experience, nor projected into the future, but are nurtured within this heart, mind, body, and life in the present.

For thousands of years people have retreated to the solitude and stillness of deserts, mountaintops, and monasteries, seeking an inner renewal, depth, and authenticity. But the great teachers who truly inspire our own journeys do so not solely because of some dramatic spiritual breakthrough experienced in solitude, but through their commitment and capacity to embody their wisdom and depth of compassion in every area of their lives.

Initially, when we face the struggles, challenges, and conflicts that are part of living, we react with the belief that they are obstacles to be overcome or subdued.

When we meet the swirls of confusion that can cloud our own minds, or the emotional storms that shatter our hearts, we are prone to believe that they are wrong or a personal imperfection. But through our own experience in meeting the difficult and challenging, we come to understand that resistance, blame, judgment, and suppression do little to bring about healing and the end of sorrow. A path of meditation, directed toward the release of our hearts and minds, encourages us to turn our attention directly toward the places of challenge and difficulty we are most prone to flee from or abandon. This is where the seeds of peace and understanding plant their roots.

Meditation encourages us to step out of the pathways of blame, judgment, and rejection, and ask ourselves where healing begins in this moment. The end of sorrow, we begin to understand, does not rely

*The practice
of meditation
illuminates our
life, inwardly
and outwardly.*

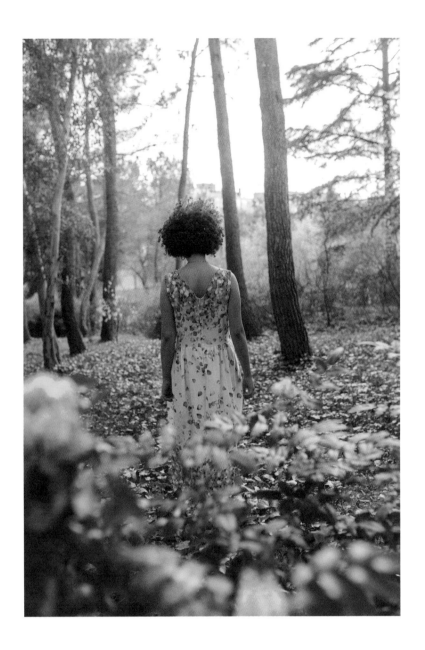

upon eradicating everything unpleasant or challenging in our lives—that is an impossible task. The end of sorrow and struggle is born of our capacity to make peace with all things and to hold the events of our life in a heart of loving kindness and understanding.

Meditation is a path of awakening, an inner journey of direct experience. It has a direction and clear sense of aspiration—serenity, balance, open-heartedness, compassion, and deep inner wisdom all lie at the heart of meditative teachings

and paths. Equally, meditation is a path of embodiment, teaching us to approach all of the events, people, circumstances, and moments in our lives with profound integrity, loving kindness, and equanimity.

Meditation is not a journey of self-improvement— it is dedicated to the relief of anguish whenever it appears. Meditation is greater and more vast than just a technique or formula for living—it is the cultivation of a heart of wisdom and a mind of calm.

LEARNING TO MEDITATE

It may come as a surprise, but genuine meditation is no stranger to any of us. Long before you undertake a formal meditation practice you will have encountered glimpses of profound peace, compassion, and serenity, moments of deep inner stillness, times of genuine connectedness with nature, other people, and yourself.

There have been times when the busyness of your mind has calmed and you have found yourself listening, seeing, and responding with a natural sensitivity and patient intimacy.

We have all experienced times when we have felt truly at ease within our own bodies, minds, and lives. Too often these moments of depth and stillness feel like random occurrences. We are inspired and touched by them and yet they feel so fleeting and are too often inaccessible to us. Meditation practice teaches a way of being present and awake at all times, to ourselves and to the world, a way of resting in inner stillness, receptivity, and understanding.

Meditation is a path of cultivation and a discipline born of dedication to peace and depth. Patient intimacy lies at its heart. It is also a path of the present. None of us can alter or recover a past that has already gone by; the future is yet to come and we cannot guarantee how it will unfold. The moment that we are in is the only moment that can be lived fully and in which we can find transformation. Meditation encourages us to turn directly toward our lives and this moment. They are the grist for awakening.

It is not a quest to find a perfect moment, but a way of cultivating balance, sensitivity, and clarity within all the joys and sorrows of our lives. We come to understand that the source of genuine happiness, joy, and peace lies within our own hearts and minds, and not within the changing events of our life.

Meditation is not a denial of past or future, but an understanding that we are writing the history of all the future moments in our lives through the way in which we attend to and experience the moment we are in.

Too often we live in a fog of confusion and busyness, governed by impulse, habit, and reactivity. We find ourselves frantically trying to do more and more each day, torn between the multiplicity of demands that compete for our attention. Our lives can be filled with lost moments—interactions, conversations, sounds, sights, and feelings that we have neglected to attend to.

Leaning into the future or floundering in thoughts of the past, we lose the richness and simplicity available to us in the present. Meditation practice is a direct way of reclaiming those lost moments— the life we can miss through neglect, inattention, and busyness.

Your meditation practice begins right where you are, in the life you are living, with your willingness to take the first steps of being attentive and present. There are a vast variety of spiritual paths, lineages, and traditions available to us. They vary in their styles, yet they share an emphasis on integrity, commitment, serenity, and wisdom. All meditative paths serve

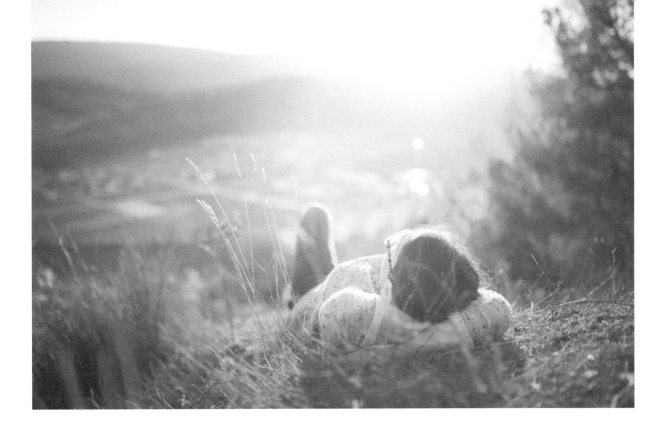

to nourish our hearts and minds, inviting us to explore the possibility of great depth, authenticity, and compassion in our lives. We nurture, through meditation practice, a climate of heart, an inner culture that is receptive to deep understanding and transformation. We learn to shed the layers of confusion and agitation that too easily cloud our capacity to live with great sensitivity.

The art of meditation

Meditation is an art, and like any other art it asks for both dedication and discipline. At the heart of every meditative path is a dedication to peace, compassion, authenticity, and freedom. Genuine discipline is not a tyrannical code governing our actions and life, but is born of our dedication to all that is truly liberating and healing. The styles, practices, and techniques of meditation are the container or discipline in which we bring to fulfillment the peace and freedom we deeply treasure.

There are two dimensions to meditation: one is the form and the other is the spirit. They are interwoven and indivisible. Meditation is much more than becoming proficient in a particular technique. The techniques of practice are ways to articulate and cultivate the spirit of awakening.

It is equally true to say that the paths and the goals of meditation cannot be separated. If we aspire to peace, understanding, sensitivity, and compassion, then we are also asked to practice meditation in their spirit. If our meditation practice is to lead to an open heart, clear mind, and greater loving kindness in every area of our lives, then it asks us to cultivate those qualities in every step on our path. Patience and dedication are key elements in the deepening of meditation.

CREATING A MEDITATIVE SETTING

Initially, as you begin to practice developing attention, it is worthwhile to create an environment around you that is supportive. A corner of your bedroom or any space in your home that is simple and quiet will serve. Find a chair or cushion that you can return to and as far as possible create in that space a meditative environment. Dedicate a period of time each day to spend in formal meditation. There is no prescribed amount of time; however long you are able to give to your meditation practice is worthwhile. Don't expect that every time you sit down to meditate you are going to have amazing breakthroughs, peak experiences, or moments of great rapture.

What you meet in your meditation is the mind and heart you bring to it. Sometimes you will be sitting with a mind of chaos, filled with the plans or memories of your day. What is valuable is making the effort to be aware of that mind, however it is. The moments of stillness you commit to each day are always worthy moments.

They are times of cultivating calm attention, awareness, and sensitivity that will begin to impact upon every area of your life. When you sit down to meditate, ensure that you turn off your telephone, radio, and television. Allow yourself to unhook for a time and care for the quality of your own heart and mind. Increasingly we feel compelled to be perpetually available and engaged. Yet meditation is a time to be engaged with stillness, an appointment we make with ourselves. It is often helpful to dedicate a period of time at the beginning and the end of the day to be wholeheartedly committed to cultivating our meditation practice. The effects of these times of stillness and focus will increasingly begin to pervade the entire day.

We will come to see that calm attention, peace, sensitivity, and open-heartedness are not random experiences or accidents we occasionally encounter in life. They live within our own hearts and minds, born of awareness and wise attention.

There is no correct posture to meditate in—you can use a chair, bench, or cushion—but find a posture that is upright and alert. In your meditation posture you are embodying the qualities of heart and mind you are seeking to develop.

Within that uprightness, also find a deep sense of ease and relaxation. Battling with bodily discomfort in meditation is not conducive to finding the well-being and sensitivity we are seeking to nurture.

If your body is particularly exhausted or distressed, it is even fine to lie down to meditate, although in this posture you may need to make a resolved commitment to be awake and present. The posture to seek is one that allows you to be at home and at ease within your body.

Approach your meditation times as moments of dedication. Commit yourself to being as fully present as it is possible for you to be. As you begin to practice, clarify your sense of intention. Take a few moments to reflect upon why you are engaging in this meditation, what this time is dedicated to.

The meditation is in the service of peace, calm, and sensitivity. Dedicate yourself to being attentive,

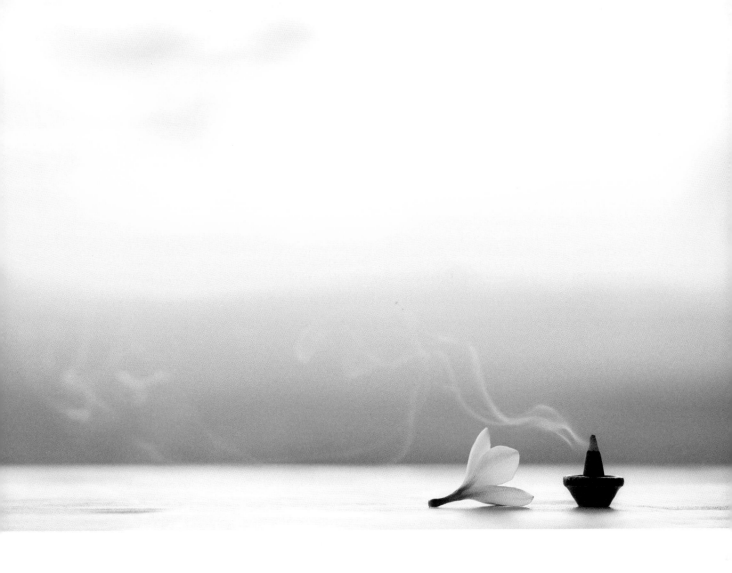

Allow yourself to unhook for a time and care for the quality of your own heart and mind.

clear, and focused. Let go of all preoccupations with the past and future. This is not a time for planning and rehearsing the future, nor for recycling thoughts about the past. Beginning your meditation with a clear sense of intention is an encouragement to establish yourself in the present. Meditation is a time of caring for your well-being and cultivating serenity and depth.

Meditation can introduce us to moments of great joy and opening. It will also make us increasingly aware of the places where we react most habitually and close down most persistently. Through sustained and dedicated practice we learn to embrace the difficult and the delightful, the joyful and the sorrowful with the same welcome, interest, and inner balance. In essence, meditation teaches us to be awake and present in the midst of all things. This is the home of genuine understanding and depth.

CULTIVATING ATTENTION

Attention is the key that opens the door to inner peace and awareness. Without attention we live only on the surface of life. The song of a bird, the beauty of a sunset, the cries of someone who needs us are lost to us. To love and to live fully, we need to be present and awake. If we are to live with compassion, balance, and generosity, we need to cultivate the art of attentiveness.

Observing our own minds, we see that they seem to be filled with a cascade of thoughts, obsessions, memories, and preoccupations. Attention teaches us to calm this busyness and agitation. The art of clear, focused attentiveness is finding calmness in the midst of agitation, serenity in the midst of chaos, simplicity in the midst of complexity. We do not need to flee the world to discover this profound inner calm; we do need to learn how to release ourselves from fragmentation and distractedness.

Interest is the primary building block of wise attention. Wherever there is interest in our lives, energy and attention naturally follow. Attention is the common thread that runs through every meditative discipline and art. Through calm and gentle attention we learn to cultivate the clarity and sensitivity that allow understanding and stillness to deepen. Wise attention is a gesture of kindness to ourselves, and it is cultivated through learning to focus upon one object, one moment at a time. Learning to attend wholeheartedly to that object, we illuminate it, forming a bond of connection. It becomes our anchor in the present moment. Whenever our attention drifts away, we learn to come back, renewing our connection with that anchor.

Cultivating attention requires great patience, and in the practice of developing attention we need to bring a deep sense of ease and relaxation, yet also to balance that ease with a committed perseverance and dedication.

Attention is the art of cultivating happiness and well-being, and it awakens us to ourselves and to everything that comes into our world. There are a variety of ways of learning to develop attention and calm in our lives. Spending time on a daily basis in formal meditation cultivating a focused and single-pointed attention will have a significant impact upon the quality of our lives. Learning to bring that wise attention to all the contacts and interactions we engage in daily will deepen and enhance our capacity to live with spaciousness and calm. It is important that meditation does not become yet another task to add to a list of things we must do. It should be approached as a time of deep ease, of reconnecting with our capacity to rest with calmness and wakefulness in all the moments of our lives.

The concentrated mind

• Find a posture for your body that is as balanced and relaxed as possible. Gently close your eyes. Take a few moments to be aware of your body, bringing your attention to all the places where your body makes contact with the ground, cushion, or chair. Bring your attention to your breath just at the point where it enters and leaves your body. Focus your attention calmly yet fully on the area of your upper lip and nostrils.

• Inhale and be aware of the sensations that arise—the coolness of your breath, tingling, whatever sensations appear in the area of your upper lip and nostrils. Sustain your attention in that area, until you sense your out-breath at your upper lip and nostrils as you exhale. Be aware of the warmth of your out-breath as it leaves your body.

• Let your attention rest clearly and gently in the area of your upper lip and nostrils. You might find that your breath becomes almost imperceptible. If this occurs, let whatever sensations are present at your upper lip and nostrils be the focus of your attention. Don't try to make your breathing fuller or deeper, just let the sensations of the breath entering and leaving be the point where your attention rests.

• If there are moments when your attention is drawn to a thought or bodily sensation, just notice this and gently return to focus once more on the area of your upper lip and nostrils.

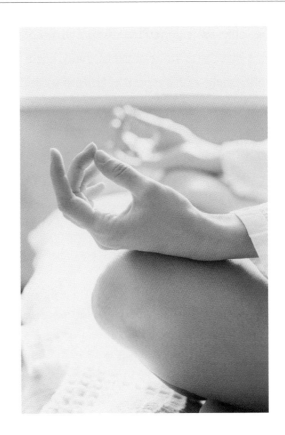

• As you focus on this area, notice how the sensations change, at times becoming very subtle. Sense the ease and simplicity that come with deepening attention. Let yourself rest within that ease. As your concentration deepens further, notice the deeper calmness and spaciousness that begin to pervade your body and mind. When you are ready, open your eyes and come out of the posture.

Your capacity to be at peace with yourself begins with your willingness to let go.

RELEASING STRESS

When we use the word "stress," everyone immediately knows what it is we are talking about. Yet stress is a generic term that attempts to describe a multidimensional and complex experience. It is not just a static state of mind, but a process that describes the way we are interacting and interfacing with the world around us and within us.

We can feel stressed by work pressures, goals, the needs and expectations of others, and by time. Stress is what happens when an overburdened mind adversely impacts upon our bodies and incapacitates us in our ability to meet life calmly and wholeheartedly.

Stress is symptomatic of an underlying disharmony in ourselves and in our lives. It is a messenger asking us to examine what we are neglecting or not giving attention to. Much of the stress we experience may be more optional than we initially believe. We can all learn to attend to our life with greater wholeheartedness, to let go with more ease, and to care more for the moment we are in.

A meditation teacher was once asked about the right amount of time to give to meditation. His answer was that half an hour was fine except in times of exceptional busyness, then an hour was needed. Too often we misinterpret stress as a signal to do and accomplish more, or another reaction is to simply flee and hide from what we believe is causing the stress we feel. Yet we need to listen to stress as an indicator of our need to slow down, to attend to each moment with greater care, and to release the haste that has come to govern our minds and lives. We cannot afford to ignore the signals that it is sending us—tension, agitation, and anxiety.

Meditation is not a quick-fix solution for stress. Ease, clarity, effectiveness, and sensitivity in our lives will not arise from a mind and heart that are overburdened. Thoughts, choices, words, and actions born of an agitated mind will invariably be themselves agitated and anxious, and rarely bring the consequences or results we are seeking.

Stress and ease both lie within how we perceive and respond to everything that life brings to us. Stress is what happens when the multiplicity of events in our lives and our reactions to them mass together into a form of inner gridlock. Eventually we find ourselves stuck in an inner paralysis—unable to respond well to even the smallest details. Life feels impossible—everything appears to be too much to respond to. We feel we are facing an impenetrable mass of needs, demands, and pressures.

This is in truth a state of mind and not a description of reality. We need to learn to unpack the solidity of that perception. We can pay attention to one moment, one event, and one impression at a time. We can learn to calm our bodies and explore with attention what it is we might be able to let go of in our minds. We can learn to pay attention to the beginnings and endings that are part of all our internal and external events.

Listen to stress as an indicator of our need to slow down, to attend to each moment with greater care.

Releasing stress

• Find a position for your body in which you feel deeply relaxed and at ease. Let your eyes gently close and for a few moments just focus on your breathing, noticing the beginning of each breath and the end of each breath.

• Follow each out-breath to its very end, sensing it dissolving into space. Let yourself rest in that momentary pause between the end of one breath and the beginning of the next.

• Expand your attention and listen to what is happening in your body and mind in that moment. Notice how many of your thoughts are preoccupied with events, people, meetings, and experiences that are not actually present in that moment. Sense this without judgment or resistance and see whether it is possible for you to gently release those thoughts and return to an awareness of breathing.

• Notice the waves of agitation, tension, or anxiety that arise with the thoughts of the past and future and how they may be impacting your body.

• Come back once more to an awareness of your breathing.

• Resting in calmness and ease, consciously invite into your mind an event, person, or experience that you have been preoccupied with or obsessing about. Surround that thought with a mindful attention. Look at it directly. Can you see it as just a thought, an event in the mind?

• Sense how that event in your mind is coexisting in this moment with countless other events—sounds, sensations in your body—and how they are all arising and passing together. Move your attention between the thought, the sounds, and the bodily sensations that are present in this

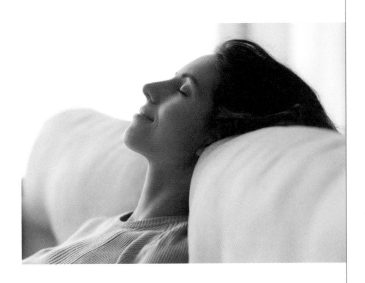

moment. Notice how they all appear, last for a time, and then begin to fade or turn into something else.

• Sense the natural rhythm of this arising and passing. Notice how when any of these events are surrounded by aversion, agitation, or resistance, their life span is extended. When the surrounding reactions are released, the events find their place again in the natural rhythm of arising and passing.

• Attend mindfully not only to the events that appear in your mind and body, but also to those subtle pauses and places of stillness between events. Just as you are able to notice the momentary pause between an out-breath and the next in-breath, sense what is present after the fading away of a sound, a thought, or a bodily sensation.

• Allow yourself to rest in the pauses and sense the possibility of resting in all the events that arise in your mind and body. When you are ready, let your eyes open and move out of the posture.

ESSENTIAL OILS TO AID MEDITATION

Aromatherapy essential oils are perfect to help evoke different moods when you're meditating, whether you want to feel alert and uplifted, or relaxed and calm. Different aromas can have different effects on your mood and how you feel.

One of the most popular ways of using essential oils is to pop a few drops of your chosen oil, or a combination of scents, into water in an essential oil burner to diffuse slowly. Another option is to make up an essential oil room spray by adding a few drops of oil to a small spray bottle of water, so that you can spritz it around your meditation space before you start practicing.

Oils for clarity and concentration

SANDALWOOD can help with grounding, bringing more clarity to your meditation practice. It may help to calm the inner chatter of your mind and make you feel calmer and more relaxed.

VETIVER has a dry, earthy, woody scent that helps relax the body and clear the mind to support concentration.

ROSEMARY can help ease mental exhaustion and give your concentration a boost.

Oils for calm and relaxation

LAVENDER'S floral scent is inherently calming and can help you reach a relaxed state. It's particularly useful if you're meditating at night, as it can aid sleep.

CLARY SAGE is an earthy scent with fruity and herbal notes. Diffuse before meditating if you're feeling stressed and tense.

CHAMOMILE is another good choice to help promote a sense of relaxation.

Oils to aid grounding and dispel negative energy

SAGE is used in various cultures to help cleanse spiritual places of negative energy, so use this in your meditation space before commencing.

YLANG YLANG can help to dispel negative energies, such as anger and frustration, and uplift your mood.

CEDARWOOD has a woody aroma and can help promote a sense of grounding, particularly if you have worries and negative thoughts.

Oils to uplift and stimulate

JASMINE'S exotic floral scent is uplifting and stimulates the senses. It's a good oil to diffuse for a morning meditation to get the day off to a good start.

BERGAMOT can help uplift your spirits and aid with focusing the mind.

Oils to create a spiritual atmosphere

FRANKINCENSE has been traditionally used to help evoke a spiritual atmosphere and increase spiritual awareness.

The floral scent of lavender is inherently calming and can help you reach a relaxed state.

Creating your own essential oil blends

As you experiment with different essential oils, you will discover particular scents that make you feel good, or that you particularly like the smell of. As well as using the oils individually, they can be combined to create blends. They can be grouped for a common purpose, such as providing mental clarity, or by type of scent, such as floral or woody.

When you're creating oil blends, take care not to use too many drops. All oils are highly concentrated, so you will need only a few drops for a good effect, plus some scents can be stronger and more overpowering than others. Aim to put a maximum of 2–3 drops per oil into your blends as this should be sufficient to scent a room. Make a note of any combinations so that you can re-create them later.

Some oil blends that may be useful for practicing meditation include:

LAVENDER, NEROLI, AND YLANG YLANG for a blend to help you relax. Add 3 drops of lavender and neroli, but only 2 drops of ylang ylang as this scent can be stronger.

FRANKINCENSE, VETIVER, AND SAGE for a blend to help you feel grounded and clear of your intentions. Add 2 drops of each oil.

ROSEMARY, PEPPERMINT, AND EUCALYPTUS blend together well to help clear your head and boost mental concentration. Add 2 drops of each oil.

BERGAMOT, SWEET ORANGE, AND LIME for a blend to uplift and stimulate the senses. Add 3 drops of bergamot and sweet orange oil, and 2 drops of lime.

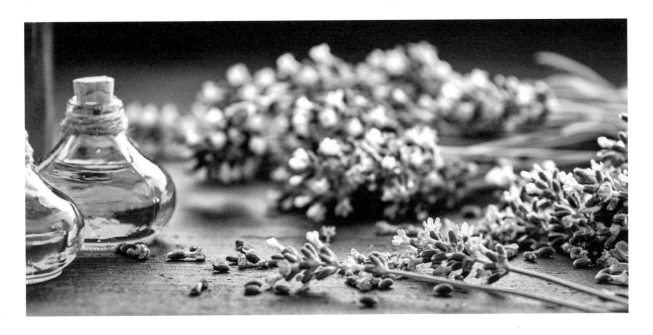

CRYSTALS TO AID MEDITATION

If you have an affinity with crystals or crystal energy, these natural gemstones can be used to aid meditation practice in several different ways.

Holding a crystal while you meditate

Choose a favorite crystal to hold as you meditate, or one that feels comfortable in your hand. Different crystals have different properties, such as helping with stress relief, relaxation, clarity, or the release of negative energies, so you could tailor the crystal you choose to hold to the outcome you'd like from your meditation. Crystals can be rough and in their natural state, or shaped and polished. Polished palm stones are designed to be held flat in your hand and can be pleasant to hold during meditation, or you could look for tumbled gemstones, which have a smooth finish.

Looking at a crystal while meditating

If you find it hard to clear your mind of all thoughts, it can be useful to look at an object while you meditate. A candle is traditionally used, with the idea that you look at the flickering flame, but a crystal with interesting facets is an option, too. You'll need to position it in front of you, perhaps on a table or small stool, so that your gaze is naturally drawn to the crystal when you're seated in front of it.

Having crystals in the room while you meditate

It's good to create a sacred space in which to meditate, and many people like to have a few special items in the room to evoke a sense of peace and calm, such as crystals. Choose your crystals carefully, selecting the ones that are most appropriate to your needs, and cleansing them by running them under fresh water before placing them in your meditation space.

Meditating in crystal grids

Crystal grids are geometric patterns that are laid out to enhance the use of crystals for healing purposes. The same patterns can be used on a larger scale—sometimes referred to as crystal nets—whereby you sit in the center of the grid with the crystals mapped out around you in a specific pattern. Meditating within a crystal grid can amplify the effect of the crystals and could create a deeply transformative meditation experience.

Placing crystals on your body while meditating

Crystals could be placed on your body while you meditate. For example, if you're carrying out a chakra healing meditation you could add to the experience by putting crystals in the corresponding chakra colors onto the appropriate chakra location on your body.

Using crystal mala beads while meditating

Mala beads originate from India and are traditionally used for prayer and meditation, in a similar way to a rosary. Mala necklaces have 108 beads, as this number is believed to be significant and represents spiritual completion, and they are often made from hand-

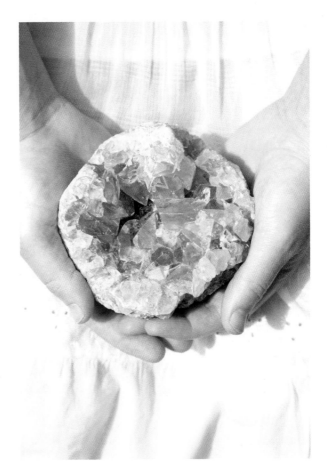

Celestine

carved crystals. You simply hold the necklace in one hand while meditating and use the thumb and finger of your other hand to touch each bead. Each touch of a bead can represent one breath, or you can repeat a mantra or affirmation as you touch each bead. Using a mala necklace in this manner may help improve your focus and concentration while meditating.

Crystals to use with meditation

Any crystals can be used for meditation purposes, although there are some that are particularly appropriate.

CLEAR QUARTZ is perfect for use with meditation practice as it can amplify energy (both yours and that of other crystals) and help evoke a sense of clarity. It's good to hold if you're feeling bewildered or uncertain, as it may help clear doubts and distractions.

SELENITE is another good choice for meditation as it can help to clear your mind and let your body relax. The crystal can help release negative energy and is an excellent stone to help cleanse other crystals.

BLACK TOURMALINE is a grounding stone, so it's a good crystal to have on hand to help ensure your energies remain grounded during meditation. It has protective properties and may help to dispel negative energy in a room.

CITRINE can help lift your mood and ensure you have a joyful meditation. The positive energy of this sunny stone is associated with good fortune so could also be useful for prosperity meditations.

ROSE QUARTZ is affectionately known as the stone of love. This pink crystal has a soothing and calming energy and can be good to have on hand to remind you of the importance of self-care and compassion, as well as when working on healing past relationships or trust issues.

AMETHYST is a stone of intuition and healing. Used in meditation, it may help to calm your thoughts, clear your mind, and allow you to become more in tune with your inner feelings.

CELESTINE can be placed or held at the throat chakra to promote communication. A cluster of these blue crystals can aid mental clarity and encourage calm and positivity as you meditate.

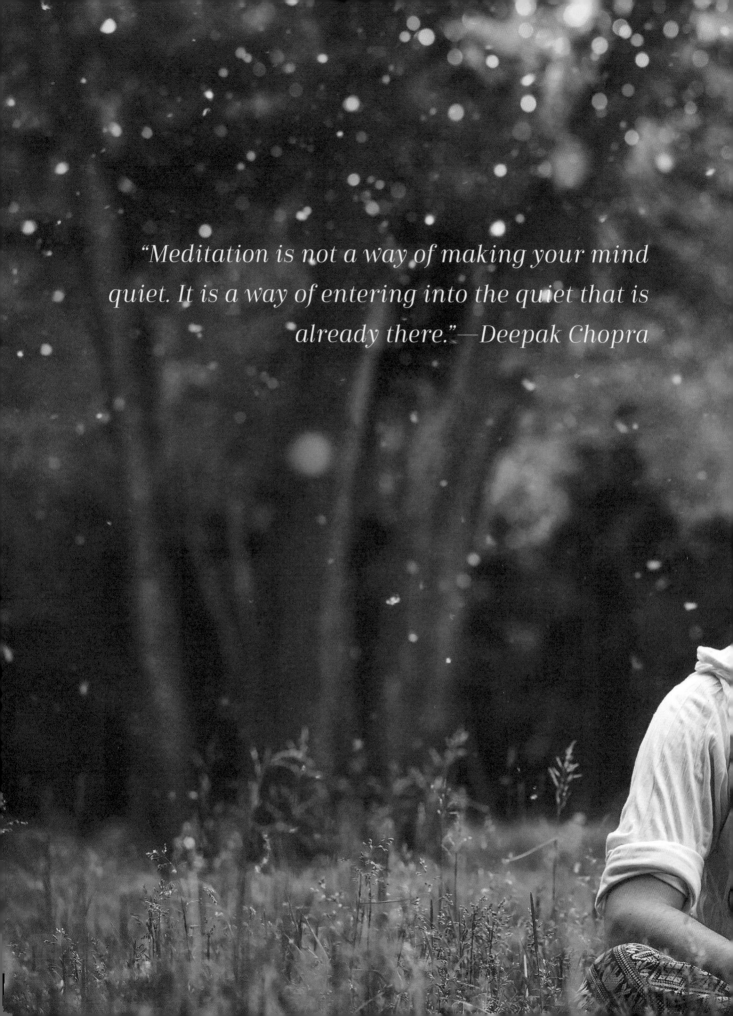

"Meditation is not a way of making your mind quiet. It is a way of entering into the quiet that is already there."—Deepak Chopra

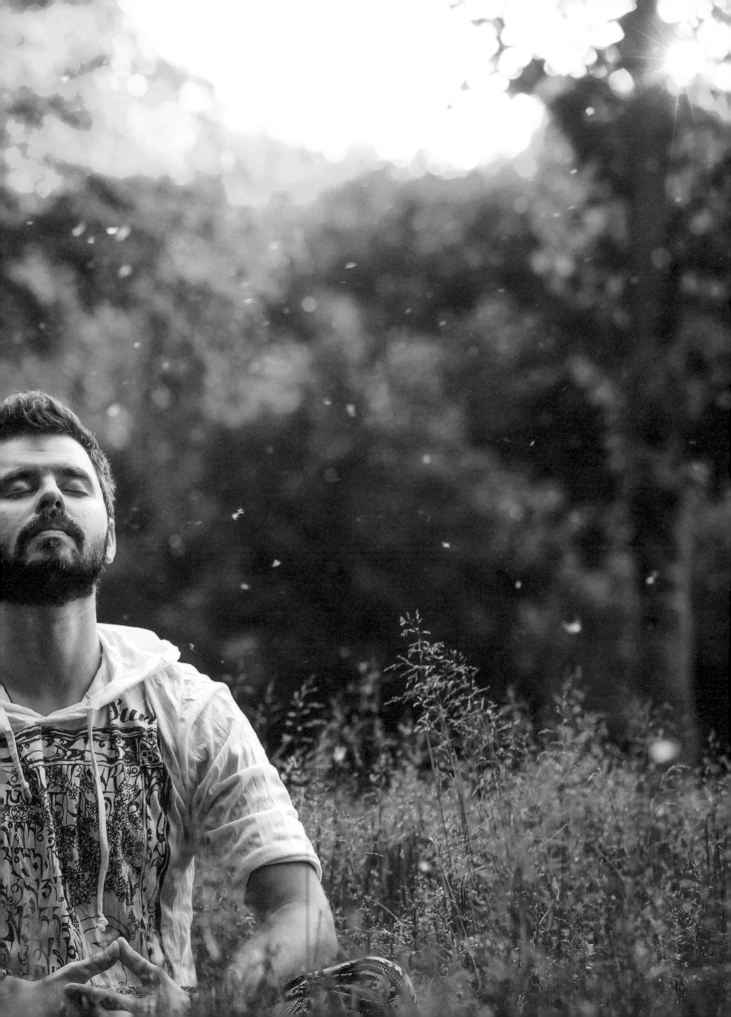

MINDFULNESS

When life is busy and you're trying to juggle family, work, relationships, and a social life, it's easy to stop taking notice of the world around you. But taking some time to still your mind, recognize how you're really feeling, and appreciate the small details can be highly therapeutic for your physical and mental wellness. Mindfulness is a technique designed to help you reconnect with both awareness of yourself and how you feel, and awareness of the wider world. It encourages you to be calm and focus on the present moment, accepting it without judgment, with the idea that this could eventually help you understand yourself better.

Mindfulness can be practiced formally and informally. With formal practice you set aside time to specifically try out mindfulness exercises which, in time, you'll get better at doing. Informal mindfulness is simply attempting to be more mindful in everything that you do, for example on your commute to work, sitting on the bus, when you're cooking, gardening, or spending time with your kids. It's an adaptable method that can fit into your life in the way that suits you best. It's also free (unless you specifically want to attend a class or have training), can be practiced by anyone of any age, and has lots of potential health benefits in store.

Mindfulness versus meditation

Mindfulness is often confused with meditation, but although they have some similarities (and confusingly there is a form of meditation commonly called mindfulness meditation), at their core they are different techniques.

The biggest difference is in how the techniques are practiced. Whereas mindfulness encourages you to focus on the present moment and acknowledge any thoughts that come into your mind, meditation involves trying to clear your mind of all thoughts. Another way to think of it is as mindfulness being the awareness of "something" and meditation the awareness of "nothing." If you find it tricky to get thoughts out of your head, which is a common issue when trying to meditate, mindfulness might be a better option for you.

Whereas meditation really needs to be practiced somewhere quiet without distractions, it's possible to practice mindfulness anywhere, anytime. Of course, it helps to set time aside for it, but as your skills develop and you become more engaged in being fully present in your life, you'll find yourself it becomes easier and more natural.

There are many different types of meditation, including transcendental meditation, chakra meditation, zen meditation, and meditation practices linked to religions and spirituality, and each form has its own aims and approach; mindfulness is simply one practice that focuses on increasing awareness.

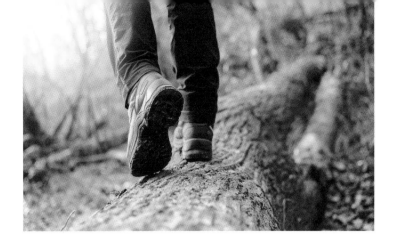

The benefits of mindfulness

Research into mindfulness has found a variety of benefits for your physical and mental health; it can also help bring about positive changes to your thinking, attitude, and behavior.

Studies have shown that practicing mindfulness regularly can help people to manage common mental health conditions such as stress, anxiety, and depression by helping to instill a sense of calm and balance. With its focus on awareness, it may help you to identify and manage your emotions and feelings in a better way. For example, you may be less likely to dwell on past regrets or worry about the future, instead feeling happier and content to live in the here and now.

One study found that mindfulness may help to boost memory and allow you to think more clearly. This is thought to be due to the process of mindfulness helping you to focus your attention and become more able to deal with shutting out thoughts that interfere with this.

It could have benefits for your physical health, too, as studies have found mindfulness may help to lower blood pressure, reduce chronic pain, and improve sleep.

Mindfulness may also help you learn to become more mindful of other people, accepting of flaws and imperfections, and more empathetic, which are all good skills to have.

With all these varied benefits for your well-being within reach, it's surely worth having a go at mindfulness? In the following pages you can discover some easy ways to get started.

Mindfulness is simply attempting to be more mindful in everything that you do.

MINDFULNESS AND BREATHING

When you sit down to practice mindfulness, there are times when you find yourself with a mind that is overfull with thought, distraction, and busyness. Your first reaction to this may be to feel that this is the wrong time for you to be mindful. In reality, times of agitation in our lives are the times that most urgently invite us to cultivate calm and simplicity. Finding it difficult to be with ourselves and to explore our inner landscape is a cue that signals the immediate need to find a sanctuary of inner calm.

Discovering our capacity to nurture even a little serenity and attention in the midst of chaos will enhance our confidence in ourselves and rescue us from further agitation.

Rising and falling

• Take a few moments to relax into an upright and alert posture.

• Let your eyes close gently and your whole body soften and relax.

• For a few moments, take some slightly fuller breaths, paying particular attention to your outgoing breath and releasing it fully.

• Let your breathing relax and find its own natural rhythm.

• Bring your attention to rest in your abdomen, noticing how it responds to each inhalation and each exhalation.

• Sense the rising and falling of your abdomen with each breath.

• With each movement of your abdomen, make a quiet mental note to mark what is happening.

• Note "rising" with the in-breath and "falling" with the out-breath.

• Ensure that the mental noting is directly linked to what is actually occurring in your abdomen.

• Let your attention rest within the noting and the movement in your body—rising, falling, rising, falling.

• Sometimes you may find it helpful to place your hands gently over your abdomen as you are practicing. This will enable you to feel more fully connected with the movement of rising and falling as it happens, moment to moment.

• At times your attention will move away, into past, future, images, sensations. As far as possible just notice those departures and note where your attention has gone with simplicity and calmness.

• Return your attention to your abdomen, once more noticing the rising and falling with each breath.

• Sense your breathing calming and your attention focusing. Sense yourself letting go of busyness and agitation, moment to moment.

• When you are ready, open your eyes and come out of the posture.

Mindfulness of breathing

• Find a posture that is as relaxed and comfortable as possible.

• Gently close your eyes. From the top of your head to the tips of your toes, gently and systematically move your attention down through the whole of your body. As you do so, consciously relax any part of your body that is registering tension or agitation. Soften any knots of tightness that you become aware of. Pay particular attention to your face, shoulders, and hands, allowing them to soften and relax.

• Let your hands rest on your legs or rest together lightly. Focus your attention for a few moments on the palms of your hands, being aware of whatever sensations are present. Let your body relax into a sense of ease, consciously being still in your posture. Gently bring your attention to rest within your breathing. Be aware of the whole movement of your breath from its beginning to its ending. Be aware of the expanding and relaxing of your chest and abdomen with each breath.

• Now make your breath slightly deeper and fuller, sensing the movement of the in-breath as it moves into your abdomen. Don't exaggerate the movement of your breath too much, just deepen it slightly.

• Bring your attention to the movement of your out-breath. Follow your outgoing breath to its very end, sensing when it has fully left your body.

• With each breath you take, give particular attention to the out-breath, to the release of your breath and your body relaxing. Sense yourself breathing out tension and agitation.

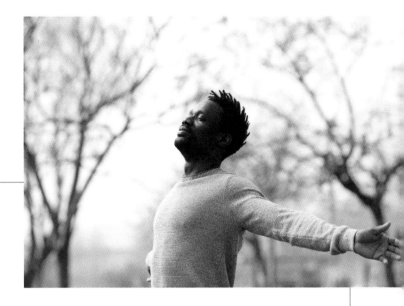

• When your mind is agitated, thoughts will clamor for your attention. Each time your attention is drawn into the thoughts or images that appear, just notice them, not pushing them away but also not becoming lost within them. Give them the barest of attention, acknowledging them but knowing that this is the time for cultivating stillness and calmness.

• Gently bring your attention back to be fully aware of the next out-breath. Breathe out the agitation. You may notice that the pressing thought patterns have an impact on your body, making it feel restless. If this happens, just consciously recommit yourself to being still and relaxed within your body.

• Continue focusing upon your breathing, keeping it just slightly fuller and deeper than it would normally be.

• Let yourself be fully present within each out-breath, staying with it until the beginning of the next in-breath. Notice the slight pause between the ending of one out-breath and the beginning of the next in-breath.

• Let yourself rest calmly within that pause.

• Sense the beginning of the next breath and your body's response. When you are ready, open your eyes and come out of the posture.

THE FIVE SENSES

Mindfulness is good to try when you want to feel calm. Taking a few minutes of time out to focus on your needs and to bring your awareness into the present, away from worries and stress, can have a calming effect. It's easy to practice and can be slotted into your day when it's convenient to you. If you have a sense of balance and inner calm, you're more likely to be emotionally resilient and less likely to be affected by stress, anxiety, or worry. Being calm helps to reduce the risks of high blood pressure, heart attacks, and stroke and gives you a degree of inner strength. If something unforeseen occurs, having a sense of calm helps with the ability to remain unflustered, think clearly and logically, and make the necessary decisions to help you tackle the situation.

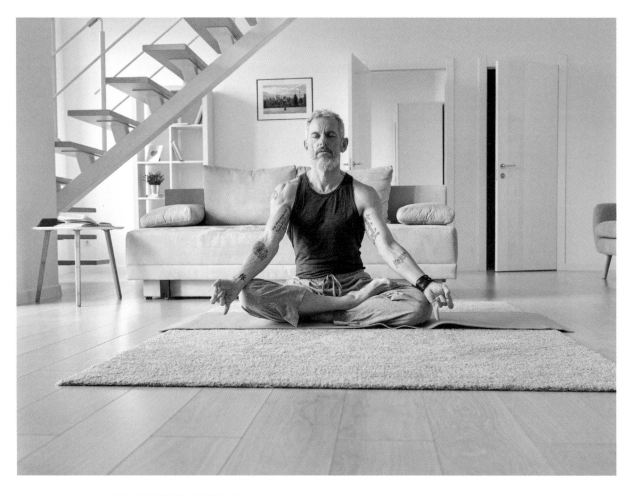

The little things in life are just as important as the big things.

The five senses mindfulness exercise

The idea of the five senses exercise is to focus your awareness on each of the five senses in turn, and to use each sense to highlight things that you can see, hear, feel, smell, and taste. This is an easy exercise that can be practiced at home or work and helps bring your attention to the little things in life that are just as important as the big things. The key thing to remember with mindfulness is to be kind to yourself. It's normal for your thoughts to wander, so don't be critical of yourself when they do. Just nudge your awareness back to the exercise in question and focus on the present moment.

Find a quiet space and somewhere to sit where you won't be disturbed so you can concentrate solely on the exercise.

1. Focus your awareness on five things that you can see. There will be obvious objects or items in your vision, like a desk, chair, or window, but look for the little details that you don't see instantly. For example, is there a cobweb on the ceiling? Maybe there's a leaf blowing in the wind, or can you see a crease in the fabric of your sofa?

2. Focus your awareness on four things that you can hear. Take time to become aware of the things that you can hear. Perhaps you can hear the sound of birdsong, of traffic going past, the ticking of a clock, or the gentle hum of office equipment.

3. Focus your awareness on three things that you can currently feel. Take time to become aware of these three things. For example, perhaps you can feel the texture of fabric on the clothes that you're wearing, the feel of the ground or carpet underneath your feet, the feeling of air against your skin, or the feel of your tongue in your mouth.

4. Focus your awareness on two things that you can smell. Take a few moments to become aware of things you can smell that you don't normally focus on. Perhaps there's a faint smell of perfume or aftershave on you or other people nearby; maybe you can smell the scent of blossom from trees, or of coffee wafting from the kitchen.

5. Focus your awareness on one thing that you can taste. Perhaps you have a lingering taste of toothpaste in your mouth, faint traces of what you ate or drank last. If you can't taste anything, have a taste of something now, such as a drink or a fruit, and notice what that taste is like.

By practicing this mindfulness exercise, your thoughts and awareness will have become more focused. It gives your mind a break, highlights the smaller details and sensations going on that can easily be overlooked when you're busy or stressed, and, ideally, you should feel calmer by the end. Take this sense of calm with you as you carry on with the rest of your day.

EVERYDAY MINDFULNESS EXERCISES

One of the benefits of doing mindfulness exercises is that they can be practiced on a daily basis and don't need to take up loads of time. In fact, the more you practice being mindful each day, the better your skills will become.

These exercises are designed to be simple and encourage you to focus all your attention on one aspect at a time, so that you learn to move your mind into the moment and focus on the present. It might sound easy, but it can be tricky at first and your concentration may wane; if your mind does wander at any point, just stay calm and bring it back to focusing on the exercise in hand.

The raisin exercise

For the raisin exercise, you'll need one dried raisin. Find a quiet spot in which to sit down and relax. Pick up the raisin, hold it in your hand, and pretend that you're seeing a raisin for the very first time. Now you're going to use all of your senses to explore the raisin.

Look at the raisin in detail. Examine its shape, size, color, its ridges, and areas of light and dark. Concentrate solely on the raisin and try to pick out all the details.

Touch the raisin and explore its texture with your fingers. How does it feel? Is it soft or hard?

Smell the raisin. Hold the raisin up to your nose so you can smell it properly. What does it smell of? Does smelling the raisin make you feel hungry?

Taste the raisin. Place the raisin in your mouth, but don't chew it right away. Spend time concentrating on exploring the raisin in your mouth and noticing how it feels on your tongue. Move it around in your mouth, feeling the texture of the raisin. Take a small bite of the raisin and notice what it tastes of and how

the rest of the raisin now feels, but don't swallow it just yet.

Hear the sounds you make as you chew the raisin and then swallow it. How do you feel after eating the raisin?

Once you have exhausted exploring raisins, why not find some more foods with interesting textures, smells, or tastes to practice with?

Three-minute mindfulness exercise

This three-minute mindfulness exercise is ideal to practice on a daily basis. You can set a timer for the three minutes if you wish, or simply go with the flow and estimate the minutes. If you choose the latter, you may find in due course that you're able to concentrate on this exercise for more than three minutes.

Find somewhere to sit quietly for three minutes, preferably in an upright position, without being disturbed. Either close your eyes or focus on a spot on a wall in front of you. Take a deep breath and spend one minute simply being in the present

In fact, the more you practice being mindful each day, the better your skills will become.

and noticing how you are feeling right now. What does the chair you're sitting on feel like, how do your clothes feel against your body? What's the temperature like, can you feel any drafts of air?

Spend the second minute relaxing and noticing whatever thoughts are in your mind. Observe and acknowledge them and how they make you feel, but try not to react to them.

For the final minute, focus on your breathing. Be aware of how you breathe, how your breath moves in your body, and notice whether your chest or stomach rises as you breathe in and out.

At the end of the exercise, open your eyes if they were closed, bring your attention back to the room, and acknowledge the whole experience and hold everything in your awareness.

Mindful seeing exercise

This exercise is good if you're out and about and have somewhere to sit and observe, or if you have a window with a good view. Take a seat and focus on looking at everything there is to see. Notice the colors, textures, and patterns of everything.

Pay attention to the movement of leaves on trees, grass, birds, vehicles, or the sea. Try and look at the world you're viewing from the perspective of someone who hasn't seen it before. Don't be critical, just observe.

If your mind wanders or you become distracted, draw your mind back to the view and focus on the shapes and objects ahead of you.

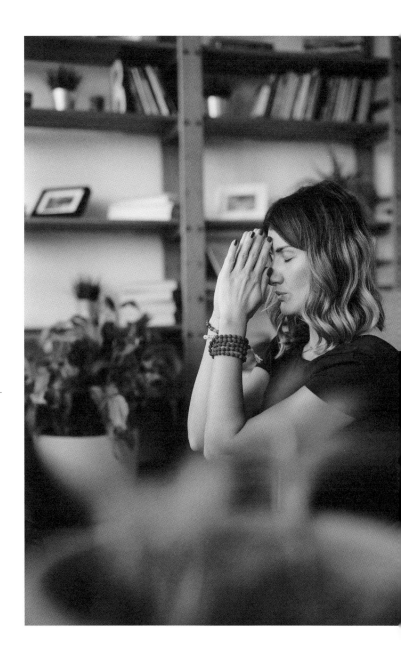

HOW TO GET THE MOST OUT OF MINDFULNESS

Here are some tips and ideas to help you get the most out of practicing mindfulness.

Persevere

It can be tricky to get the hang of mindfulness, so don't give up without giving it a proper go. If you can't focus during your first attempt, don't worry—it's perfectly normal for your mind to wander. Likewise, if you don't like the mindfulness exercise you've tried, it doesn't mean the whole technique is wrong for you; it might just be that exercise that doesn't resonate with your needs. Look for an alternative exercise and give it another try.

If you have mental health issues and are often plagued by worrying thoughts about the past, present, or future, it can seem counterproductive when practicing mindfulness to focus on your thoughts. But it's also true that the more you try and avoid thinking of them (as you would if you were trying meditation), the more difficult it is to get them out of your head. So mindfulness at least gives you the chance to sit calmly and acknowledge those thoughts in the present moment. In fact, it may even allow you a bit of space to be able to reflect better on your thoughts and worries.

Be prepared to acknowledge your thoughts

At the heart of mindfulness is the ability to learn to be more aware, and this includes acknowledging and accepting your own thoughts. It may sound straightforward, but in a life where you may often be too busy to stop and take note of how you're feeling, it can be hard to learn to accept how you really feel.

It's worth it though, and you could come out the other side with a much greater knowledge of yourself and a better ability to deal with your feelings.

Practice regularly

It goes without saying that one of the best ways to get the most out of mindfulness is to practice it regularly. A lot of mindfulness exercises are quick and easy to do, so can be incorporated into your daily routine. Set yourself a goal to do one short exercise a day, or if it works better for you, twice or three times a week. Routine and regularity can be beneficial, especially if you're juggling a lot of other demands, so allocate yourself a set time of day to do it and try to stick to it. For example, if you're a morning person, first thing in the morning or on your way to work might suit you, or you could try during your lunch break or in the evening. Experiment and find times that work best for your needs.

Practice with a friend

Practicing mindfulness with a friend or colleague may help you get more out of the techniques. You have the accountability that you've agreed with someone else that you'll both practice, and it can be more motivating to know you're not doing it alone. You don't necessarily have to be together as you do it; you could each be mindful on your own and get together to share your experiences later over a cup of coffee.

Set yourself a goal to do one short exercise a day.

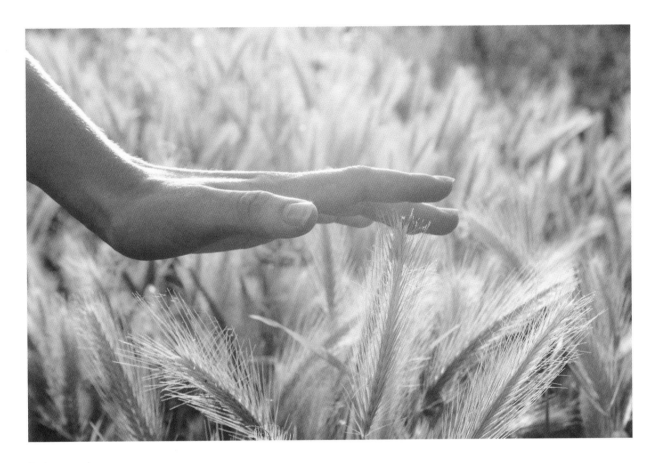

Join a class

To help keep you motivated, you may find it beneficial to join a mindfulness class. The sessions will help you learn new skills and provide you with plenty of different ideas that you can take away and use at home when you're practicing. They're also a way of connecting with people who share your interest in mindfulness, and for helping your wellness regime.

If you can't find any suitable classes near you, look online instead. Some organizations run online mindfulness sessions or podcasts that can be downloaded and enjoyed in your own time. You may also be able to find discussion groups online where you can ask for help with your practice.

MIND–BODY HEALING

In natural healing, the mind and body are inherently connected in a holistic manner—healing one may help to heal the other. Traditional medicine takes a slightly different view from modern medicine on how to go about treating and healing illness and disease, but together traditional and modern ideas and practices can complement and balance each other.

The mind–body connection

The mind and body might seem like separate entities, but in terms of health and well-being, they are very connected. Mental states, such as thoughts, beliefs, emotions, and attitudes, can affect how you feel physically, both in a positive and negative manner.

If you feel low, fed up, and negative about yourself and are not able to deal properly with your emotions, physical illnesses may develop. In contrast, if you feel happy and enthusiastic about life, and are able to cope with things, you are more likely to feel energized and well.

What you do physically, such as exercising and eating healthily, can affect your mental state and how you feel about yourself, too. If you have a poor diet, lack of exercise, and sleeping problems, you are more vulnerable to experiencing depression and other mental health problems.

Ideas of traditional and modern medicine

Traditional Chinese, Ayurvedic, and complementary holistic medicine take a different approach from modern medicine when defining and treating disease and illness.

Traditional approaches focus on looking at the person as a whole, and not just their symptoms. They recognize that the mind and body are connected. They acknowledge that an imbalance or illness affecting the mind can cause physical symptoms in the body, and vice versa.

A complementary practitioner works to find the underlying cause of the illness and then treats it on an individual basis—one person presenting with the symptoms of a cold will not necessarily receive the same treatment as another person.

On the other hand, modern or conventional medicine looks first at the symptoms of illness, then diagnoses the problem and provides treatment. Rather than focusing on the whole body, modern medicine often homes in on the specific part or organ of the body that is affected. Medical practitioners often specialize in particular areas, rather than covering the whole person, and standard treatments tend to be prescribed for certain ailments, such as ulcers.

Although the two approaches are inherently different, they can be used successfully alongside each other. Used well, they can balance each other and provide support and healing in different ways.

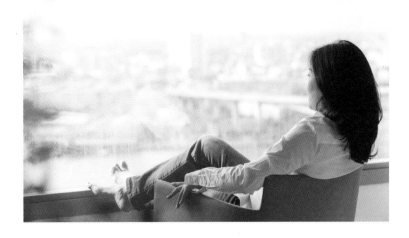

The placebo effect

The term "placebo" comes from the Latin words for "I will please" and refers to an inactive medication that is given in place of a working medication. The person receiving the placebo does not know it is inactive, but because they expect the drug or medication to work, sometimes they feel better after taking it. Clinical drug trials often include a placebo, so they can test the true effectiveness of actual treatments. In randomized double-blind research studies, neither the patients nor the researchers know which are the real treatments and which are the placebos, helping to rule out any element of bias.

The placebo effect highlights the true natural healing power of the body and especially the important part the mind plays in certain aspects of health, well-being, and healing.

The effects of stress

Stress describes the feelings you have when the demands made on you, or that you feel are being made on you, are more than you are able to fully cope with. Stress can affect all ages and is a normal reaction to pressure.

It can be caused by external stressors, such as work, life experiences, family, or finances; or internal stressors, such as thoughts and feelings of inadequacy, uncertainty, or low self-esteem.

Sometimes the effect of stress can be positive, for example if it acts as encouragement or motivation to get on with the task at hand. This is because stress is a physical response, causing your body to move into the fight-or-flight mode. As it does so, the body releases a mix of hormones and chemicals, such as adrenaline, cortisol, and norepinephrine, that prepare your body for action. That is what causes physical symptoms such as a pounding heart, a rush of energy, and fast breathing, which can prove to be exhilarating and motivational for some. However, stress is healthy and positive only when it is short-lived. Stress becomes a problem when you experience too much of it, causing it to become overwhelming and resulting in both physical and mental exhaustion. Too much cortisol can also affect your immune system, making it less efficient.

Stress can also cause emotional and behavioral changes. You may be plagued by feelings of anxiety, fear, anger, depression, and frustration, and lack concentration, sleep, and the ability to make decisions. In turn, a buildup of all these feelings can produce physical symptoms, such as heart palpitations, headaches, and aches and pains.

Stress can be a highly unpleasant experience, and an important part of tackling stress is to accept you have a problem. As well as identifying the root causes and making lifestyle changes, exploring ways to release your stress, relax your mind, and rebalance your body are some of the key ways of combating it.

TAKING CARE OF YOUR MIND

The first step to physical and emotional well-being is a clear, unstressed, and positive mindset. When it comes to healing the mind, there is a wealth of possibilities to explore, from meditation and mindfulness, to art and music, talking, and ecotherapy.

Some therapies can easily be practiced on your own, while others are best carried out in classes or on a one-to-one basis with a professional therapist, but they all share the common goal of helping to harness the healing power of your mind. Many of the therapies can be successfully combined, offering an even better boost to your mental and physical well-being. If troubling or negative thoughts and feelings are overwhelming or affecting your ability to live your daily life, consult with your health-care provider about next steps.

Giving thanks and breathing

Sitting quietly to say a prayer of giving thanks can ease the mind. You may choose to pray for yourself or for others, or to focus on being thankful for all the good things in your life. You do not need to be religious to give thanks, and it is a technique that you can try at any time, on your own or in a group.

Controlled breathing techniques can also help you to relax and manage stress. Diaphragmatic breathing helps you learn how to breathe slowly and deeply from your abdomen and is particularly useful for dealing with panic attacks. Even if you think you breathe properly already, trying a class can be an eye-opener into your breathing habits.

To get an idea of the technique, lie flat on your back, with your knees bent and your head on a pillow. Place a hand on your upper chest and the other just below your rib cage. Slowly breathe in through your nose so your stomach moves out against your lower hand. Now tighten your stomach muscles as you exhale through pursed lips. Throughout your inhalation and exhalation, the hand on your chest should remain as still as possible.

Biofeedback

Biofeedback is a form of noninvasive therapy that helps to promote relaxation. A series of electrodes are attached to your skin and send signals to a monitor via a biofeedback device. Beeps, flashes, and images appear on the monitor, giving details on your heart rate, breathing, blood pressure, muscle activity, and temperature.

As your heart rate and other bodily functions change when you are under stress, you can see them as they happen and then get feedback to learn to control them better yourself. Biofeedback is typically done in a therapist's office, but there are computer programs available that connect the biofeedback sensor to your own computer. Other mind–body healing methods can be combined with biofeedback to help improve relaxation, such as mindfulness and deep breathing.

Art and music therapies

Art, music, dance, and drama therapies are often recommended or provided by psychotherapists and counselors. It can sometimes be hard to express your feelings, especially if you are confused about them yourself, so these therapies allow you to go beyond words to express how you feel and what you are going through.

One of the benefits of these therapies is that you do not need any prior experience or artistic skills. The key aim is to be guided to create something, such as a play, dance routine, piece of music, or painting; to express yourself in a way you feel comfortable with. Arts therapies can be physically relaxing and open up another outlet for mind–body healing.

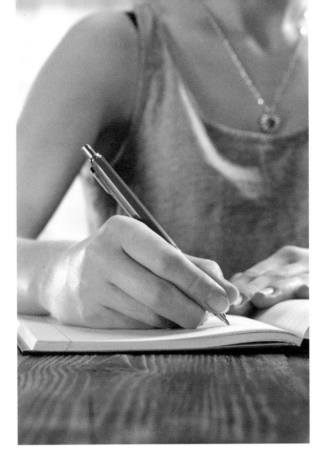

Journaling

Journaling or keeping a diary can be therapeutic as it gets your feelings down on paper in the form of words. This can sometimes be easier than saying them out loud and gives you a private place in which you can express yourself in a way that feels right to you. There's no right or wrong way of journaling and you can write as much or as little as you like. At a basic level, you could start by just writing your feeling of the day—even just one word—at the beginning or end of each day. You don't have to journal every day; it's fine to dip in and out of your journal as you see fit. If you feel you could benefit from some journaling prompts, there are websites with lots of ideas. Or you could invest in a journal that has prompts and ideas provided.

Ecotherapy

Ecotherapy is a relatively new term in treatment programs, but the idea behind it is by no means new. Ecotherapy means using outdoor activities involving nature to help heal your mind and boost your mental and physical well-being. Ecotherapy can include activities such as gardening, exercising outside, getting involved with a conservation project, helping with animals on a farm or refuge, or cycling through woodland.

Research into ecotherapy shows that it can help with mild to moderate depression, and reduce anger and low self-esteem. It also offers the chance to connect with nature, other people, and improve your mood.

It's fine to dip in and out of your journal as you see fit.

AROMATHERAPY

Aromatherapy can be beneficial for mental wellness in several ways. First, the scent of the aromatic essential oils stimulates the olfactory centers in the brain linked with the hypothalamus, the part of the brain concerned with mood. Different scents can evoke different moods, feelings, and emotions, helping you feel more uplifted, energized, relaxed, or soporific. Second, aromatherapy massage can ease symptoms such as stress and anxiety through massaging away tension in the body.

Using an aromatherapy vaporizer

These can be electric, or a ceramic ring that is heated by a light bulb, but most are ceramic pots warmed by a small candle. They are a natural way to scent, deodorize, or disinfect a room, and are one of the best ways to use oils for enhancing mood and balancing the mind. Vaporizers are also useful for when young children have breathing difficulties.

> Basic Measurements: Add water and 6–8 drops of oil to the vaporizer. Alternatively, add the oil to a bowl of water and place by a radiator.

Aromatherapy bath

An aromatic bath is a simple, useful, and versatile way to use essential oils at home. It can be used to enhance moods, relax or stimulate body systems, treat skin disorders, and ease musculoskeletal pain. Essential oils do not dissolve in water, but form a thin film on the surface. The heat of the water releases their vapor and aids absorption into the skin.

> Basic Measurements: Fill the bath with warm water before you add the oils. For adults, add 5–10 drops of essential oil to a full bath. Use less than 4 drops for children over two, and 1 drop for babies. Stir through the water with your hand.

Massage

Massage in itself is nurturing and therapeutic, and the rubbing action releases the fragrance of the oils and ensures that they are well absorbed into the skin. When combined with the medicinal properties of the oils, massage forms a potent healing treatment that can be relaxing or energizing; it can soothe the nervous system, or stimulate the blood and lymphatic systems to improve physical and psychological functioning. It eases pain and tension from tired, taut, or overworked muscles, and lifts the spirits. Whenever possible, try to include massage in your home aromatherapy treatments.

> Basic Measurements: Dilute the essential oil in a cold-pressed vegetable carrier oil such as grapeseed, sweet almond, or sunflower oil. Use up to 5 drops of essential oil to 1 teaspoon of carrier oil for adults, half that strength for children under seven, and a quarter of the strength for children under three (but not babies). The only essential oils suitable for babies are chamomile, rose, or lavender—use 1 drop to 1 teaspoon of carrier oil.

Damascene roses are cultivated in Bulgaria and Turkey for the finest of essential oils.

Steam inhalation

Inhalations are beneficial for headaches and an effective way to use oils that could cause irritation if applied to the skin. The steam releases the vapors of the oils. Steam inhalations are not always suitable for asthmatics or people with breathing difficulties, and they are not appropriate for treating children and infants.

Basic Measurements: Add 3–4 drops of oil to a bowl of very hot water. Bend over the bowl, cover your head with a towel, and breathe deeply for a few minutes. You can also use this method as a facial sauna.

Essential oils for mental wellness

Some good examples of essential oils for mental wellness include:

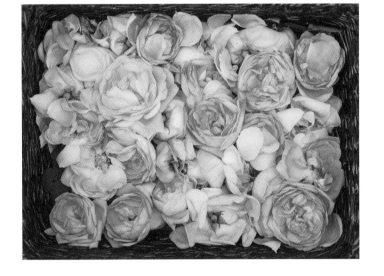

LAVENDER—this floral aroma is well regarded for its soothing and antidepressant effects. It can help calm the body and mind, reduce stress, and promote better sleep.

BERGAMOT—this citrus-scented oil has an uplifting aroma that could help to boost mood and alleviate feelings of stress.

GERANIUM—the scent of geranium essential oil can have a balancing and stabilizing effect on mood.

CHAMOMILE—the scent of chamomile essential oil may have a calming effect on your mind, helping you to get to sleep more easily at night.

ROSEMARY—rosemary essential oil has an uplifting and cleansing scent and may be useful to help relieve tension headaches.

LEMON—the fresh and uplifting scent of lemon essential oil may evoke a brighter, happier sense of well-being.

ROSE OTTO—this floral-scented oil can be one of the pricier scents to purchase, but it's worth it as the aroma may help to reduce feelings of anxiety and aid relaxation.

HEALTH, EXERCISE, AND DIET

Mental wellness can be affected by your overall health, the amount of exercise you do, and your diet. You can look after your mental health and wellness by caring for your body, developing healthy habits, exercising, and eating healthily. If you're feeling depressed, anxious, or low, it's easy for basic self-care habits such as showering or eating regularly to fall by the wayside, but keeping up with them can help you feel better.

Getting outside into the fresh air and exercising is beneficial for your health and helps lift your mood, so it's worth finding forms of exercise that you enjoy and are motivated to continue with. Even a simple walk around the block at lunchtime can have a positive impact on your health. Being active can help you to manage feelings of stress or anxiety, plus it can boost your self-esteem and improve your sleep. Sleep is vital for mental well-being, but can easily be disrupted by mental health issues. It can be a vicious circle—unless you step in and try to manage your lifestyle habits and self-care routines.

Diet for mental wellness

Eating a healthy diet is known to be good for your physical health, but it's also crucial for your mental health and well-being, too, as what you choose to eat and drink can have a profound effect on your mood and how you feel.

A healthy balanced diet should consist of:

FRUITS AND VEGETABLES—eat plenty of different varieties and colors of fresh produce. Aim to fill about half your plate at each meal with fruits and vegetables.

BREAD, CEREALS, AND POTATOES—high-fiber varieties such as brown rice and whole-wheat bread are best for your health. Aim for a quarter of your plate to be made up of whole grains.

PROTEIN—meat, fish, beans, eggs, soy products, nuts, and seeds; about a quarter of a plate per meal.

DAIRY PRODUCTS OR VEGAN ALTERNATIVES— dairy products contain many useful nutrients but they should be consumed in moderation due to their high fat content. Alternatives include nut milks and tofu, but be aware of allergies.

OILS—oils such as olive, soy, and sunflower are some healthful examples, but all oils should be consumed in moderation due to their high fat content.

FATTY AND SUGARY FOODS—should be consumed in moderation.

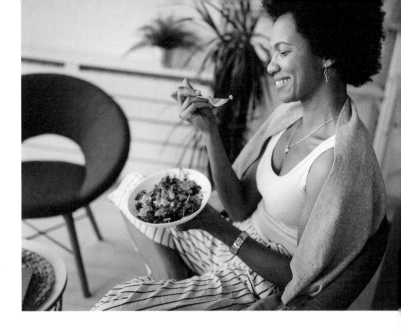

How food affects mood

Protein-rich foods help to fill you up, but they also contain amino acids, which play an important role in helping your brain regulate feelings and thoughts. Without these foods, your mood can be unduly affected.

Sugar-rich foods might give you a sudden boost of energy, but it is short-lived and the effect soon wears off, resulting in a dip in mood. Instead, it's better to eat foods that release energy slowly, such as whole-wheat bread, oats, cereals, and pasta. The benefits of energy being released slowly is also the reason why it's advised that you eat breakfast in the morning—it gets the day off to a good start, and foods such as oatmeal help keep your blood sugar levels balanced.

Although fats such as trans fats are bad for you, your body does need healthy fats as part of a balanced diet. In fact, your brain relies on fatty acids such as omega-3 and omega-6 in order to keep it functioning well. That's why it's important to include healthy fats in your diet, such as from oily fish, walnuts, almonds, olive oil, sunflower oil, milk, or avocado.

To help keep your mood balanced, it's worth trying to avoid drinking too much caffeine, which acts as a stimulant. You'll get a quick burst of energy from a caffeinated drink, such as coffee, tea, or cola, but when it wears off you may feel anxious or low. When caffeine is consumed in the evening, it can affect your ability to get to sleep. Try switching to decaffeinated drinks and remember to drink plenty of water, too (ideally, six to eight glasses a day) to stay fully hydrated. Without enough fluids, you may end up with a headache, feel fatigued, and have difficulty concentrating, all of which can affect your mood and mental wellness.

Note: If you are taking prescribed antidepressants or other medication, be aware that some foods (for example, grapefruit) may interact with your drugs. Always carefully read the information that comes with your medication and follow the guidelines.

A healthy diet and an active lifestyle can boost your self-esteem and improve your sleep.

SELF-CARE FOR MENTAL WELLNESS

Self-care involves looking after yourself and your needs. Getting into the habit of practicing self-care regularly can help boost your mental and physical wellness. It doesn't have to be taxing or take long; just a few simple changes and good habits can work wonders.

Get a good night's sleep

Sleep is an essential part of a good self-care routine, so make an effort to focus on getting a better night's sleep. Aim to try and go to bed at the same time each night so it becomes a habit. Do something relaxing before you go to bed, like getting lost in a good book or having a warm, relaxing bath, and give your eyes a rest from screens, phones, or computers in the evening—exposure to the blue light from screens can reduce your ability to sleep.

Take lunch breaks

When you're busy at work it's easy to get into the habit of having a sandwich at your desk or during a lunch meeting, but it's far better for your mental wellness to take a break. Go and eat your lunch in a different location, even if it's still in the same building, as a change of scene and the act of getting up and walking away from your desk will be beneficial. If you have time, go for a short walk to get some fresh air and to clear your head. You'll be in a better state afterward for tackling the rest of the day.

Try journaling

Some people find it helpful to write a journal, noting down thoughts and feelings for the day, experiences, or setting motivational goals. It doesn't have to be just words, you could also use art or craft techniques to express how you feel. As well as being therapeutic, by keeping a note of your moods or how you're feeling, you may be able to determine any potential triggers for your low moods and then apply methods to help reduce them.

Learn to say no

We're all guilty of it at some point, but you can't always say yes to doing everything. If you're constantly taking on new work, always seem to be the one that gets persuaded to be on committees, or are keen to help other people whenever you can, you do need to learn to say no sometimes. It's not good for your mental well-being if you're under too much pressure, and juggling too many different commitments could hinder your ability to do anything to your full ability. Think about yourself and your needs and say no to the things that you can't do.

Give yourself treats

We all deserve a treat now and again, and that includes you! Make time to give yourself a treat or spend time on your own doing something you enjoy. Perhaps you'd love to have half an hour to yourself to relax in a hot bath, get lost in a good book, have a pamper session, or indulge in your favorite hobby. Schedule in some time to spend on indulging yourself with the things you enjoy.

Laugh

There's a lot to be said for the saying "laughter is the best medicine." Having a good laugh really does help to relieve tension and stress. The act of laughing releases endorphins, decreases blood pressure, and stimulates your lungs and muscles. Laughing can boost your mood and make it easier to deal with pain and difficult situations. Why not pop on your favorite comedy show? There are even laughter classes available.

Have a digital detox

If you spend too much time scrolling through your phone, browsing on your tablet, answering emails, or looking at social media, perhaps it's time to take a break from it. Give yourself a digital detox. Try a weekend or a week free from checking emails and social media; you might even find that you enjoy it.

Spend time with friends

There are times when it can help to have some time on your own, but it's also beneficial to spend time with friends. Try and incorporate a regular catch-up with your friends over a coffee or a glass of wine.

Develop routines

Any form of routine can help you feel more organized and in control of your life. So if you feel as though things are too unpredictable and disordered, your mental well-being may improve if you establish better routines. It could be anything from a morning routine to get you out of the house on time, or a meal-cooking routine, an exercise routine, an organized time to socialize, or bedtime routines for the kids.

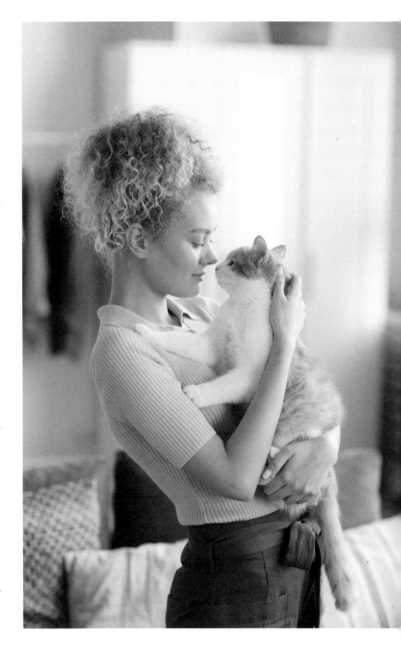

Just a few simple changes and good habits can work wonders.

CREATIVE VISUALIZATION TECHNIQUES

Creative visualization is a powerful technique to help boost your mental wellness and reduce feelings of stress, anxiety, and panic. It uses simple mental imagery (visualizations) to help you unwind, relax, and escape from negative thoughts—and by using the power of your mind in this way you may be able to begin to change the way you cope with difficult situations in real life. The technique is often used in psychotherapy.

How creative visualizations work

Creative visualizations are thought to work in part due to the element of distraction, and also as a result of the associative process. This process involves thinking of a highly pleasant scene or place that makes you feel good, which helps distract the mind from worries and stressors. By imagining creatively, you trick your unconscious mind into thinking that the happy and relaxing place is real. Over time, as you continue to use the power of your mind to transport yourself to a better place that makes you feel good, the associative process can form into learned cues or triggers that help you deal more appropriately with difficult emotions when you experience them. The technique has similarities to some forms of guided meditation, especially the idea that you can learn to detach yourself from negative thoughts. There are no right or wrong ways to practice it and you can create your own ways of visualizing according to your own needs. Relaxation techniques can be useful alongside visualization, as the more relaxed your body and mind are, the more benefits you'll gain from visualization. It's also helpful to keep an open mind, as you're more likely to benefit than if you think it's a waste of time.

As a starting point, some of the following creative visualizations may be helpful.

Trick your unconscious mind into thinking that the happy and relaxing place is real.

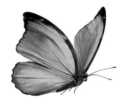

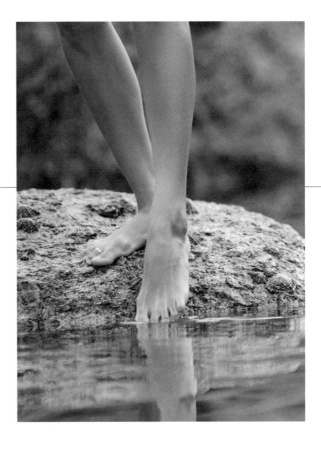

Visualization for stress and anxiety relief

• Find a quiet and comfortable spot in which to lie down, ideally on your back, and turn off your phone. Close your eyes, relax your body, and imagine that you're sitting on a sandy beach, feeling calm and happy.

• Visualize the feel of warm sunshine on your skin, the gentle breeze in the air, and the view of a gorgeous blue ocean. You can hear the gentle sound of the waves coming up the beach, of seagulls overhead, and the warmth of the sand between your toes. Visualize all of the scene in detail—are you sitting on a chair, or a picnic blanket, do you have a sunshade, are you on your own or do you have someone with you that you enjoy being with?

• Let all the tension escape from your body and focus on how calm, relaxed, and at peace you feel. Enjoy the sensations and the scene for as long as you need.

• When you're ready, open your eyes, breathe deeply, and slowly get up. At any point when you feel stressed, anxious, or worried, picture yourself back on the beach and remember how good you felt.

• If you're not fond of a beach, try imagining a green and peaceful meadow instead, perhaps with the sound of a waterfall in the distance and birdsong coming from the trees around you.

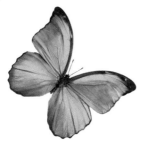

Self-motivation visualization

• Find somewhere quiet to sit comfortably, where you won't be disturbed, and turn off your phone. Close your eyes, relax, and visualize the room you're in. See it in detail in your mind—the furniture, the colors, the textures—and make it vivid. Now visualize yourself doing the tasks you've been unmotivated to do. Visualize what you're wearing, how you're completing the task, and how it makes you feel. As you watch yourself completing the task, see all the stress, anxiety, and worry you've been feeling disappear from your body. Imagine that you're realizing that even though you thought it might have been a stressful or hard task to do, it's actually a lot easier than you thought. Visualize how good it makes you feel to have done it and how other people react to the fact that you've successfully completed it.

• When you've finished and are feeling great about what you've imagined yourself doing, open your eyes and slowly get up. Remember that feeling of achievement and take it with you in your memory as you progress with your day.

LEARNING TO KNOW YOUR LIMITATIONS

An important part of mental wellness and self-care is knowing your limitations. In modern society, life can become really busy and it's easy to get piled up with responsibilities and commitments—these can include work you've agreed to do; dropping and collecting kids from clubs; and social, relationship, and family responsibilities. We're often told that we should "work hard and play hard," but taking on too much and failing to look after ourselves properly can result in burnout. In essence, we're only human and everyone has their limitations. The question is, do you know yours?

Identifying your limitations

It can be hard to admit and identify your limitations, but it's well worth giving it some serious thought. Many people find that sitting down and writing a list of what you can and can't reasonably do helps to put things in perspective. Consider all the expectations, responsibilities, and commitments you currently have and write them down, splitting them up into sections covering, for example, work, family, social, and personal commitments. Next, split up your existing commitments in terms of priority. List the things that are essential and that you have to do; the things you'd like to do; and the things that you either don't want to do or you're not so keen on doing. Look at your list of things that you don't want to do—are there items on that list that you could say no to or pass on to someone else to do? This isn't about shunning responsibilities, it's about making sure you're fully able to do the things you've committed to do. If you're feeling burned out, your ability to perform to your usual standard will suffer, and it's likely to impact on other people, too, so you need to ensure you don't take on more than you can physically and mentally cope with.

Once you've identified things that you could let go of, you need to let people know you're unable to take them on anymore, or find someone else to take your place; it's no help to anyone if you just ignore it and fail to find a solution. Normally, if you're upfront and honest about something, people will be understanding. Be prepared to stand your ground though, and don't be persuaded back into doing something that's beyond your limitations.

In the future, when you're approached or asked to do something, give it careful thought before answering or agreeing. Think about your list of priorities and imagine how it could fit in—would it be on your essential list and have you realistically got time to do it? It might be easy to fit in a one-off commitment, but anything that's going to be frequent or long term needs careful consideration. Don't be afraid to use the word "no." It's not a sign of weakness to say no—everybody has their own limitations, and we can't all do everything. They may even be asking you because they can't cope with doing it themselves.

List the things that are essential and that you have to do.

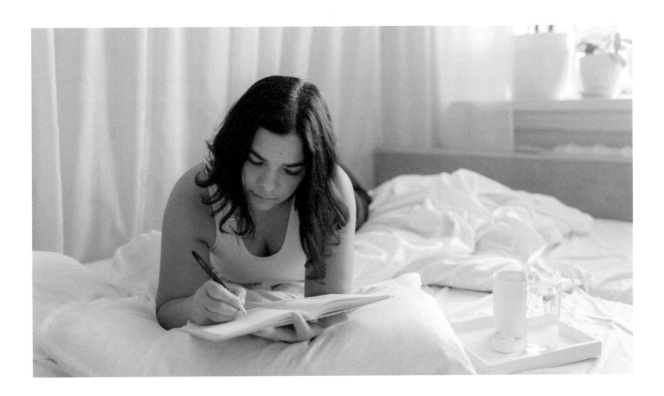

The signs of burnout

If you continually take on too much and push yourself beyond your capabilities, it will result in stress and burnout. Burnout is a state of physical, emotional, and mental exhaustion caused by pushing yourself too hard. Some of the signs of burnout include:

• Feeling overwhelmed

• Feeling trapped or helpless

• Feelings of self-doubt

• Feeling tired and drained of energy

• Feeling negative and low

• Taking longer than you normally would to get things done

To avoid burnout, it's crucial you're able to identify your limitations and work within them. It's never a cop-out to say no to other people's demands or admit you're not able to take on anything else. In fact, it's a sign of strength that you're recognizing your capabilities and not pushing yourself beyond what you can physically and mentally cope with. You have to prioritize your own wellness, and that of your family and loved ones, and when you set yourself boundaries and keep to them, you'll thrive.

TALKING THERAPIES AND PSYCHOTHERAPY

There is a lot to be gained from talking to someone else and getting a different perspective on life, and talking to a complete stranger, rather than someone you know who you fear may judge you, can be hugely beneficial. A range of different talking therapies can be used to help you understand your behavior and feelings, and learn how to cope better with overwhelming emotions, difficult life events, and traumatic experiences. If you're feeling out of sorts, struggling with your mental wellness, or are experiencing mental health issues, talking therapies are worth exploring.

Cognitive behavioral therapy

Cognitive behavioral therapy (CBT) is a form of therapy that helps you explore the different ways in which you think and act, and helps to change unhelpful behavior. CBT is used with various health conditions, including anxiety, depression, panic attacks, insomnia, and phobias.

CBT focuses on the problems and issues you are currently facing, rather than issues from the past, and offers practical ways to make positive changes. It breaks problems down into smaller, more manageable chunks, and you're given ideas for changing your negative patterns. A course of CBT normally involves several sessions, for example between five and twenty, each lasting for up to an hour. During a session your therapist will help identify your thoughts, feelings, and actions and help you understand how and why they could be unhelpful or unrealistic. Then you'll work together to see how simple changes could turn things around. Your therapist is likely to set you tasks to do as homework, so that you can practice them and talk about how you got on at your next session. Sometimes sessions are held on an individual one-to-one basis, and sometimes group sessions are available. The overall theory is that by changing the way you think and behave, you can learn new skills with which to manage your problems in an easier and more practical manner.

Psychotherapy

Psychotherapy is a form of talking therapy that can be used to help you identify problems, habits, and worries, and devise ways to find solutions. It can help with a range of conditions, from anxiety, stress, and depression, to a lack of confidence, low self-esteem, and bereavement.

Psychotherapy often explores the impact that past events or trauma have had on you. Rather than making a diagnosis, a psychotherapist will listen, be compassionate and understanding, and help support you to express your feelings and gain a better insight into the difficulties you experience. They'll help you find better ways to cope with strong emotions, worries, and fears, give you the chance to talk in confidence, and help you learn to change the way you think and behave. They'll guide you through the process and ask you questions to help you see things in a different way.

Most psychotherapy sessions are on a one-to-one basis—unless you're having a couple's or a family session—and last for up to an hour; the number of sessions you'll need will depend on your individual circumstances.

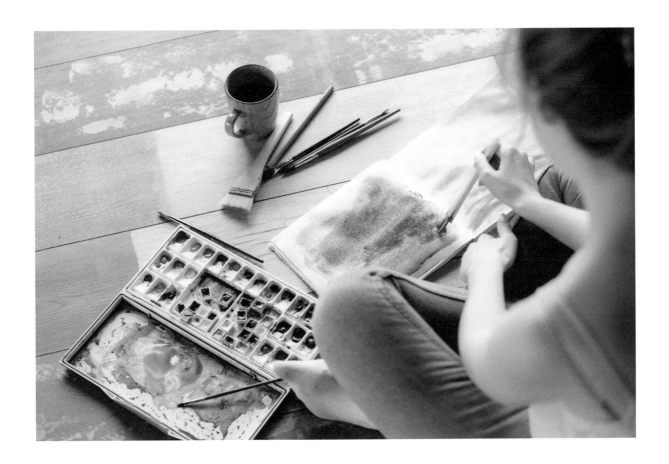

Art or drama therapy can be an alternative way of expressing deep feelings and emotions.

As well as talking, psychotherapy sessions sometimes involve the use of art, music, or drama, all with the help of a professional therapist. These methods can be an alternative way of expressing deep feelings and emotions, especially those caused by traumatic events.

Online therapy

If you're not yet ready to visit a counselor or psychotherapist in person, or circumstances are difficult, then there's also the option of online therapy. This allows you to connect with a therapist via the Internet, an app, or using your phone. It can be an easier and more accessible way to find someone you feel comfortable opening up to, and means you can fit the sessions in at times that are suitable for you. Research has shown that online therapy can be just as effective as face-to-face therapy for some people.

SUPPORT GROUPS AND NETWORKS

Everyone needs support in their life, and if you're going through difficult times it's even more important. Good friends and family are often the first port of call where support is concerned, and they can definitely be helpful, but there are times when you need other people who are more detached from the situation. Perhaps you're going through a hard time with bereavement, are struggling to manage with anxiety, or are really stressed at work. Finding support groups and networks where people understand your situation more clearly—whether they've been through it themselves, have cared for someone who has, or are trained in this area—can provide a vital source of help and understanding when you need it most.

Finding local groups

In the first instance, if you're unsure of where to look for support groups, check out your local library or community center. They typically have information about local groups and may be able to guide you as to who to contact. If it's related to a medical condition, your local medical practitioner may also be able to point you in the right direction, or you could ask friends, neighbors, or contacts if they know of any relevant groups you could join.

One of the benefits of attending groups in person is being able to meet other people who can relate to your experience. Some groups meet formally for sit-down meetings and talks, others informally for a chat over a cup of coffee, so find out the format and see what works best for you.

Phone networks

Some national organizations run phone networks, where you can speak to someone in confidence. If it's a sensitive area you're dealing with or there are no suitable groups in your local area, this is a good alternative to explore. Simply spending time on the phone talking to someone who is kind, compassionate, and supportive can make a world of difference.

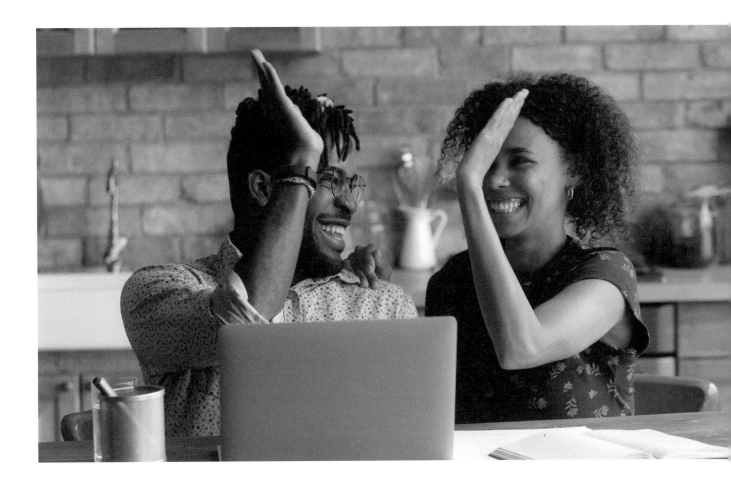

Online support groups and networks

There are numerous support groups and networks online, which can be of enormous help. Some are run by national organizations or nonprofit associations; others are set up by people who've been through similar experiences themselves who want to reach out and help others. One of the benefits of joining an online group is that it may be easier to remain anonymous. If you find it hard to talk about how you feel or what you've been through, sometimes it can be a lot easier to do so anonymously. Plus, some people may find it easier to write down their feelings rather than speak them out loud.

It's also worth searching on social media networks where informal support groups are often set up. If

you do use these, be sure to check out the privacy settings first and make sure you're aware of who can see your posts before you share personal information. A well set-up group will be secure and private and posts will only be visible to people who join the group. Your name will show on any posts you make and your posts may remain in the group even if you later decide to leave.

Whatever support you need, please take the time to search and find it. Talking, opening up, sharing, and relating to the stories of other people can be a great relief and help lighten our loads.

PART THREE

Emotional Wellness

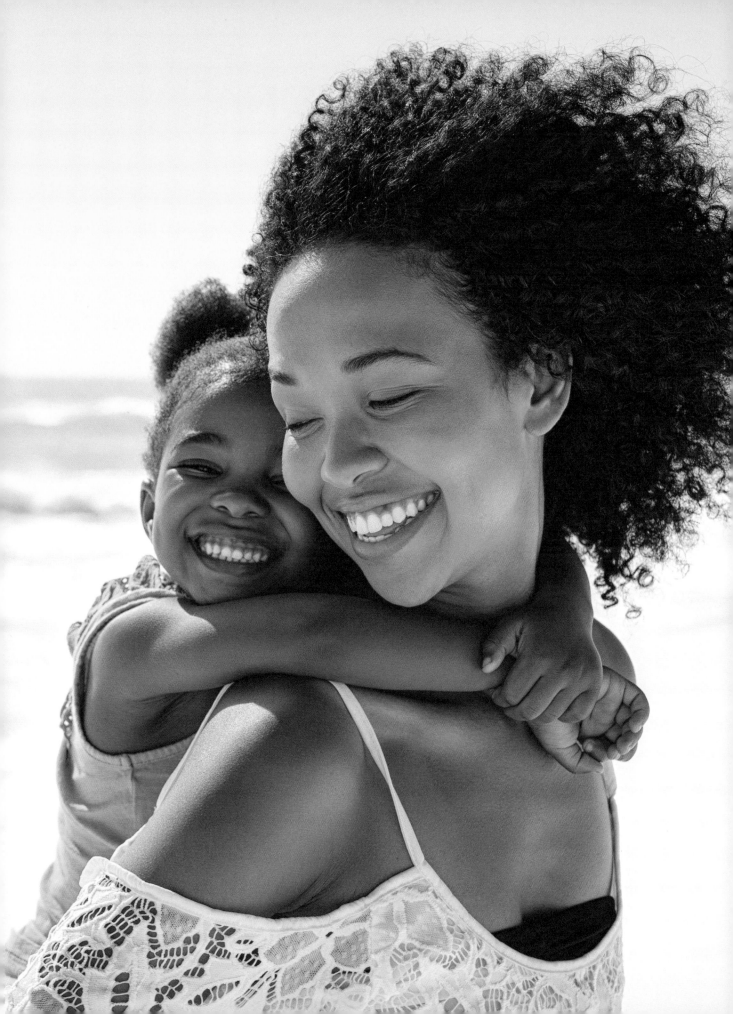

WHAT IS EMOTIONAL WELLNESS?

Emotional wellness is our ability to recognize and handle our emotions, both positive and negative. When we feel emotionally well, we can face change and challenges. We seldom recognize the importance of emotional wellness until it is under duress from stress, upheaval, or crisis. Yet building our emotional wellness has deep benefits for our relationships, working lives, and mental and physical health.

Relationships

A key step toward maintaining strong relationships, both romantic and platonic, is to understand what we are feeling and why we are feeling it. If we can accept our feelings and forgive ourselves for them, we can also begin to recognize what lies behind them. Our past experiences, in childhood and in former relationships, have an overwhelming effect on our emotions. Perhaps, for example, the root of jealousy lies not in a partner's behavior but in insecurity caused by past hurt. Anger may have its roots in low self-esteem, the seeds sown by events that took place before we can remember. Yet if negative feelings are overwhelming you or affecting relationships, knowing when to reach out for professional help is the greatest skill of all.

A major boost to emotional wellness comes from opening up to others about our feelings. If we are able to both talk and listen, we gain support, advice, and a different point of view. We can work toward basing our relationships on being able to disagree when necessary, without communication breaking down irrevocably. For most of us, a key challenge to healthy disagreement is being able to communicate our feelings clearly, calmly, and kindly. Perhaps an even greater challenge is being able to listen as others express their feelings with hasty, jumbled, or unkind words. In addition to understanding our own feelings, true emotional wellness also lies in understanding the feelings of others—to know when to accept and forgive them, or when it is time to seek help.

Work

Being able to manage stress, change, and disappointment at work is central not only to success—as business handbooks will tell us—but to contentment, self-esteem, and a good night's sleep. When faced with a setback in our working or financial lives, being able to move forward with positivity can be a deep test of our emotional resources. The great British wartime leader Winston Churchill said: "Success consists of going from failure to failure without loss of enthusiasm." While few of us share Churchill's world-changing goals or unshakable self-worth, there is still wisdom for us in his words—that it is within ourselves alone that we find the resources to build happiness. The first essential ingredient in that build is self-belief, so certain for some and so intangible for others.

As in personal relationships, it is useful to understand our emotions in the workplace, by examining what we truly want and why we want it. Being able to express ourselves clearly and calmly is as useful in relationships with coworkers and supervisors as it is with partners and friends.

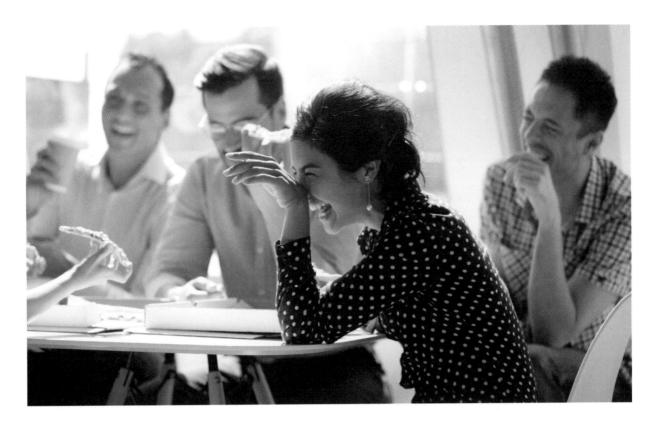

It is within ourselves alone that we find the resources to build happiness.

Yet honest communication can be as difficult within a workplace as it is within a family. In fact, many workplaces can feel like dysfunctional families! For some of us, our feelings toward authority figures in our working lives are influenced by feelings about authority figures in our family lives. Difficulties with coworkers may be rooted in the ways we—and they—learned to perceive and to express ourselves in childhood.

Mental and physical health

Our emotional, mental, and physical health are tightly interwoven. Negative emotional states are indivisible from mental stress. Together, they can impact our physical health, by lowering our immunity to infection and raising our blood pressure. Likewise, poor physical health, injury, or lack of sleep can impact our emotions, making us less able to face our days with calmness and positivity.

Managing our physical wellness is central to emotional wellness. A good beginning is regular exercise, which releases mood-lifting endorphins. We can ensure we make time for a full night's sleep, nutritious food, and relaxation. We also need to establish a balance between work and play, leaving ourselves time to pursue hobbies or connect with family and friends. It may be easiest to do this if recreational activities are scheduled, while downtime is blocked off so that all emails and phone calls are answered during work hours.

WHAT ARE EMOTIONS?

Emotions perform a vital function for our species: they help us to survive. Humans have evolved to feel emotions because they benefit us. Fear keeps us safe. Disgust prevents us from eating or touching materials that could harm us. When we work with others, feelings of happiness ensure that we cooperate for our mutual success. Love, perhaps the most powerful of human emotions, encourages us to take care of each other. Long ago, when food was hard-won and danger was everywhere, it was love that urged families and kinship groups to hold each other close, giving children—and our species as a whole—a greater chance of survival. Sadness may seem to serve no purpose in our survival, but it is sadness when we are lonely or lost that encourages us to make bonds with others. Showing our sadness through tears encourages others to be kind, strengthening cooperation.

The science behind emotions

What is an emotion? Neuroscientists have been trying to answer this question for many, many years. What we do know is that emotions are usually triggered by experiences. The "feeling" of an emotion is linked with changes in the brain and body. In the brain, chemicals called neurotransmitters are released, leading to different patterns of activity among the brain cells known as neurons. For example, the neurotransmitters serotonin and dopamine are linked with feelings of happiness. Patterns of firing neurons, running through different areas of the brain, lead to changes in thoughts and decisions, as well as, sometimes, the release of hormones. For instance, the feel-good hormone oxytocin courses through a mother's bloodstream when she hugs her baby. In addition, signals may travel from the brain along nerves to the muscles, resulting in changes to facial expression and body posture. Physical reactions may be triggered, such as laughter or tears. Perhaps, the conscious "feeling" of an emotion is a recognition of these diverse changes.

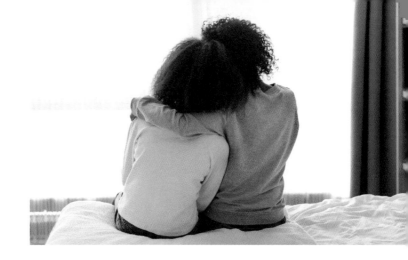

Basic and complex emotions

Psychologists have identified a number of basic and complex emotions. Both groups include positive and negative emotions. Basic emotions are those that have contributed to our survival over the course of our evolution. These include fear, disgust, happiness, sadness, anger, and surprise, while some psychologists add pride, shame, and trust to the list of basics. These basic emotions can be recognized easily by others because they have characteristic facial expressions, postures, tones of voice, and sometimes physiological reactions, which show little or no cultural variation across the world. For example, we are all familiar with these responses:

FEAR: Widened eyes, attempts to run or hide, and rapid breathing and heartbeat.

DISGUST: Wrinkling the nose and curling the upper lip, turning away, and retching or vomiting.

HAPPINESS: Smiling, a relaxed posture, and an upbeat voice.

SADNESS: Downcast eyes and lowered lip corners, closed posture, quietness, and crying.

ANGER: Frowning or glaring, a strong stance, a gruff or loud voice, and sweating or turning red.

SURPRISE: Widened eyes and mouth, jumping backward, yelling or screaming, and rapid breathing and heartbeat.

Interestingly, love is not usually considered to be one of the basic emotions, but is listed among the complex emotions. Many theories of the emotions position the complex emotions as mixtures of the basic emotions, in the same manner that the secondary colors (purple, green, and orange) are mixtures of the primary colors (red, blue, and yellow). According to this theory, love can be defined as a mixture of happiness and pride. Jealousy can be seen as a mixture of anger and disgust, while submission is a mix of fear and trust.

The complex emotions are harder to identify in others because they do not usually have characteristic facial expressions, postures, or tones of voice. Grief may not reveal itself by physical changes, or it may give the appearance of sadness or anger. Likewise, jealousy has no characteristic physical expression, but may be expressed as anger. Perhaps for these reasons, complex emotions are also more difficult to spot in ourselves. We may wrongly identify them as one of their constituent emotions, truly believing for days or months that we are angry rather than grief-stricken. In addition, many complex emotions are more culturally conditioned than basic emotions, with the occurrence and expression of emotions such as shame, guilt, and hope highly dependent on both social and familial mores.

BUILDING EMOTIONAL INTELLIGENCE

Emotional intelligence is the first—and largest—step on the road to emotional wellness. It is the ability to identify and understand our emotions. It is also the ability to use emotions, both positive and negative, to soothe and inspire ourselves; to communicate with and empathize with others; and to deal with change and challenges.

Identifying your emotions

Emotional intelligence begins with being able to identify our own emotions. Many of us have been taught to shut down or disconnect from our emotions. Yet to manage our emotions, we must be able to examine them. Try practicing the following techniques, which will encourage you to become more aware of your feelings:

• Observe and name your emotions. As you go through the day, notice which emotions you feel, name them, and note what has triggered the feeling. This goes for both positive and negative emotions. For example, notice that you feel proud when a coworker praises your work. Notice that you feel relaxed when you take a coffee break. Notice that you feel frustrated when you are stuck in traffic.

• Choose one emotion, then track it over the course of a day. Practice this exercise with both positive and negative emotions. For example, choose the emotion of happiness, noticing that you feel it when you receive kind words, when you finish a dull chore, or when you walk the dog. Then choose a less positive emotion, such as disappointment. Notice that you feel this emotion when you are overlooked at work, when your partner messages to say they will be home late, or when your children do not want to share stories about their day.

Recognizing how you suppress emotions

Most of us have been taught that expressing negative—and even positive—emotions is not acceptable. To varying extents, we have all absorbed the lesson that negative feelings are wrong. As a result, many of us shut down our emotions. Notice the ways in which you try to suppress your emotions:

• Distraction: Do you overeat, drink alcohol, gamble, clean, or obsessively watch TV or scroll social media to distract yourself from how you are feeling?

• Shutting down: Do you try to protect yourself from powerful emotions by disconnecting from them, so that you feel numbed or entirely emotionless?

• Shielding: Do you make the same stock, rehearsed emotional response to events—such as making jokes or shouting—no matter how the event truly makes you feel?

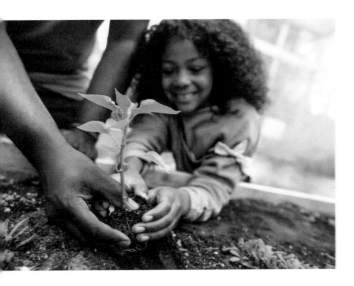

Managing your emotions

Recognizing how emotions affect our behavior is the first step to managing both the emotions and the behavior. A good start is "noticing" yourself as you go through the week:

• Notice how emotions affect your thoughts and behavior, so you can gain an awareness of your strengths and weaknesses. For example, you may notice that sudden demands from others make you feel stressed and frightened.

• Notice when impulsive feelings lead to impulsive behavior. For example, notice when sudden anger leads to lashing out.

• Notice triggers, which lead to the same cycles of emotion and behavior, again and again. For example, notice how mild criticism may always lead to feeling threatened, leading to angry words or withdrawal.

Harnessing your emotions

In order to harness your emotions, it is essential to recognize that all emotions can be beneficial, even negative ones. Fully understanding this fact can help us not only to tolerate negative emotions but to harness them. Emotions carry a message. Negative emotions are warning lights, which alert us to the need to pay attention, both to what is happening inside ourselves and in our environment. Negative emotions allow us to understand ourselves, to learn, and to gain wisdom. If we can understand the message carried in our emotions, we can begin not only to soothe the emotion, but to take positive action:

• Anger can mobilize, inspiring positive, carefully considered action.

• Anxiety can give us the energy and urgency to problem-solve.

• Shame can inspire us to make careful choices or to question the social values that are hampering our choices.

• Jealousy can make us work harder, be kinder, and empathize.

• Sadness can encourage us to get in touch with ourselves and to build connections with others.

Choose one emotion, then track it over the course of a day.

ANGER

There is nothing wrong with feeling angry! It is a natural reaction to life's events, both large and small. However, anger is a warning sign that an issue needs to be addressed. If we can address that issue calmly and positively, then anger has served its purpose. Anger becomes a problem only when it is so intense that it makes us lose rationality, or control over our behavior. When anger leads to unpredictable behavior, violence, self-harm, or addictions, we need to seek help. A visit to your primary care doctor is the first step toward managing overwhelming anger.

Is anger justified?

If you are feeling angry regularly or continually, examine your anger and its causes. Ask yourself if your anger is justified. This requires profound emotional honesty. If you believe your anger is fully justified, the next step is to consider—carefully and calmly—whether you can bring about change so the causes of your anger are removed or mitigated. If another person's behavior is provoking your anger, can you find the words to tell them, with empathy and without unkindness?

If your anger is not fully justified or if it is directed toward someone who cannot take full responsibility for their actions, such as a child or teenager, examine why you are feeling as you do. Is your anger a mask for another emotion that you find harder to face, such as feelings of inadequacy or hopelessness?

Sometimes anger is the result of intense emotional distress, caused by grief or abuse. Anger may also result from illness, pain, or chronic exhaustion. In these cases, your primary care doctor can address any physical causes, make referrals for further treatment, and direct you to support groups.

Managing anger

While it is not possible to magically cure anger, we can work toward managing its effect on us. We can also strive to become less reactive to situations that make us angry. Cognitive behavioral therapy techniques for anger include:

• Identifying situations that trigger anger, so they can be avoided or managed.

• Examining the thoughts and behaviors that follow an anger trigger.

• Recognizing negative thought patterns that lead to anger, including: overgeneralizing when faced with a single annoying instance (examine your internal monologue for words such as "everyone," "always," and "never"); being preoccupied with notions of justice and injustice; always looking for someone to blame; taking things personally; and black and white thinking (not recognizing that people's behaviors are never entirely good or bad—a friend can sometimes behave badly without being bad through and through).

• Replacing negative thought patterns with positive ones, including: looking for the best in people and situations; accepting imperfection; seeing things from different points of view; and not taking events personally.

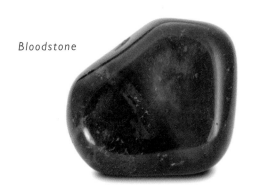

Bloodstone

Anger management exercise

Anger provokes immediate physiological effects, including quickened heart rate and breathing, as well as tense muscles. When anger is triggered, try to reverse those effects while also taking a moment to calm your thoughts:

1. Take slow, deep breaths, making sure you exhale for twice as long as you inhale. Count to four as you breathe in, then count to eight as you breathe out. Focus on your breaths, the air entering and leaving your lungs as your ribs and lungs expand, then return.

2. Roll your head gently toward one shoulder as you exhale, then back to the center as you inhale. Repeat on the other side.

Key crystals

The placing of suitable crystals, when performed along with meditation or mindfulness exercises, can ease anger and direct us toward positive action.

LAPIS LAZULI—place on the throat chakra to help release repressed anger that is bubbling up under the surface.

BLOODSTONE—place on the heart chakra to help release impatience, aggressiveness, and irritability. This crystal's energies can calm the mind and bring better logic to decision-making.

BLUE LACE AGATE—place on the throat chakra to help cool hot-headedness and neutralize feelings of anger.

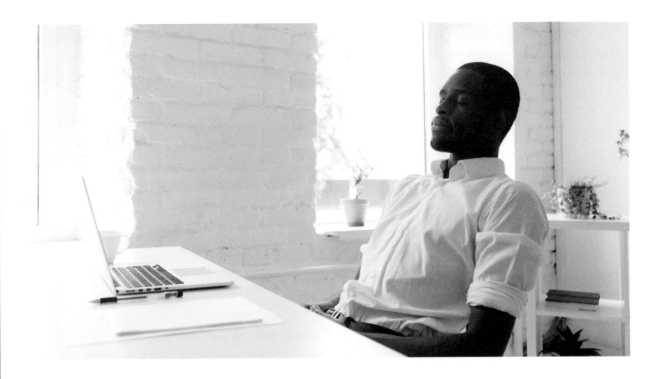

GRIEF

The pain of losing someone you love can feel overwhelming. Grief is a natural response to both death and nondeath losses. We will all experience grief during our lives and there is no one way—and certainly no right way—to feel it. Examining the nature of grief may help as we journey through the greatest of life's challenges—and can help us support those who are grieving.

The nature of grief

Everyone experiences grief differently. Some say that grief feels like a roller coaster, with deep, long lows at the start of the journey. As time goes by, lows may be briefer and less intense. Yet many years—even a lifetime—later, an event or memory can trigger feelings of intense loss. Some people feel that grief is a series of stages, although everyone experiences each stage differently or not at all:

1. Denial: A person tries to avoid facing the inevitable by refusing to believe in the loss.

2. Anger: Bottled-up emotions may reach the surface as anger, often in a hunt for someone to blame: doctors, God, yourself, or the person themself.

3. Bargaining: Searching for a way out, a grieving person may make a deal—with God, or with themselves—"I will do anything if this can be undone."

4. Depression: Deep sadness, despair, emptiness, and loneliness may be long-lasting.

5. Acceptance: A way is found to move forward, bringing peace.

Many people experience other emotions after a loss, all of them normal. Among the most common are relief, if the person has died after a long illness; guilt, for things that were not said and done; and fear, about facing life alone and about one's own mortality.

Self-care

Although grief for the loss of a loved one is often coupled with a lack of desire to take care of oneself, there are self-care steps that help reestablish emotional wellness as time goes by. This is also useful for those experiencing a nondeath grief, such as divorce, or loss of a job or friendship.

• Take care of your physical health: Emotional and physical health are closely bound, so remember to eat well, get regular sleep, and exercise.

• Acknowledge your feelings: Trying to numb your feelings will only lengthen the grieving process. Continual suppression may lead to depression, misuse of alcohol, or physical illness.

• Don't tell yourself how to feel: Allow yourself to laugh, cry, and howl when you want to or need to. No one else has the right to tell you how to behave.

• Connect with others: Although grief often leads to a desire to withdraw from the world, try to spend time with friends and family.

• Get involved: Find an outlet for your feelings in hobbies, writing about your emotions, or even organizing photos of your loved ones.

• Recognize triggers: If places, people, events, and anniversaries are likely to trigger overwhelming feelings, make a plan about how you will manage these triggers. Seek the support of friends or family.

Allow yourself to laugh, cry, and howl when you want to or need to.

Flower remedy for shock

The star of Bethlehem flower remedy is said to calm and comfort us through the effects of shock. Put 2 drops into a glass of water and sip regularly. The star of Bethlehem plant, known scientifically as *Ornithogalum umbellatum*, has delicate white flowers shaped like six-pointed stars. A prepared remedy can be bought online or the remedy can be prepared at home:

1. Place freshly picked star of Bethlehem flowers in a small glass bowl filled with water.

2. Leave the bowl in direct sunshine for three hours.

3. Filter the flowers from the liquid.

4. Pour 1½ fluid ounces of the water into a 3-ounce bottle containing 1½ fluid ounces of brandy. This is your "mother tincture," which will keep for many years and can be used to prepare stock bottles. To prepare a stock bottle, put 2 drops of mother tincture into a 1-ounce dropper bottle, then top up with brandy.

Key crystals

AMETHYST—wearing an amethyst crystal can support you as you deal with the physical, emotional, and mental pain of grief.

ROSE QUARTZ—the gentle energies of rose quartz can soothe, calm, and reassure as you process grief and shock. Keep plenty of rose quartz near you for its loving vibrations.

APACHE TEAR—the vibration of Apache tears is gentle and soft, helping to ground and protect as you grieve. Hold an Apache tear to provide strength and healing.

RHODONITE—keep rhodonite in your first-aid box of crystals to reach for in times of crisis and shock. Place on the heart chakra, or make an elixir, to help calm and soothe emotional wounds.

OBSIDIAN—place on the root chakra to help ground and stabilize, mentally and physically, after experiencing shock.

Star of Bethlehem

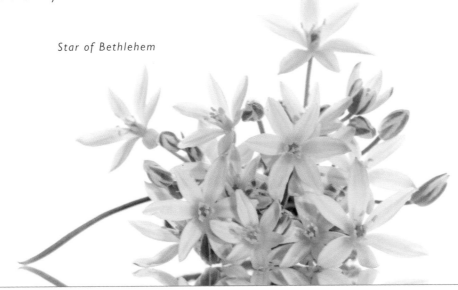

FEELING OVERWHELMED

Everyone feels overwhelmed at some point in their life. It feels as if an intense emotion has swamped us. We find it hard to think and act rationally. It may feel difficult to get through the day. Common causes of feeling overwhelmed are caring for young children, a demanding job, financial problems, life changes, and abuse. The feeling may also be caused by illness—physical or mental— lack of sleep, or a very poor diet.

Key symptoms

The key symptoms of being overwhelmed are feeling submerged by negative emotions and persistent thoughts. These emotions may be fear, guilt, anger, anxiety, or despair. Problems feel insurmountable to the point where action becomes impossible. This may result in a feeling of being frozen, unable to make decisions or see a way forward. Significant self-doubt and feelings of helplessness may infiltrate all thought processes. Sometimes the feeling of being overwhelmed is short-lived, but it can persist. Responses to, and manifestations of, being overwhelmed are often the result of an increase in the stress hormone cortisol. Symptoms may include:

• Frequent or inconsolable crying

• Increased irritability

• Irrational worrying

• Lashing out verbally

• Sleeplessness

• Loss of appetite or overeating

• Panic attacks, characterized by some or all of the following symptoms: dizziness, faintness, headaches, chest pain, stomach pain, nausea, chills, numbness, tingling, shortness of breath, shaking, sweating, and pounding heart. All of these symptoms can also be signs of physical illness or a medical emergency, so always seek medical help.

Try to examine what lies at the heart of your feelings.

Easing the feelings

To alleviate unmanageable feelings, the first step is to address the cause. This may be possible by asking friends, family, or coworkers for emotional support, advice, or practical help. Seek the help of your primary care doctor, too. In the meantime, try the following techniques:

• In particularly stressful moments, breathe deeply, using the exercise on page 174.

• Do not attempt to squash your feelings, but welcome them as the warning lights they truly are. Try to examine what lies at the heart of your feelings, whether it is physical exhaustion, fear of failure, or any other unaddressed physical, mental, or emotional issue.

• Notice your negative thought processes, which may include irrational worries, self-defeating ideas, and catastrophizing. Try to replace these processes with positive thought processes, focusing on positive outcomes.

• If fears for the future are causing your distress, focus on the now. Take pleasure in joyful moments. Try to break down seemingly insurmountable tasks into small, incremental steps, so you can tackle the indigestible in bite-sized pieces.

• Recognize how your emotions are affecting your decision-making, by hampering your ability to focus on solutions and make concrete plans.

• Practice yoga (see page 46), meditation (see page 146), or mindfulness (see page 162), which will help you build a store of resilience.

• Exercise regularly, even if it feels as if there is no time in the day. As well as offering a moment to decompress, going outside for a short walk can offer thinking time—with the fresh air opening the mind to new possibilities and ideas.

Flower remedy for feeling overwhelmed

The English elm flower remedy is helpful to those suffering temporary feelings of inadequacy. It helps us through periods of despair and loss of confidence. This flower remedy restores faith in abilities and helps us to balance our responsibilities with our desire for perfection, and to move on with fresh energy. Put 2 drops in a drink of your choice, then sip regularly. The remedy can be bought online or prepared from the tree's flowers and twigs, although the English elm is rare today, due to the ravages of Dutch elm disease. The leaves and twigs should be simmered for 30 minutes, before preparing the remedy as described on page 201, steps 3–4.

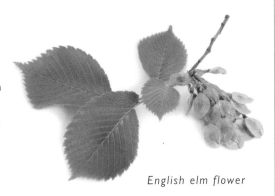

English elm flower

HOPELESSNESS

Hopelessness is a powerful emotion characterized by pessimism and a lack of interest in life. A person overwhelmed by hopelessness may feel there is no possibility of happiness, success, or improvement in their future. Although feelings of hopelessness may arise independently, they may also be a symptom of depression, anxiety, post-traumatic stress, bipolar disorder, and eating disorders. Hopelessness may lead to suicidal ideation, so seek help if feelings are not short-lived.

Facing hopelessness

Someone who is feeling hopeless may feel like giving up. They may feel that no one can help them and there is no way out of their current situation. As their mood darkens, they may lose interest in other people and in activities. Their sense of the world, of other people, and of themselves may change. Hopelessness may be linked with feelings of abandonment and loss.

Mild feelings of hopelessness can be helped by taking the following steps:

• Ask for help from friends and family. Talk with them to gain a new perspective.

• When the future feels dark, focus on the moment. Find joy in the now (see page 244) or practice meditation (see page 146), mindfulness (see page 162), or journaling (see page 246).

• Change what you can and try to forget the rest. Focus on what can be improved rather than overwhelming yourself by focusing on the issues that are beyond your control. For example, if you are experiencing job loss, try volunteering or learning a new skill.

• Rekindle your passions and interests. Connect with friends, pick up an old hobby, or go hiking.

• Remember that positive changes take time. Most changes are made in small steps, hesitant at first—and with a few setbacks along the way—but growing in stride and confidence.

Moderate feelings of hopelessness may be helped by cognitive behavioral therapy. A therapist may suggest exercises such as the following:

• Take note of negative thought patterns and assumptions. These may include the belief that it is too late to make changes.

• Examine the accuracy of these assumptions.

• Replace negative thought patterns with positive ones, such as the fact that change is always possible and that the future is not predetermined.

When to seek immediate help

It is essential to seek immediate help if you or anyone else talks or writes about killing themself; accesses the means to kill themself; engages in risky behavior; definitively withdraws from friends and family; or talks about seeing no way out or having no reason to live. Call 911 in an emergency.

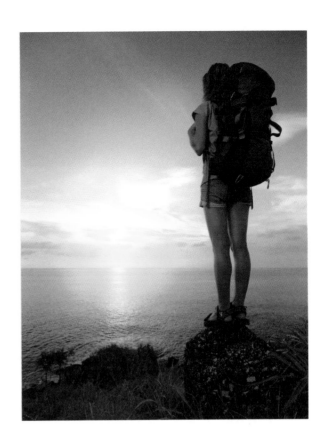

Rekindle your passions and interests. Connect with friends, pick up an old hobby, or go hiking.

Flower remedy for hopelessness

The gorse flower remedy can be taken as 2 drops in a glass of water by those who are suffering moderate feelings of hopelessness or despair. It gives the courage to try again, to hope for the future, and to strive. The remedy can be bought online. Alternatively, the yellow scented flowers, which appear almost year-round, can be picked—with care—from the prickly *Ulex europaeus* bush, which is found on stony soils and heaths. The flowers should be prepared by the sun method, described on page 211.

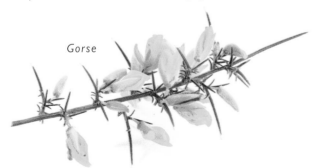

Gorse

Key crystals

Many crystals that offer help in periods of moderate hopelessness are red. These chime with the root chakra, where our drive for love, success, and happiness is centered. Unblocking and stimulating this chakra can offer renewed hope and motivation.

SPINEL—place spinel by the bed or under the pillow to awaken with fresh strength, positivity, and hopefulness.

RED JASPER—hold red jasper or wear as a pendant for protection and support. It enables us to find the right path to take at times of hopelessness and indecision.

RED CALCITE—place at the third eye chakra to gain insight into fears, but place at the root chakra for the courage to face them.

MAHOGANY OBSIDIAN—meditate with this stone to sow the seeds of hope and resourcefulness.

JEALOUSY

Jealousy is a feeling of envy or suspicion about relationships or possessions. Jealousy may take the shape of unfounded distrust and possessiveness of a partner. We may also experience jealousy as an angry or unhappy feeling of wanting to have what another person has, whether that is possessions, physical appearance, or financial or emotional success. Jealousy has many causes, including insecurity, feelings of inadequacy, and a history of past loss.

Managing jealousy in a relationship

Everyone experiences passing moments of jealousy, but if unfounded jealousy is intense and ongoing, it may be damaging to both the relationship and emotional wellness. When jealousy is focused on the fear that a partner may like or be liked by someone else, this emotion may manifest itself in behavior such as frequent accusations or possessiveness, or grasping the partner tightly to prevent them from being taken away. Try the following steps to reestablish emotional balance:

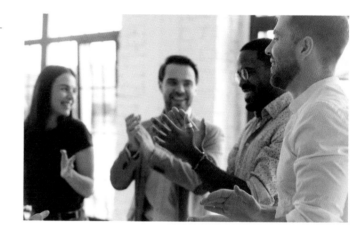

• Recognize your feelings as being rooted in jealousy. Examine how this emotion has arisen. It may be caused by experiences in past relationships. It may have its roots in childhood, if key relationships were unstable, challenging, or absent.

• Take responsibility for your feelings. Only you can manage your feelings of jealousy, through being honest with yourself, forgiving yourself, and learning to value yourself as someone worthy of being loved. Try talking with trusted friends or accessing therapy.

• Tell your partner how you feel and why you are feeling it. Remember that your partner cannot make you feel better with reassurances or changing their behavior. However, honesty and compassion are key to maintaining a relationship of loving trust.

Managing jealousy of what others have

Jealousy can be focused on wanting what another person possesses, an emotion often described as envy. Everyone feels envious from time to time, but intense envy can impact on emotional wellness. It can manifest itself in self-criticism, anxiety, sadness, and the desire to undermine others' successes. Jealousy may arouse intense feelings of hostility to the object of the envy. The first step is to acknowledge the emotion:

• Acknowledgment that what you are feeling is jealousy. This acknowledgment requires the emotional strength to admit our own feelings of inadequacy.

Honesty and compassion are key to maintaining a relationship of loving trust.

• Replace boosts to self-esteem with compassion. Trying to boost your self-esteem by reminding yourself about your own enviable traits and possessions only reinforces the idea that there is a hierarchy of enviable and unenviable people. Instead, forgive yourself for your self-doubt while also recognizing that everyone—even the object of jealousy—feels that self-doubt. By reminding ourselves that we are all human, and all suffering but striving, we can be accepting and kind.

• Count true blessings. By learning to be grateful for what is truly valuable in our lives—family, friendships, good health—rather than on outward trappings, we can break free from jealousy. Jealousy may also be a spur to genuine self-improvement, if it drives us to work harder at the relationships and projects that truly matter. However, if jealousy has arisen because of the things that we cannot change about ourselves, self-compassion—not "self-improvement"—is key.

Flower remedy for jealousy

Holly is the ideal flower remedy for addressing powerful negative feelings, such as jealousy, vengefulness, and suspicion. It is beneficial for those who may have other intense emotions that they feel afraid to express. This flower remedy helps us to address these negative emotions and to open our hearts to giving and receiving love. The holly bush (*Ilex aquifolium*) is known for its spiked leaves and red berries, but its inconspicuous flowers appear during spring and early summer, depending on climate. The flower remedy can be bought online or made at home. The flowers should be simmered for 30 minutes, before preparing the remedy as described on page 201, steps 3–4.

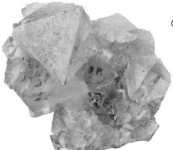

Green fluorite

Key crystals

Many green crystals can help us to work through jealousy. These crystals are particularly resonant at the heart chakra, where they can help us to manage and to harness negative emotions. When jealousy is overwhelming, they help us to find balance, within ourselves and in our relationships.

PERIDOT—sleep with peridot under the pillow to awaken refreshed and cleansed of negative emotions.
PRASIOLITE—meditate with prasiolite to find the true cause of jealousy, then the strength to move forward with love and honesty.
LIZARDITE—carry or wear lizardite daily in order to slough off damaging feelings and repetitive thought patterns, just as a snake rubs away its old skin.
SERAPHINITE—place inspirational seraphinite on the table when using journaling or other creative projects to work through jealousy.
GREEN FLUORITE—place at the heart chakra during meditation to free yourself from negative feelings about loved ones.

GUILT

Although our experience of feeling guilt is negative, appropriate guilt is a healthy emotion. Appropriate guilt is our moral compass. We feel guilt when we sense that we have done harm or we have breached a moral code, whether that code is our own or we have absorbed it from family, society, or religion. When guilt is excessive, turns to shame, or is irrational, it can damage our emotional wellness.

The difference between guilt and shame

In a 2015 study published in *Cognition and Emotion*, psychologist Matt Treeby and colleagues studied the different emotions and behaviors of people who are guilt-prone and people who are shame-prone. The study revealed that people who perpetually feel guilty (whether they have genuinely done "wrong" or not) were experts at reading other people's emotions. It was not clear whether their tendency to feel guilty caused their ability to recognize emotion or whether their sensitivity to the emotions of others led to them feeling guilty more frequently. What was clear was that, when these guilt-prone people felt they had done something wrong, they voiced a desire to do better next time.

In contrast, people who were prone to feeling shame at their own mistakes, real or imagined, responded to feeling they had done wrong by wanting to hide or punish themselves, rather than wanting to try harder. These people showed no greater than average sensitivity to others' emotions. One of the lessons of this study is that guilt can be a healthy emotion, if it leads us not into punishing or disliking ourselves but toward respect for others' feelings and the desire to learn from our mistakes.

Managing appropriate guilt

Most people feel guilty frequently, for letting down a friend, for not spending time with their family, for leaving a colleague to shoulder a burden. This guilt is useful, as it encourages us to try harder. For some of us, the reason for our guilt may be more serious and less easy to put right. Overwhelming guilt can cause insomnia, anxiety, and depression. All of us can benefit from the same approach to managing our appropriate guilt:

• Keep your mistakes in perspective. We are all imperfect and we all make mistakes.

• Learn from your mistakes and make amends. If it is not possible to make amends directly, find a way to do good elsewhere.

• Do not torture yourself. Constantly focusing on past mistakes, disliking yourself, or punishing yourself cannot undo mistakes or help you make amends.

• Try mindfulness, meditation, journaling, and regular exercise to calm and soothe.

• Seek the help of a therapist or counselor, who can examine guilty feelings, find perspective, and address the guilt productively.

Keep your mistakes in perspective. We are all imperfect and we all make mistakes.

Managing irrational guilt

Irrational guilt is when we falsely take responsibility for a problem we have not caused, or when we overestimate the harm that a minor transgression has caused. We may also feel irrational guilt or shame for transgressions of a code with which we do not consciously agree, imposed on us by an authority figure from the past or present. Overwhelming irrational guilt may be linked with depression, anxiety, and obsessive-compulsive disorder.

If irrational guilt has become overwhelming, visit your primary care doctor, who can offer referrals for appropriate therapy.

Flower remedy for guilt

The pine flower remedy may be beneficial for those suffering self-reproach and guilty feelings. It is soothing for those who never feel they are good enough and blame themselves for events that are beyond their control. Pine gives us the strength and freedom to examine, address, and move on from guilt. The remedy can be bought online or prepared by simmering the young twigs of Scotch pine (*Pinus sylvestris*) before preparing the remedy as described on page 201, steps 3–4.

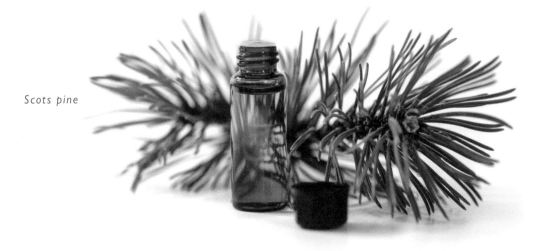

Scots pine

LONELINESS

Loneliness is a feeling of sadness because one feels a lack of true friends and company. Loneliness may be caused by social isolation, but it can also be felt by someone who is surrounded by family, friends, and coworkers but still feels as if they have no one with whom they truly connect.

Reasons for loneliness

Social isolation may be the result of life changes, such as divorce, the death of a partner, a move to a new area, or loss of a job. Isolation may also be caused by long-term illness or disability. It may be the result of being a single parent or caring for someone who is ill. For some, isolation is the effect of discrimination due to sexual orientation or race. Isolation may also be brought about by difficulties with forming lasting relationships due to social anxiety, abuse, trauma, mental health problems, and other challenges to emotional well-being.

Emotional loneliness can be felt by someone who is surrounded by others, but feels the lack of meaningful relationships or a sense of belonging. The teenage years can be a time of emotional loneliness, but this feeling can be suffered by anyone at any time in life. Loneliness can also arise from the feeling of having too few good-quality relationships, as may happen in middle age or the senior years, when there seem to be fewer opportunities to form new friendships.

Making connections

Everyone feels lonely at times, but if loneliness persists it can lead to stress, insomnia, low self-esteem, and depression. Since loneliness has so many causes, no one strategy can end it, but a combination of the following steps can benefit those who want to form new and deeper connections with others:

• Seek the support of your primary care doctor, who can help address and offer referrals for underlying physical, mental, and emotional issues.

• Talking therapies offer a way to address the emotional issues that stand in the way of satisfying relationships.

• Cognitive behavioral therapy can help to address social anxiety or low self-esteem, by focusing on how your thoughts and feelings affect your behavior. A therapist will offer coping strategies for different situations.

• Join a group or club based on your interests, just watching from the back at first if this feels overwhelming. A peer support group for people in similar social situations may also be helpful. Over time, new friendships will grow.

• Try volunteering in your local area, which is an ideal way to meet new people and build self-esteem.

• If you have friends and family but do not feel close to them, try opening up to a sympathetic person about how you are feeling.

• Take good care of your physical health by getting the right amount of sleep, eating well, and exercising regularly.

• Steer clear of social media, which gives a false impression of other people's happiness. People share only what they want to share on social media; few are brave enough to post that they are feeling lonely or low.

Loneliness can be suffered by anyone at any time in life.

Flower remedy for loneliness

The water violet flower remedy is for those who isolate themselves by putting up barriers from fear of hurt. Those who benefit from water violet often feel left out because they hold themselves back. They solve problems alone. Water violet encourages us to form connections with others, to open ourselves to friendship and love. Water violets can often be found in ditches, where they remain submerged for most of the year, their delicate lilac flowers appearing above the surface only in summer. The flowers should be prepared by the sun method, described on page 205.

THE SUN METHOD

A 3 fl. oz. bottle of mother tincture will last the average family many years. This recipe can make more, up to six bottles. Each 3 fl. oz. should contain ¼ cup of brandy and be made up as follows:

18 oz. spring or mineral water

Plain glass bowl

Natural and unbleached filter paper

3 fl. oz. amber bottle(s)

¼ cup brandy

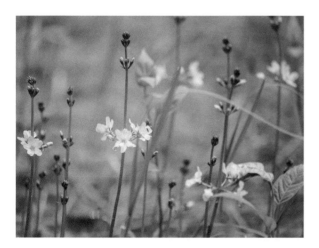

Decide beforehand on the plants, where to pick from, and where to place the bowl (as close to the plants as possible, but away from shadows and possible contamination), then wait for a suitable sunny day.

The best time for harvesting the plants is between 9:00 a.m. and midday. Put the water in the bowl, pick the flowers, and put them in the water as quickly as possible. Float the flowers on the water until the whole surface is covered. Use a twig or leaf to arrange them, not your fingers. Leave the bowl out in the open where it will receive direct sunshine for 3 hours.

Remove the flowers with a twig or leaf and filter the liquid. Pour ¼ cup of the water into a bottle with the brandy. Shake and label with the name "flower essence mother tincture" and date. This mother tincture will be used to prepare stock bottles, and it will keep for many years. To prepare a stock bottle, put 2 drops of mother tincture into a 1 fl. oz. dropper bottle, and top up with brandy.

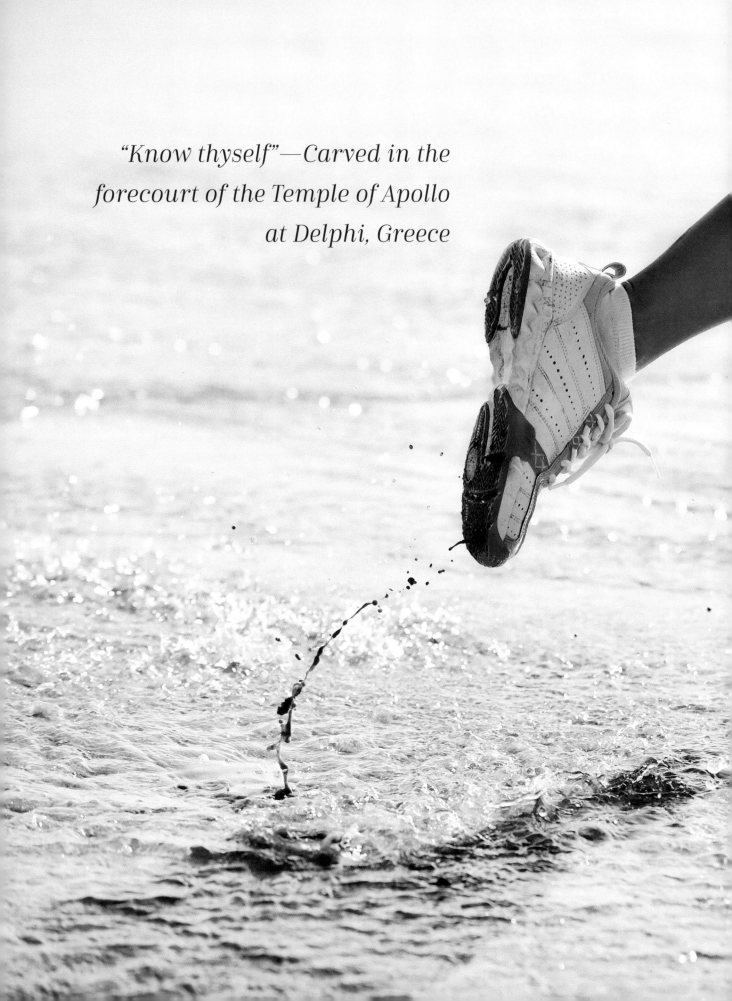

"Know thyself"—Carved in the forecourt of the Temple of Apollo at Delphi, Greece

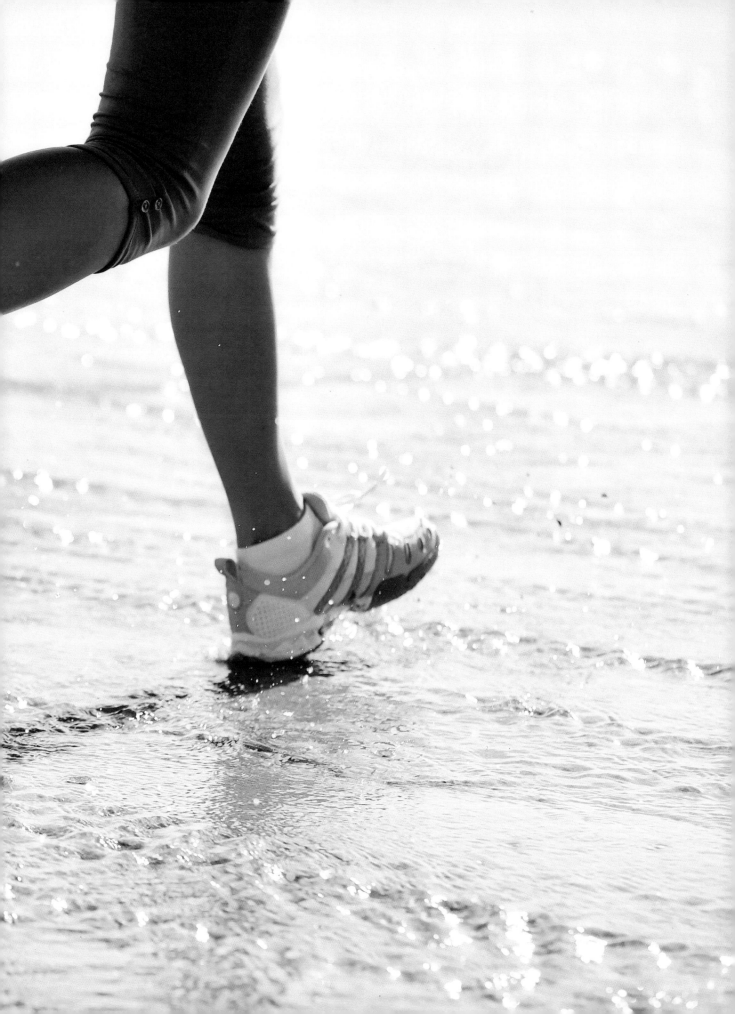

MEDITATION FOR EMOTIONAL WELLNESS

Facing and releasing negative emotions

Meditation can bring inner peace and calm when we feel overwhelmed or troubled by emotion. In the short term, meditation frees the mind of the repetitive thoughts that churn when we are in the grip of negative emotions. In the longer term, with frequent practice, meditation allows us to release negative emotions. As the mind stills, meditation may also give us greater clarity about the true causes of our troubling feelings. Different forms of meditation may be helpful for calming, managing, or releasing negative emotions:

• Guided meditation: When we are suffering from overwhelming or agitating emotions, the visualization of a relaxing place or situation will slow the breathing and heartbeat, ease repetitive thoughts, and calm the mind. You may choose to focus on a place where you have felt positive, calm emotions, such as a garden where you have felt contented and peaceful.

• Mindfulness meditation: This form of meditation teaches us to focus on the present moment, while being aware of our breathing and heartbeat. As you breathe, you will become aware of your emotions and thoughts, but allow them to flow through without judgment.

• Mantra meditation: The repetition of a calming word or phrase can be a helpful tool in anger management or to prevent jealous, resentful, or frustrated thoughts from moving toward destructive actions. Choose a mantra that suits your own emotional needs. Common mantras for moments of anger include: "I breathe in calm and breathe out anger" or simply the repetition of "Peace, peace, peace."

• Qigong: This traditional Chinese combination of meditation, breathing, and physical movement is particularly helpful when emotion is taking its toll on physical health. In qigong, it is believed that emotions can be regulated by harmonizing the body, breath, and mind, and released through movement. Rhythmic movements, related to five animals—dragon, tiger, leopard, snake, and crane—can release emotions pent up in the body, including fear, grief, anger, low self-esteem, and sadness. For help with finding a local qigong practitioner, turn to Resources on page 296.

Awakening positive emotions

The following pages offer guided meditations for awakening and nurturing positive emotions, such as forgiveness, kindness, and compassion. They also offer meditations that build resilience and fearlessness. The regular practice of such meditations can not only benefit emotional wellness, but every aspect of our lives. A research paper by Barbara Fredrickson, Michael Cohn, Kimberly Coffey, Jolynn Pek, and Sandra Finkel, published in the *Journal of Personality and Social Psychology*, examined the results of loving-kindness meditation. The researchers concluded that loving-kindness meditation not only engendered positive emotions but built personal resources, including increased purpose in life, better life satisfaction, improved social support, decreased illness symptoms, and reduced depressive symptoms.

Guided meditation: facing difficult emotions

This meditation allows us to face a troubling emotion rather than suppress it. This may be helpful for those who numb or distract themselves rather than acknowledge their feelings. Facing a difficult emotion is an essential step toward understanding and managing it.

• Sit comfortably. Breathe deeply for a few minutes, in through your nose and out through your mouth, letting your breath enter your lungs and leave your lungs, enter and fill, leave and empty. Relax any tension in your body, letting it flow from your neck, your back, your temples.

• Think of a difficult situation that you are going through, a situation that causes you to feel an emotion that embarrasses, saddens, or frightens you. Now focus on your desire to push away the emotion and to reach instead for an easy retort or whatever you customarily use to distract yourself, such as a snack, a phone, or a glass of wine.

• Turn toward your difficulty, toward the emotion that troubles you. Face your emotion. Name it if you can. You may feel your breathing and heartbeat start to speed, so focus on your breathing until it stills, inhale and exhale, fill and release. Now invite the spirit of love, compassion, and forgiveness to wrap you in its arms and hold you. You may choose to imagine a motherly figure, an earth goddess, a great bird with wide, soft wings. Let the spirit of love speak to you, with kind, calming words: "You can do this, you are strong, you are loved."

• Turn back to your emotion, name it, welcome it, then repeat the same loving statements as many times as you need. Each time you return to your emotion, it will become easier to acknowledge without the need of distraction or numbing.

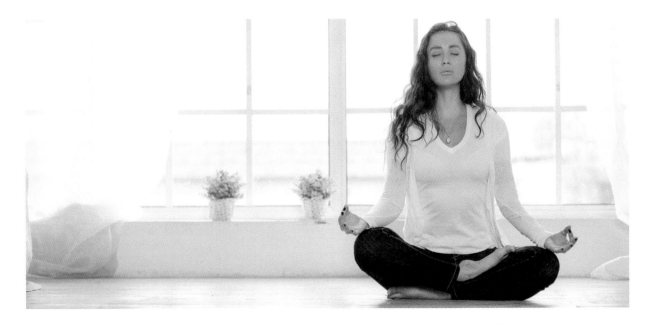

FINDING FORGIVENESS

Our hearts and minds can be tormented by storms of hatred, anger, resentment, and fear. They can equally be healed by the power of forgiveness. Our common bond as human beings is our capacity both to be hurt and to hurt others, but we also share the unique ability to forgive.

Why we need to forgive

In our life we will face difficult situations in which we may be insulted, humiliated, dismissed, or rejected. These are all painful experiences that can fester in our hearts, poisoning our capacity to trust and care, and leaching joy from our lives. We can carry these moments of pain through the whole of our lives. Fearing and resenting those who have harmed us, in truth we often think more about them than the people we love. We can expend considerable energy planning strategies of retaliation or self-protection.

We can find ourselves obsessing about experiences that have long passed, while those who have harmed us may be oblivious to the impact they have had upon us. We can live our lives in regret and bitterness,

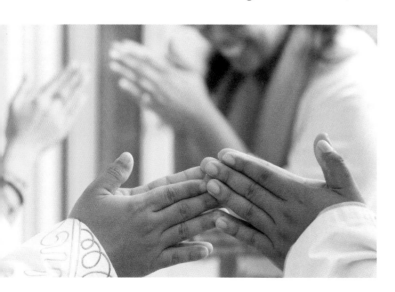

which is often to forget to live at all. A wounded heart and all the fears and apprehensions born of that hurt can seem to create an eternal prison. And though the pain may have been inflicted upon us by another, we are perhaps the only ones who can release ourselves from that prison of resentment and fear. We may also encounter times in our lives when it feels deeply difficult to forgive not only others but also ourselves. We may have harmed another person through our words, actions, unconsciousness, or insensitivity, and we sense the divide of mistrust, fear, and anger that now separates us from that person.

We cannot undo the acts that have been done, we cannot take back the words that have been spoken. So guilt, regret, and remorse become part of our lives. Storms of thought are born, beginning with the phrases "if only" and "I wish," and taking up space in our minds. Forgiveness does not condone or justify the unjust, harmful, or unacceptable. But with wise forgiveness may come the resolve never to permit any past harm to be repeated in the present or future. It is not easy to forgive, but it is less painful than continuing to carry the burden of a painful past into all the remaining moments of our lives.

So forgiveness is a way of releasing our own hearts from pain. It allows us to live a life in which we no longer carry the burdens of the past or endlessly

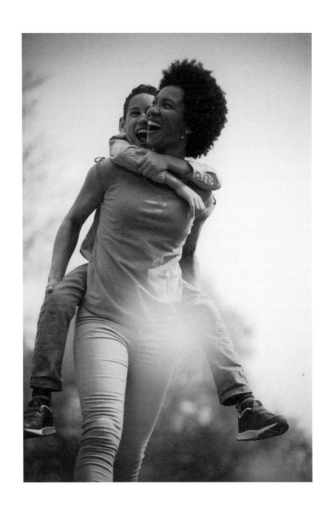

replay the past in the present. We are released into a present that is no longer defined by the past. It is here that we find peace and the capacity to live with openness and trust. Forgiveness is built upon patience, tolerance, and acceptance—qualities we extend to both ourselves and others. In doing so, we do not erase the imprints of pain from our own hearts or the hearts of others.

Forgiveness is often a long journey that asks us to meet the hurt of betrayal, loss, and anger over and over. In each of these meetings we see the choices we face—we can linger in what has gone by and suffer, or we can meet that pain with understanding, compassion, and courage, and find a heart of ease. The forgiving heart is also a free heart.

Willow infusion for forgiveness

An infusion of willow encourages a more positive and mature attitude. Do not take willow bark when pregnant or breastfeeding.

• Add 2 heaping teaspoons of dried willow bark to 2 cups of water. Simmer for 10 minutes. Strain.

• Add honey to taste, then drink.

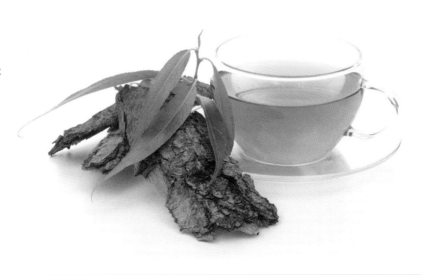

FORGIVENESS FOR OURSELVES

Forgiveness for ourselves

In our lives we can harm and abandon ourselves in countless ways—physically, emotionally, and psychologically. Through feelings of worthlessness, habit, and self-judgment we forget how to care for ourselves. For many people it is easier to care for others than to care for themselves. We need to forgive ourselves for all the harm or hurt we may have inflicted on ourselves. We must also learn to forgive ourselves for the harm we have done to others. Out of unconsciousness, fear, and anxiety we can speak, think, and act in ways that hurt others, that make others fear us.

Yet we can do what is possible to reconcile ourselves with the person we have hurt and forgive ourselves for our past insensitivity. Forgiveness for ourselves rests upon our capacity to let go of what has already gone by and find a new beginning in the present.

Guided meditation: forgiveness for ourselves

• Find a posture of calmness and ease. Let your eyes close and consciously soften all the parts of your body that feel tight or contracted.

• Let your breathing relax and find its own natural rhythm.

• Let your attention rest in the center of your chest, in the area of your heart, and just sense the life of your body in that area, cultivating a sense of calm.

• Take some moments to reflect on the ways that you may harm or hurt yourself through thought, word, or action.

• Receive with kindness the images, memories, or bodily feelings that may arise, even if they are deeply painful.

• Sense how those images, memories, or feelings belong to actions, words, and thoughts that have already passed.

• Let go of any form of self-judgment, guilt, or anxiety over what has in truth passed. Reflect on what forgiveness might mean in this moment, what it might mean to release the burden of the past and all that you regret.

• Let these phrases rest softly in your attention and your heart:
"I forgive myself."
"I forgive myself for the words, actions, or thoughts that caused harm to myself, whether intentional or unintentional."
"I forgive myself for any way that I have hurt myself through fear, pain, or confusion."

• Continue for some minutes to rest your attention in these phrases.

• Sense in your heart the possibility of letting go of the past, of learning new pathways of respect, kindness, and compassion for yourself. Memories and images laden with regret may arise. You can also allow them to pass and return to a forgiving heart.

• When you are ready, open your eyes and come out of the posture.

At times our inaction can cause as much pain as our actions.

Asking forgiveness from others

Out of confusion, fear, and pain we can hurt others both through action and inaction. In fear and anger we can strike out at another as a way of trying to protect ourselves. Lost in confusion, we don't always appreciate the hurtful impact our words or actions have on the heart of another, except in retrospect.

At times our inaction can cause as much pain as our actions. We remember the times when we failed to reach out to another in need; we recall the words of comfort we never said and the times when we turned away from a person in pain out of fear or a sense of inadequacy. Just as we need to forgive ourselves for those moments of neglect, so we can also ask forgiveness from another. Asking for forgiveness from others can be a powerful way of recommitting ourselves to sensitivity, integrity, and care in the present.

Guided meditation: asking forgiveness from others

• Let your body relax into a posture of ease and balance, and close your eyes if it enables you to focus better.

• Spend some moments focusing on your breathing. With each out-breath, sense the release of any agitation or busyness within your mind.

• Let the memories, images, and emotions arise in your heart of the times when you may have wounded, hurt, or neglected another.

• Sense the heaviness of those images and feel your own sorrow and regret.

• Silently forgive yourself, letting these phrases of forgiveness rest in your heart:
"I forgive myself."
"I forgive myself for any hurt or suffering I may have caused you by my words, actions, or thoughts."
"I forgive myself for neglecting to care for you when it was asked of me."

• Let your attention rest in the phrases for a time and then turn your attention to those whom you would ask forgiveness of. Think about anyone from the past or present you feel you have hurt, whether intentional or unintentional. Invite them into your meditation and let your attention rest in these phrases:
"For any way I have caused you pain or hurt, I ask your forgiveness."
"For any way I have neglected you, I ask your forgiveness."
"For any way I have made you fear me, I ask your forgiveness."

• As you rest your attention in the phrases, try not to become lost in the story of past pain and hurt. Come back to the present and the phrases.

• Let go of the guilt or regret as you recommit yourself to kindness and integrity in the present.

• When you are ready, open your eyes and come out of the posture.

FORGIVENESS FOR THOSE WHO HAVE HURT US

It is not easy for us to forgive those who have caused hurt or suffering to us or to others. It is not easy for us to sense the anger, fear, and confusion that drive those acts and words that can so deeply damage.

It is truly challenging to open our hearts to those whom we fear, despise, and judge for the pain they have caused. Yet forgiveness asks us to cultivate understanding; it is an invitation to intimacy rather than alienation.

A path of healing

The incidents, words, and acts that have wounded us deeply may belong to a distant past, yet they can continue to dominate our present. We can find ourselves endlessly replaying them. Forgiveness releases us from this prison of fear and anger and sets us on a path of healing. Forgiving those who cause pain is in truth a way of protecting and healing ourselves. Forgiving those who hurt us does not mean, however, that we should ever place ourselves in situations of danger or peril, nor does it mean justifying or condoning actions or words that are clearly harmful. We all need to find the courage and clarity to bring about the end of anything that violates and damages our world. We also need to find the mercy and compassion to embrace and understand those who cause pain. Then the wall of anger, hatred, and fear that can so powerfully divide us from one another can begin to melt in the light of forgiveness.

Forgiveness for those who have harmed us asks for a powerful generosity of heart. It is often helpful to begin with a case where the barriers of fear and anger do not feel so solid. We need to find deep inner resources of balance and courage to approach those who have most deeply wounded us.

Sometimes we are simply not ready to reach out with forgiveness and understanding to a person who has hurt us deeply. But we can forgive ourselves for that reluctance and fear until a time comes when we feel more inwardly healed and renewed and we are able to forgive another.

Forgiving those who have harmed us is in fact a profound act of compassion for ourselves. It allows us to move on, unburdened by fear and anger, and embrace our present wholeheartedly. In forgiveness we are releasing ourselves from the tortured world of blame, anger, and hatred. As we forgive those who cause suffering, what we are in truth forgiving are the powerful forces of confusion, ignorance, fear, and anger that can blight any of our lives.

In cultivating forgiveness we need to respect the limits of our own hearts. It may be too soon for us to forgive. We may still be too wounded to open our hearts to someone who has hurt us. At these times we can learn just to visit the places where our hearts feel most raw or painful, to acknowledge the need to heal these tender places of division and pain, and to learn the kindness and power of forgiveness for ourselves and for all those who, through ignorance and confusion, cause pain.

In cultivating forgiveness we need to respect the limits of our own hearts.

Calming and uplifting massage blend
As you reach forgiveness, this aromatherapy blend will boost your mood.

> • Add 4 drops of rose essential oil, 2 drops of frankincense oil, and 4 drops of chamomile oil to 3 teaspoons of sweet almond or grapeseed oil.

This blend encourages positivity, acceptance of others, and joyfulness.

Do not use rose essential oil during the first three months of pregnancy and not at all if there is a history of miscarriage.

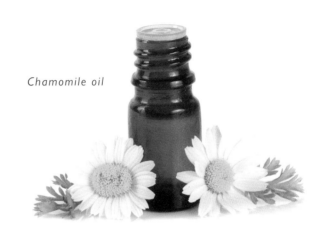

Chamomile oil

Guided meditation: forgiveness for those who have caused pain

• Find a position for your body that is relaxed and free from tension and gently close your eyes. Bring your attention into your body, consciously softening any places that feel tight or contracted.

• Pay particular attention to your face and jaw, your neck, shoulders, and hands, letting them relax fully.

• Bring a gentle and calm attention to rest in your chest, in your heart area.

• Invite into your attention someone who has hurt you, whether in small or deep ways.

• Hold that person in your attention and sense the array of images and emotions that arise, without judging any of them. Let them rest in your heart and mind without grasping hold of any of them.

• Sense the ways in which you have felt harmed or abandoned, intentionally or unintentionally, by that person. Feel the pain you carry with you from this past and sense that it may be time to lay down this burden.

• Holding the difficult person in your attention, gently begin to offer the intention of forgiveness with the phrases:
"I forgive you for the pain you have caused."
"I forgive the anger, confusion, and ignorance at the heart of your harmfulness."
"To you who have hurt me, I offer forgiveness."

• As you rest your attention in the phrases and intentions of forgiveness, sense whether even the tiniest glimmers of release or opening may be possible.

• Sense the new beginnings that may be possible for you as you release the weight of the past.

• You may find it difficult to stay connected with the image or memory of someone who has hurt you deeply. If this happens, just return your attention to your body and breathing. Let your body relax and soften, and when you are ready, come back to the phrases, again offering forgiveness.

• When you are ready, open your eyes.

FINDING INNER PEACE

Peace is not the absence of challenge or difficulty, but the release of judgment and fear. It begins in our own hearts, minds, and lives. We cannot control or govern the hearts and minds of another, but we can reclaim our own capacity to be at peace with all things, including ourselves. Learning to make peace with ourselves is the first step in understanding what it means to be at peace with all things. It is not difficult for us to see that our relationships with other people frequently mirror the kind of relationship we have with our own bodies, minds, and hearts.

Making peace with ourselves and others

Peace in our lives is not separate from our capacity to make peace with ourselves. Serenity in our lives rests upon our capacity to make peace with the inner struggles that devastate the calmness of our own hearts and minds. Peacemaking begins with our capacity to release ourselves from the conflicts and struggles we carry in our relationship to ourselves.

If we are prone to be judgmental or dismissive of others, it may be worthwhile to explore the ways in which we are judgmental or dismissive of ourselves. The impatience, frustration, expectancy, or blame that may sabotage our relationships with all those who are part of our lives will likely have their roots in the ways in which we relate to our own inner world.

If we wish to nurture relationships of kindness, understanding, and intimacy in our lives, it may be important to acknowledge that our relationship with ourselves is the classroom in which we learn the arts of generosity, tolerance, care, and tenderness. Wherever we go in this life, whether alone or with others, we can never divorce ourselves from our own hearts and minds. Our longings for intimacy, oneness, and friendship with others rest upon our capacity to cross the abyss of distance and fear that can separate us from ourselves.

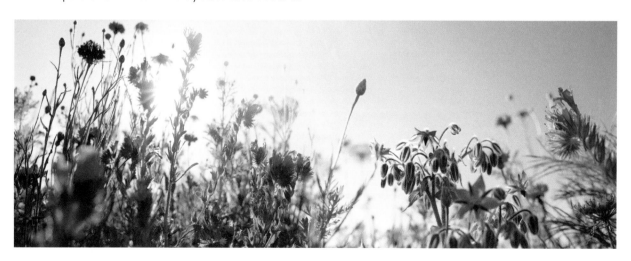

Our relationship with ourselves is the classroom in which we learn the arts of generosity, tolerance, care, and tenderness.

Guided meditation: inner peace

• Settle into a posture that is as relaxed and alert as possible, and gently close your eyes.

• Take a few moments to be aware of your body, releasing any areas of tension.

• For a few moments, focus your attention on your breathing. Be particularly aware of your out-breath, following it with your attention until the very end of the breath.

• Rest your attention in the brief moment between the ending of an out-breath and the beginning of the next in-breath.

• Take a few moments to reflect on where you most repetitively battle with yourself. Sense the places you are most judgmental of yourself, the places where you extend to yourself the greatest unkindness or blame, the places that trigger feelings of shame or self-consciousness.

• You may be aware of carrying events or acts from the past in your heart and mind that are laden with guilt or regret. You may be aware of recurring patterns in your present, in speech, thought, or action, that cause pain or alienation and that you wish to be free from.

• As you reflect on these patterns or events, sense what happens in your body and mind.

• Sense how simply bringing these places of pain into your attention may trigger feelings of contraction, tension, or resistance in your body. You may be aware of the rhythm of your breathing changing, becoming shorter or tighter. If this happens, bring your attention to the part of your body that is registering distress or discomfort and let it soften and relax.

• Sense the aversion you have for these places in your own heart and mind. Sense your wish to be free from them. Be aware of how the aversion and resistance themselves are the energy of struggle and inner estrangement.

• Reflect on what you may need to cultivate or nurture to make peace with yourself.

• Reflect on what difference it would make to those places of rejection and alienation to cultivate a greater kindness, acceptance, or compassion.

• Can you offer to yourself the forgiveness and generosity of heart to embrace the places of greatest difficulty and unease in your own heart and mind? Are you able to stay present with those places in yourself that you are most tempted to flee from? Reflect on what it might mean to befriend yourself, to offer to yourself the openness and understanding you would both wish to offer to others and to receive from others.

• Sense that your capacity to make peace with yourself may not depend upon denying anything.

• With a wholehearted and gentle attentiveness, explore those places in your heart and mind that are the source of the greatest struggle and pain.

• Sense how it may be possible to bring calmness, gentleness, and care to those places without any expectation.

• When you are ready, open your eyes and come out of the posture.

BUILDING EMOTIONAL RESILIENCE

The phrase "emotional resilience" refers to how you cope with and adapt to stressful or negative situations. If you have strong emotional resilience, you're likely to be able to cope easily, adapt to the changes that the situation brings, and sail on with your life. But if you have a low level of emotional resilience, you're likely to find life a lot harder, perhaps taking things to heart and finding the situation difficult to move on from.

Cultivating emotional resilience

Levels of emotional resilience can change over time and be affected by the situations you've experienced and the circumstances you've found yourself in. If someone has a higher level of emotional resilience than you, it doesn't make them any better than you, it just means you deal with things differently.

The good news is that you can learn how to boost your emotional resilience, so you're better placed to deal with unexpected situations or sudden changes. To do so, you need to identify how you tend to react to things now, then focus on ways in which you could change this response to be more positive or keep things in perspective, rather than succumbing to being anxious.

Jasmine massage for inner strength

• Add 4 drops of jasmine oil, 4 drops of clary sage, and 2 drops of lavender oil to 5 teaspoons of sweet almond oil.

• Start the massage by sliding your hands from your hips across your abdomen in a clockwise direction, sliding one hand after the other.

• Move gently over your chest.

• Stroke your hands up and around your hips, and around to the small of your back. Repeat.

Cultivating fearlessness

Fear is one of the most debilitating and paralyzing emotions in our lives. It is often the root of a wide spectrum of other emotions.

Cultivating fearlessness does not presume that fear will never arise in our hearts and lives. Fearlessness is not living without fear, but turning directly toward the fears and anxieties that do arise. When we are willing to do this, we learn that it is possible to embrace fear with a gentle and loving attention rather than being governed by it.

Flower essences for fear

• Mimulus may help with the everyday fears of known things, such as spiders or flying.

• Aspen is for those vague, unknown, dark fears that hover and play on the imagination.

• Rock rose should be added when the fear is turning into terror and perhaps even panic.

• Cherry plum is for the fear that everything will fall apart.

• Red chestnut is for fear for another's safety.

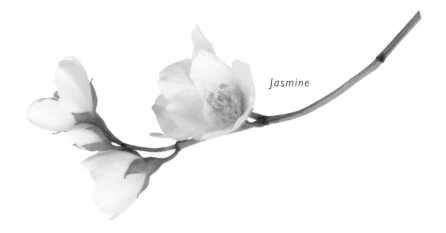

Jasmine

Guided meditation: exploring fear

• Sit comfortably and allow your body to relax fully. Bring a gentle attention to any places in your body where there is tightness or discomfort. Gently and consciously soften those areas, allowing your whole body to relax.

• Close your eyes and for a few moments pay attention to your breathing. Give particular attention to your outgoing breath. With each out-breath, relax more deeply, and consciously release any of the turmoil or busyness in your mind. Follow each out-breath with your attention until its very end.

• When you feel calmer, consciously invite into your attention and heart something that makes you afraid. Initially, don't focus upon anything you feel terrified or overwhelmed by, but upon a dimension of your life that you may habitually flinch from or avoid. It might be a fear of speaking honestly, a difficult person who is part of your life, making changes, or relationships you tend to turn away from.

• Let yourself feel the fear that arises in the face of the object, situation, or event you resist or feel anxious about.

• Sense where the fear is in your body and explore that with your attention. Cultivate a curious attention, sensing how the feelings change and move. Allow yourself to rest within those sensations. If they become overwhelming, come back to your breathing for a few moments, connect deeply with each out-breath, and allow your mind and body to calm once more.

• As you invite the object or situation of anxiety into your attention, be aware of the different emotions, memories, or images that arise. Let them rest in your attention without trying to get rid of them or becoming lost within them. They may be uncomfortable, but you may also begin to sense that they are not intrinsically threatening.

• Sense that fear and all its associated images and reactions may be uncomfortable yet in itself need not be threatening or overwhelming.

• Move your attention back and forth between the fear and your breathing, cultivating a calm steadiness moment to moment.

• Sense the way that avoidance deepens and perpetuates fear. Sense, too, how fear diminishes in the light of calm attention.

• Throughout the meditation, continue to check in with your body, relaxing and softening any tightness or tension that appears.

• When you are ready, open your eyes and come out of the posture.

Check in with your body, relaxing and softening any tightness or tension that appears.

LETTING GO

Life continues to teach us the direct relationship between peace and our willingness to let go. No matter how tightly or fearfully we hold on to something, inwardly and outwardly, it will change and we will be asked to let it go. The art of being able to let go fully and freely in every moment of our lives is the art of finding balance and serenity. Fear makes us hold tightly to countless things in our lives; trust and understanding teach us how to let go.

How to let go

Learning to let go will never be born of willpower, forcing, or striving. Commanding ourselves to let go will only set up new standards and judgments of success and failure that harm our well-being.

Letting go is born of calmness, compassion, and understanding. These are qualities we cultivate moment to moment in our meditation practice and our lives. Each day of our lives invites us to let go in countless moments and encounters. We learn to let go not in order to make ourselves suffer, feel deprived, or bereft, but to bring about an end to suffering, to feelings of deprivation and fear. Letting go is the art of happiness and contentment. Finding a greater simplicity in our lives has the inevitable companion of learning to let go.

As we become increasingly sensitive to our inner life we begin to see the ways in which we are imprisoned by whatever it is we are clinging to most tightly. The times when we feel least free, connected, and open in our lives are when we are desperately trying to make life conform to our wishes and expectations. At these times we are lost in identification and holding. The times of greatest freedom are when we can embrace each moment, person, and encounter in our lives just as it is, free of demand and expectation.

Meditation practice invites us to bring a wholehearted attention to all the places where we struggle and suffer most deeply. We often discover that these are the places where we are holding on most tightly. Opinions, expectations, roles, identities, fears, objects, goals, and desires are all fertile ground for holding and clinging, so become the places of greatest distress in our lives. Yet it is in the places where we hold on most fiercely that we can also discover the greatest freedom as we learn to loosen the hold of clinging.

It is not always difficult for us to see the places in our lives that are inviting us to learn to let go, but there are many ways in which we learn to let go freely and completely. When our mind is calm and attentive, letting go is often effortless and easeful. And the more we are able to let go, the more generosity, compassion, simplicity, and freedom we discover in our lives.

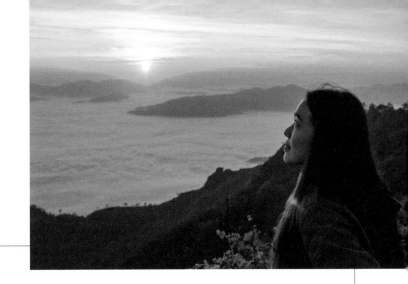

Guided meditation: letting go

• Let your body relax into an alert and upright meditative posture, and gently close your eyes.

• Focus your attention for some moments on your breathing, consciously following each out-breath with your attention until its very ending.

• Sense the letting go within your breathing—letting go of preoccupation, busyness, and turmoil.

• Settle into calmness and simplicity, being fully present in just this moment.

• When you find yourself present and calm in your breathing, open your attention and invite into it the most recent memory of a moment, an event, or conversation that was burdened by struggle, anxiety, or resistance. Hold that memory or image gently and calmly in your attention, without being tempted to justify, condemn, or explain it. Ask yourself what it is you may be being asked to let go of to find greater ease, peace, and simplicity. Is it expectation, judgment, fear, anger?

• Hold the question gently in your attention and sense the response that may intuitively arise from your heart.

• If you find yourself becoming lost in the story, return your attention to your breathing for a few moments, releasing each out-breath fully, until once more you find yourself calm and relaxed.

• You might invite into your attention another recent time when you have been embroiled in confusion, argument, or discord with another person. Again, hold that image or moment simply in your attention.

• What are you being asked to let go of, to release to bring the disharmony or argument to an end?

• Sense how you may walk down familiar pathways of judgment, blame, or self-hatred. Is it possible to bring some wise restraint to those pathways, to walk new pathways of compassion, tenderness, and loving kindness?

• Whenever your attention gets caught in a memory or story, return to be aware of your breathing. Sense that your willingness to come back to your breath, to be fully present in just one breath and one moment at a time, is in itself a way of letting go. It is releasing the story and the sense of imprisonment.

• Hold lightly in your attention the question: "What can I let go of to find greater simplicity, peace, and freedom in my life?" Allow an intuitive response to emerge, sensing the spaciousness born of being able to let go.

• When you are ready, open your eyes and come out of the meditation.

When our mind is calm and attentive, letting go is often effortless and easeful.

COPING WITH CHANGE

Some changes are positive, such as a promotion or a new baby, but others—such as job loss or divorce—can feel painful. Even positive changes can disturb our equilibrium, leaving us feeling unmoored. The most difficult changes to adjust to are those that are out of our control, those that are sudden and unexpected. We may resist the change by refusing to cooperate with it, but in the end learning to cope with the change will be the better route to take for the sake of our emotional wellness.

Accepting change

When faced with change, some of us cope by escaping and some by controlling. Escape coping is rooted in avoidance of acknowledging the change. We may ignore warnings that our job is at risk or simply numb ourselves with alcohol, social media, food, or whatever calms us in the short term. In contrast, control coping is about acknowledging the change and the feelings that it engenders. It is about finding strategies to move along with the change, positively and proactively. When challenged by change, most of us swing between these two modes, escaping and controlling. By moving toward the latter, making ourselves a participant in change rather than a victim, we can reestablish emotional peace.

When confronted by change, we may experience shock, anger, fear, or even grief. If we allow ourselves to accept and examine those emotions, they can be managed. Suppressing emotions such as fear and anxiety will not quell them, but can impact our mental and physical health, resulting in insomnia, irritability, angry outbursts, and—over time— lowered resistance to infection.

As soon as we come to terms with the new reality, we can move forward. We can help ourselves through this process of acceptance by examining what the change truly means for us and seeking out reliable information and support. It may be helpful to write out a mission statement, with goals and an action plan for reaching them. Ensure that your goals are achievable through small, incremental steps.

Key crystals

LEPIDOLITE—hold or wear lepidolite to help you cope with changes in your life. This crystal helps us to accept what is beyond our control, then to adapt.

DANBURITE—place on the heart chakra to heal fears and help you come to terms with changes. The energies of this crystal are calming and reassuring.

As soon as we come to terms with the new reality, we can move forward.

Guided meditation: embracing change

• Sit comfortably. Note any places in your neck, your back, your temples, your hands, where there is tension. Relax those areas, allowing tightness to ease and flow from your body.

• Close your eyes and pay attention to your breathing. With each outgoing breath, release the anxiety and churning of your mind. As you inhale, take in calmness from the air, and strength from the forests and mountains across our beautiful planet.

• When you feel calm, think of the change that you are facing. Let yourself feel the fear, the sadness, the stress that well up in the face of this change. Note the thoughts and worries that flow through your mind. Let these emotions and thoughts rest in your attention without trying to get rid of them or becoming lost in them. Although these feelings and ideas are uncomfortable, they cannot do you harm.

• Move your attention back and forth between thoughts about the change and your calm, steady, strong breathing. Relax any tightness in your body.

• Sense the way that avoidance of change perpetuates fear and sadness. Note how these emotions shrink and fade in the face of calm, steadfast attention.

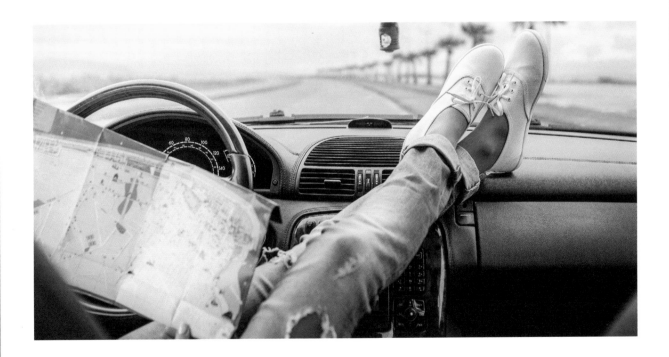

BUILDING SELF-CONFIDENCE

There are two types of self-confidence: true self-confidence and relative self-confidence. Relative self-confidence is based on comparing ourselves with others. Boosting relative self-confidence is achieved easily by reminding ourselves of our achievements, intelligence, or good looks. However, such a boost can never be unconditional or long-lasting. True self-confidence is based on acceptance of one's own worth. It is centered on a connection with our own goodness.

Understanding self-confidence

Low self-confidence may be based in low self-esteem. This may have its roots in childhood, when you received the message that you were not good enough. Many life events—including bereavement, job loss, and even childbirth—can also lower our belief in ourself.

Visiting a cognitive behavioral therapist can be the first step to boosting true self-confidence. A therapist may suggest some of the following exercises:

• Identify situations and relationships that you find hard to face or that habitually dent your self-confidence. These may include a challenging relationship with a partner, parent, or coworker. A common trigger is a major life change. Many people find their self-confidence challenged by activities such as public speaking or meeting new people.

• Notice the thoughts and assumptions that run through your head when you face these situations. These may include believing you are not good enough, putting yourself down, focusing on negatives, and believing in failure as a certainty. You may find it helpful to write down these thoughts in a journal. Ask yourself when you first started to believe these things.

• Replace these negative thought processes and assumptions with positive ones. These may include believing that you are more than good enough, giving yourself credit for achievements and changes, focusing on the positives, forgiving yourself for mistakes, and being hopeful of success.

• Returning to your journal, write down some positive facts about yourself and your true worth. These may be facts like: "I am kind to my friends," "I notice when other people are unhappy," or "I try to be generous."

• When you feel ready, set yourself a challenge to do something that, in the past, would have made you anxious. This need not mean giving a speech in front of a thousand-strong crowd or taking a vacation on your own, but perhaps try joining a new class or speaking up during a work meeting.

Replace these negative thought processes and assumptions with positive ones.

Key crystals

Black, brown, and gray crystals offer inner strength, self-acceptance, and self-confidence. They find resonance at the earth and root chakras, where they bring both grounding and comfort.

ANDRADITE—when entering a challenging social situation, wear andradite close to the body for the self-confidence to build new bonds.

SMOKY QUARTZ—meditate with smoky quartz for help with accepting yourself as you truly are, both physically and mentally.

BROWN ZIRCON—zircon jewelry is useful for anyone who is struggling with low self-worth and negative body image.

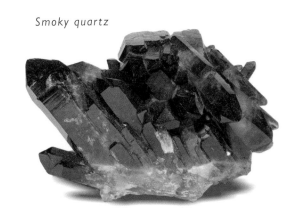

Smoky quartz

Guided meditation: boosting self-confidence

• Sit comfortably and close your eyes. Focus your mind on your breathing as you inhale and exhale. Relax your neck, shoulders, arms, and hands. Let the breath fill your lungs, then flow out into the air.

• Feel the beating of your strong, good, brave heart. Sense the flow of blood and strength through your body, down your arms and legs, to every finger and toe.

• When you feel calm, allow yourself to think of a situation when you feel small, alone, or frightened. Allow yourself to note all the emotions and thoughts that race through your mind. You may feel your breathing and heartbeat begin to

speed. Gently refocus your mind on your breathing. Feel your heart pumping strength around your body. When you feel ready, return to the situation that troubles you. Know that the situation cannot reverse the beating of your heart and the flow of goodness through every part of your body.

• Repeat to yourself: "I am good, I am strong, I am worthy." Feel the words flowing through your body as your heart beats with strength and love. Know that you are strong.

• When you are ready, take a deep breath and let it go.

EMBRACING KINDNESS AND COMPASSION

Loving kindness embraces the qualities of acceptance, generosity, friendliness, and warmth we long to receive from others. It describes an unconditional warmth and care that we are able to extend to all those who are part of our lives—those we cherish and love, those we are indifferent to, those we feel most separate from, and our own selves. Cultivating loving kindness, we discover that the walls of mistrust and fear that can so painfully separate us from others can also begin to crumble. In developing our own capacities for fearlessness, tenderness, and benevolence, our lives are lived with greater ease and connectedness. The small gestures of love we receive from others nurture and heal us, while the gestures and words of love and kindness we are able to offer to others bring depth and intimacy to all of our relationships. Loving kindness awakens and gladdens our hearts.

Kindness is liberating

We all know the power that ill will, anger, and fear have to damage and scar our lives and our world. Individuals, communities, and nations are divided by mistrust, fear, and rage. Our whole world cries out for greater generosity, tenderness, and love. Its divisions and conflicts will not be healed by yet more formulas, prescriptions, and strategies, but through a radical change in each of our hearts. We share with all living beings the longing to be happy and free from pain and fear. We share with all living beings the yearning to be accepted, loved, and cared for. In the face of anger our tendency is to withdraw, close down, or disconnect from the person before us. Gripped by the rage or hurt present in our own hearts, we are prone to strike out, to harm another, or exile them from our lives. The division, mistrust, and alienation that follow scar our lives and relationships.

Our own anger and fear will lead us to commit countless acts that are born of unconsciousness and reactivity and lead to sorrow and alienation. Loving kindness meditation teaches us how to find a refuge of calm openness within our own hearts. It is a refuge that protects us from fear, anger, and turmoil. With loving kindness meditation we learn to remember, honor, and cultivate the capacity each of us has to touch our world with warmth and friendliness.

We nurture a sanctuary of balance and strength within ourselves that allows us to turn toward pain and adversity and heal division. In loving kindness meditation we cultivate, again and again, the intention to embrace all moments with generosity and warmth.

Yet loving kindness is not sentimentality, or even a particular kind of feeling. Simply in each moment we nurture our capacity for intimacy and understanding. Loving kindness meditation is a practice of happiness.

Loving kindness meditation is a practice of happiness.

Guided meditation: loving kindness for a friend

• Relax into a calm and upright posture, closing your eyes gently.

• Bring your attention to rest in the center of your chest, in the area of your heart. Be aware of your body expanding and relaxing with each breath.

• Begin your meditation by extending a genuine sense of loving kindness toward yourself, letting your attention rest easily within each phrase:
"May I be free from fear and danger."
"May I be happy."
"May I be peaceful."

• When you are ready, invite into your heart and your attention someone who is dear to you, a friend you treasure.

• Again, if possible, visualize their face or remember a contact you have had with them. As you bring them into your attention, sense the qualities of the friendship that bonds you with that person—the trust, acceptance, tenderness, and love that you cherish.

• As far as possible, sustain the connection, offering to that person your heartfelt wishes for their well-being:
"May you be free from fear and danger."
"May you be happy."
"May you be peaceful."

• Continue to rest your attention in the phrases, extending loving kindness, warmth, and care.

• If you wish, you can alternate your attention between your friend and yourself, sensing your mutual wish to be free from pain and to be happy.

• Stay present with the phrases of intention, aware of the warmth, tenderness, and happiness that can begin to emerge in your heart and mind. Let them pervade the whole of your body and mind.

• If your attention wanders, come gently back to the phrases, nurturing your capacity for profound loving kindness and sensitivity.

• When you are ready, open your eyes and sense the calmness and happiness that might continue to pervade your body and mind.

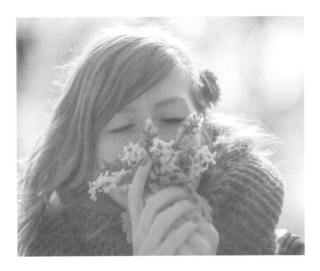

KINDNESS FOR YOURSELF

Traditionally, loving kindness begins with ourselves. We learn to offer an unconditional warmth, acceptance, and tenderness to our own bodies, minds, and hearts. Many people find it easier to extend love and care to others than to receive it or to offer that same generosity of heart to themselves.

Love yourself

Historical feelings of worthlessness or inadequacy at times make us feel we are undeserving of love and tenderness. By meditating on loving kindness we can heal those historical wounds that impair our capacity to offer to ourselves the boundless generosity, acceptance, and tenderness that make our hearts sing. In learning to extend loving kindness to ourselves we discover the freedom of heart born of letting go of painful judgments, expectations, and demands.

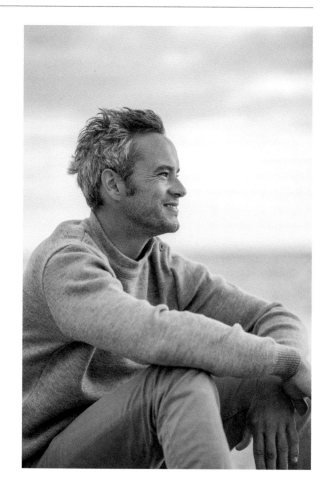

Cultivating loving kindness for ourselves is also the training ground for learning the lessons of the patience, attentiveness, tolerance, and warmth that we would wish to pervade all of our relationships. Classically, loving kindness is developed through establishing our attention using a few simple phrases that embody the intentions for the happiness and well-being we treasure. The phrases remind us of the possibility of making our inner home in a place of fearlessness, warmth, and balance instead of one of confusion or ill will. The practice is not a mechanical repetition of empty words, but a genuine offering of kindness and love in each moment. Loving kindness meditation can be developed in a dedicated posture and time; it can also be cultivated in all the moments and circumstances of our lives that ask for healing and connectedness and invite us to nurture a loving heart.

Many people find it easier to extend love and care to others than to receive it.

Guided meditation: loving kindness for oneself

• Find a position that is relaxed and comfortable. You can develop this practice in any posture, though you may find that sitting upright helps you to be more alert and attentive.

• Let your eyes close and take some moments to consciously relax your body, softening any areas of holding or tension.

• For a few minutes focus a gentle, alert attentiveness on your breathing, letting your mind and body calm with each out-breath. Bring your attention to rest in the center of your chest, in the area of your heart.

• Silently repeat the simple phrases of loving kindness, sensing the meaning of each one:
"May I be free from fear and danger."
"May I be happy."
"May I be peaceful."

• Let each phrase rest gently in your heart and mind, taking care not to hurry the words, simply offering to yourself your heartfelt wishes for your well-being and happiness.

• Don't expect that any particular feeling will arise. Simply allow the phrases and their meaning to fill your heart and mind.

• If you wish, you can alter the words so that you are using phrases that have a personal meaning for you.

• Expand your attention to be aware of your body, sensing all the pain and well-being your body can experience in this life. Youth, aging, health, illness, birth, and death are held within all of our bodies. Holding your body in your awareness, continue to rest your attention in the phrases:
"May I be free from fear and danger."

"May I be happy."
"May I be peaceful."

• Expand your awareness to sense the life of your mind, with the spectrum of experiences it can undergo—confusion, calm, agitation, serenity, contractedness, spaciousness, busyness, and stillness. With loving kindness befriending your mind, gently repeat the phrases:
"May I be free from fear and danger."
"May I be happy."
"May I be peaceful."

• Expand your awareness further to embrace the life of your heart, sensing all the joy and sorrow that can live there. Anger, love, fear, trust, anxiety, and happiness touch all of our lives. We can learn to befriend them all without exception; we can learn to embrace the world of our emotions without fear.

• Continue to rest your attention in the phrases. It is not unusual in this practice for buried feelings of confusion, pain, or anger to arise. Do not try to banish them; simply touch them with the intention to welcome them, accept them, and befriend them.

• Stay with the phrases for as long as you wish. If they become an empty repetition of words, let them go for a few moments and reflect upon what it is that brings meaning, richness, and depth to your life, and upon all the qualities of heart you long to bring to fruition. Then, on the foundation of that reflection, return your attention to rest in the area of your heart and begin once more to offer the phrases of intention to yourself.

• When you are ready, open your eyes and come out of your posture.

KINDNESS IN THE MIDST OF INDIFFERENCE

The people we love and the people we despise both evoke powerful emotional responses in us. Yet as we move through our lives and our days, we are surrounded by countless beings with whom we share no common story or history. We walk down a crowded street, sit on a train, or stand in line in a store, and all around us are those who, like us, long to be happy and free from pain. Yet we often feel neutral toward these people; we feel separate and apart from them. We easily sink into feeling indifferent toward them. They become invisible to us.

Universal kindness

Indifference is the first building block of passivity and disconnection. A homeless man once said that the greatest curse of homelessness was not the obvious lack of a home or security—it was that most people would not look him in the eye. No matter our history, identity, race, or circumstances, we are all connected in our longing for happiness, intimacy, safety, and peace.

No one wants to suffer. All of us wish to be happy. Loving kindness meditation roots itself in the mutuality of these longings—it is where we are all connected. Loving kindness meditation can bring a renewed depth to our relationships of care and intimacy. It can heal the wounds of fractured and painful relationships. On a deeper level it can awaken our hearts so that no one is dismissed or felt to be separate from ourselves. Cultivating loving kindness, we learn to embrace everyone who comes into our life with respect, sensitivity, and friendliness.

In focusing loving kindness upon a neutral person, we learn to cultivate an unconditional friendliness that has no expectation of anything in return. We are nurturing a profound inner generosity that can freely offer warmth and care without investment in result or preference. We discover that our capacity to bring caring attention to all the people we encounter in our lives lifts our hearts and we form bonds of connection and care that are rooted in sensitivity and generosity.

It is a fascinating exploration to go into each day of our life with the intention to receive each person we meet with unconditional warmth and friendliness. Cultivating the intention to ignore no one, to dismiss no one, awakens our hearts and brings only joy. When our words and actions are born of loving attention, our hearts become saturated with friendliness. There are countless opportunities for us to experiment with cultivating loving kindness for the neutral person, and a single word or gesture of care and friendliness can transform our day. Indifference turns to affection, distance turns to warmth, and separation turns to connection. Cultivating loving kindness is learning to smile upon our world.

Loving kindness meditation can be cultivated and deepened in formal meditation practice; it can also be nurtured in all the moments of our lives. Experiment with this practice in the situations and circumstances where you feel the most separate and isolated from others. Sense the feeling of vitality it brings.

Cultivating loving kindness, we learn to embrace everyone who comes into our life with respect, sensitivity, and friendliness.

Guided meditation: kindness in the midst of indifference

• Settle your body into a posture of alertness and ease.

• Gently close your eyes and rest your attention in the center of your chest, in the area of your heart. Bring a sensitive attention to your breathing. Be aware of your body expanding and relaxing with each breath.

• With each out-breath, consciously release anything that is preoccupying your mind—thoughts of the past, the future, and anything you are anxious about in the present.

• Begin your meditation by inviting into your attention a person you feel affection and tenderness for—a good friend or loved one. Visualize their face or remember your last contact with them. Offer to that person your heartfelt wishes for their well-being with the same phrases you previously used:
"May you be free from fear and danger."
"May you be happy."
"May you be peaceful."

• Sense the warmth and friendliness that may arise. Continue for some minutes to rest your attention in the phrases of intention. Now expand your attention and bring to mind a person you feel quite neutral toward. It may be someone you work with, the teller in your bank, the driver of your bus, a person in your neighborhood you frequently pass yet do not know. If possible, remember their face or the last time you encountered them.

• Begin to offer to them the same warmth and friendliness you feel for the person you are most affectionate toward, using the phrases:
"May you be free from fear and danger."
"May you be happy."
"May you be peaceful."

• Sustain your connection with the neutral person for as long as you are able, with your attention steadily rooted in the phrases of intention. Don't anticipate the arising of any particular emotional responses.

• If your attention begins to waver, return your focus to the person you feel closer to for a time. When you are ready once more, switch back to the neutral person, remembering the phrases:
"May you be free from fear and danger."
"May you be happy."
"May you be peaceful."

• Sense whether it is possible for you to offer the same depth of warmth and care to the neutral person as to the person who is dear to you.

• When you are ready, open your eyes and come out of the posture.

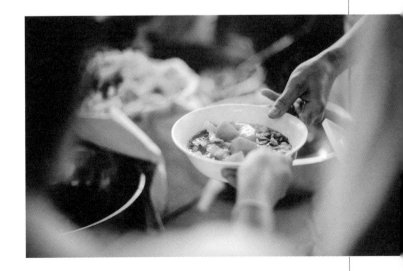

KINDNESS IN THE FACE OF DIFFICULTY AND FEAR

The greatest challenge we face in our lives is learning to be present and receptive to those we fear or dislike. Yet the most direct way to transformation is to turn toward the moments and people in our lives we resist most strongly.

Healing forgiveness

When we are hurt by or afraid of another person, our tendency is to strike out in anger or to disconnect through fear. But it is not difficult for us to see that anger is not healed by anger, and that ever-deepening division and conflict are the children of fear.

We think a lot about the people we dislike and fear in our lives. They can govern our hearts and minds. Cultivating loving kindness for these people does not mean trying to force an artificial affection or tenderness. We do, however, discover that our capacity to turn toward the people from whom we habitually recoil begins to loosen the grip of aversion and fear. We may, through loving kindness meditation, begin to find a way to calm the turmoil and anxiety in our own hearts and minds.

We may begin to discover the possibility of greater forgiveness, tolerance, and patience.

The difficult person sometimes lives within our own hearts and minds in our relationship to ourselves. We see inner tendencies of judgment, harshness, blame, or anger that damage our well-being and impair our capacity to live with happiness and peace. We can learn to approach those areas of inner struggle with care and sensitivity and heal that inner division. As you approach dimensions of your life where there is estrangement and struggle, whether inner or outer, take care not to expect some immediate transformation or inner emotional shift. Be patient—it is enough to find the willingness to embrace with kind attention any area of your life that has previously been banished from your heart.

Take care not to expect some immediate transformation or inner emotional shift.

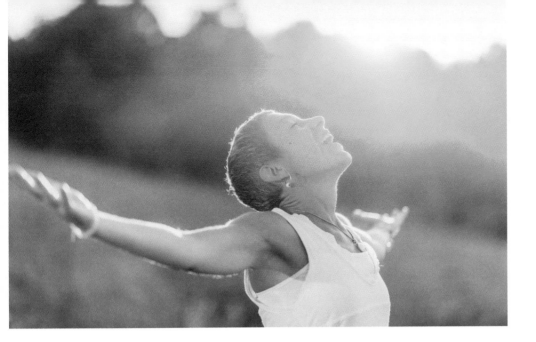

Guided meditation: loving kindness in the face of difficulty and fear

• Find a posture for your body that is as relaxed and tension-free as possible.

• Gently close your eyes and bring your attention once more to rest in the center of your chest.

• Remain present with your breathing for a few moments to let your mind and body settle in the present.

• Begin to offer the phrases and intentions of loving kindness first to yourself:
"May I be free from fear and danger."
"May I be happy."
"May I be peaceful."

• Extend your attention and invite into your heart and mind the image or awareness of someone you have had difficulty with. Let them rest in the center of your attention.

• Offer them a genuine wish for their well-being and peace:
"May you too be free from fear and danger."
"May you too be happy."
"May you too be peaceful."

• If it is difficult to stay connected, bring your attention once more back to yourself for a time and then open again to the difficult person, using whatever phrases have meaning for you.

• You may wish to focus your phrases and intentions upon parts of your own emotional or psychological being that bring pain or harm to yourself.

• Find just a few phrases that embody your wish for healing and peace:
"May I find acceptance."
"May I find peace."
"May I find healing."

• After some time you may want to expand your attention to embrace all beings in our world—the people you are close to, those you struggle with, and those you feel indifferent toward.

• Open your attention even further to include all those in the world you don't know, all the animals and creatures on the earth, in the seas and in the sky:
"May all beings be free from fear and danger."
"May all beings be happy."
"May all beings be peaceful."

• Let your attention rest for a time in that open, warm attentiveness.

• When you are ready, open your eyes and come out of the posture.

COMPASSION FOR BLAMELESS SORROWS

Sorrow, loss, and pain will be part of all of our lives, and at some time we will all meet people in the midst of great physical, emotional, or mental pain and distress—a child with a terminal illness, a friend grieving a loss, a person whose world has been shattered by violence. We see, too, endless images of people caught in famine or desolation, or brutalized by wars they do not even understand. There is suffering in this world that is blameless, and compassion is the response.

The power of compassion

Faced with situations of severe distress, our first response is often to feel stunned. We desperately search to find the "right" words or actions, yet often feel they are inadequate. Confronted with great pain and our own feelings of helplessness, we may be tempted to withdraw to protect ourselves.

Alternatively, we may be tempted to throw ourselves into a frenzy of busyness, searching for solutions that can fix the suffering we see before us. Yet there is not always a solution for a broken heart, an illness, or unexpected losses.

Compassion asks us to be still in the face of immeasurable pain, not to blame or judge, or try to control or fix. Blame and judgment can be mechanisms we use to console ourselves in our own despair and helplessness. The heart of compassion is willing to surrender both numbness and the desperate desire to try to control the world. With compassion we can learn to open to pain and in so doing find a deep inner steadiness that can embrace the anguish we face. We can find the empathy within ourselves to dissolve the separation between ourselves and another. We can discover a way of being awake and receptive in the face of pain without being shattered or overwhelmed.

Sometimes anguish feels bottomless. Compassion, too, can be bottomless. Our world and all those in it who live on a daily diet of deprivation, fear, and pain cry out for compassion. We do not need to hold grandiose thoughts of healing the world—we would break beneath the weight of that expectation—but we can commit to opening our hearts to the moments in each of our days when we meet sorrow and pain, whether in ourselves or in another. All of us have experienced times in our lives when compassion is our immediate and natural response to suffering. At such times the walls of distance melt and we see ourselves in the eyes and life of another person.

These are powerful moments of connection and healing. Compassion meditation encourages us not to look upon that heartfelt response as a random accident. We can commit ourselves to finding compassion in all moments of our lives.

Compassion asks us to be still in the face of immeasurable pain.

Guided meditation: compassion for blameless sorrow

• Find a posture that is relaxed and comfortable for your body.

• Let your eyes gently close.

• Take a few moments to be aware of your body, its stillness, and the life within it.

• Bring your attention to rest in the center of your chest, in the area of your heart, and for a few moments be aware of your breathing.

• Let your mind relax and calm. Invite into your heart and attention the image or awareness of a person who is in the midst of great physical, emotional, or mental pain. It might be someone close to you, but it can also be someone you don't know personally. Let the image settle in your attention. Sense the struggle and sorrow that person is living with. Reflect on their hardship, heartache, or pain.

• With an open heart filled with empathy and sensitivity, offer to that person your heartfelt wishes for their healing and well-being:
"May you find healing."
"May you find peace."

• Let these phrases rest in your heart and mind. If you find that you begin to become lost in despair, pity, or anxiety, just come back to your breathing for a few moments to steady your heart and mind. You may need to find words and phrases that are appropriate to the person you are

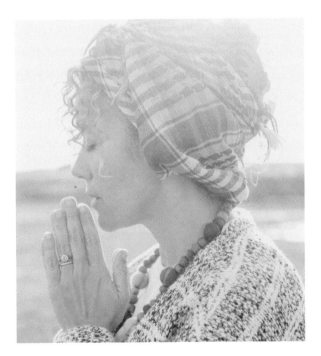

connecting with. You might use:
"May you find acceptance."
"May you find ease."

• Stay with the phrases as long as you wish. Before coming out of the posture, extend the scope of your compassion to embrace all beings:
"May all beings find healing."
"May all beings find peace."

COMPASSION FOR YOURSELF

Many people in this world find it easier to extend compassion to others than to receive it or to offer it to themselves. Aware of the pain that pervades the lives of so many people, we may feel it is inappropriate to reflect on the pain or sorrow in our own life. We may even believe that it is self-indulgent to care for our own broken hearts, ailing bodies, or confused minds.

If we are able to surrender our tendency to flee from pain, we discover an inner balance that is not shattered by change and loss. In our relationship to our own bodies, minds, and hearts we learn the lessons of patience, tolerance, equanimity, and receptivity. In the world of our body, mind, and heart we sense the world of all bodies, minds, and hearts—moments of joy and despair, health and illness, fear and trust. Compassion invites us to be intimate with this universal story and deeply acknowledge the essential interconnectedness and interdependence of all life. The lessons of healing we learn within our own story are the lessons we bring to our lives.

Compassion in grief and loss

Our capacity to form bonds of intimacy with people in our lives inevitably means that all of us will experience the sorrow of loss and separation. Grief is our very human and heartfelt response to death and the endings of the relationships that have gladdened our hearts. In the midst of grieving it can feel that it will be endless, as if the fabric of our lives has been torn apart. In the pain of grief we may find ourselves lost in a cascade of memories, replaying the endless stories of our relationship with the person who has died. Our hearts can fill with an overwhelming sense of injustice, particularly when someone we care for deeply dies unexpectedly and unpredictably. Part of our grieving in those moments may be to shut out the world, to seek causes we may never be able to find or understand, or to blame ourselves for not preventing the death.

Grief is a territory in which we feel rootless and bereft. It can seem a time of such darkness, sorrow, and uncertainty that there is nowhere we can find a place of rest. Meditation practice is not a device to make grief disappear, but it can offer a way of discovering a sense of refuge and ease. We can learn to find a home for ourselves in the present, one moment at a time, rather than being lost in stories of the past or fears about the future. Grief has no predetermined timetable, but within it we can discover a way of caring for ourselves. The times of greatest sorrow in our lives are those that ask for the greatest compassion. Compassion has its roots in listening, the capacity to receive sorrow without fear or anxiety. In grief, being listened to by others is part of our healing. Our capacity to listen deeply to our own hearts and minds is equally part of the fabric of our healing.

Guided meditation: compassion in grief and loss

• Take a few moments to settle into a posture that is as relaxed and comfortable as possible. Gently close your eyes and be aware of your whole body.

• Let your breathing relax. Consciously take a few slightly fuller breaths, and as you breathe out, be aware of releasing the out-breath fully.

• With each out-breath sense your body relaxing more and more deeply.

• Bring your attention to your heart area, the center of your chest, and the sensations or feelings that are being held in that area of your body.

• Your heart may feel heavy, contracted, or painful. Let your attention rest there without demanding that it should feel different.

• Offer to yourself heartfelt compassion and care:
"May I find ease within this sorrow."

"May I find peace within this sorrow."
"May I find healing."

• Thoughts and memories may flood your mind, bringing their own waves of grief. Embrace them with the same compassionate attention. Discover that it is possible to be present with these thoughts and memories without becoming lost.

• Bring your attention gently back to the phrases of compassion:
"May I find ease within this sorrow."
"May I find peace within this sorrow."
"May I find healing."

• Stay with this practice as long as it is comfortable for you. In the moments of greatest heartache you may discover that it is possible for you to find some sense of refuge and ease within the phrases of compassion.

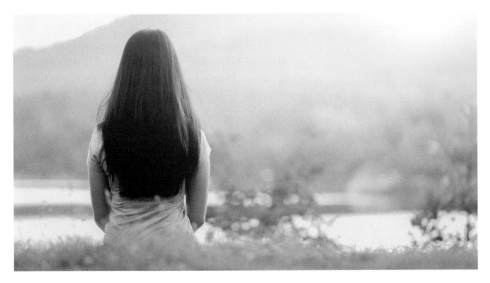

"May I find healing."

FINDING JOY EVERY DAY

Teaching ourselves to find joy in the moment makes us feel happier right here and now. But if we make this habit ingrained, psychologists tell us it can lead to a long-term reduction in symptoms of depression, stress, and anxiety.

How to find joy

Appreciating the present moment prevents us from worrying about the future or regretting the past. Psychologists also tell us that the more often we engage with positive emotions, the more frequently we *can* feel them. In this way, finding joy now, today, can help you through tomorrow, no matter what it brings. Here are some tips for finding joy every day:

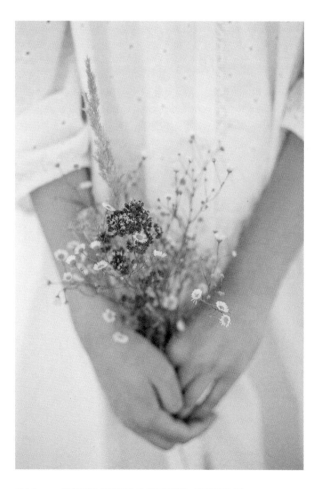

• Find joy in the little things, such as a warmly held hand, the smell of a cookie, or the pink clouds at sunset.

• Go outside, to take a walk or pull some weeds. If possible, exercise vigorously, which will release endorphins to boost your mood.

• Talk with family, friends, or even strangers. It is our connections with other people that create the truest happiness. The more we laugh, the happier we feel. And the happier we feel, the more we laugh.

• Be kind! Being kind leads to joyful feelings. Show kindness to a friend or family member, volunteer at a local group or school, or donate to charity.

• Avoid reading negative news stories, particularly first thing in the morning (when they can color the day) or immediately before going to bed (when they can spoil sleep).

Be kind! Being kind leads to joyful feelings.

Developing a daily gratitude habit

Gratitude is the act of feeling grateful, happy, and blessed for the good things in our lives, both large and small. Feeling grateful encourages us to look for the positive rather than dwelling on the negative. It teaches us to appreciate the people and activities in our lives that make us truly happy.

The act of feeling grateful can have deep benefits for emotional, mental, and physical well-being. A study by psychologists Robert Emmons, of the University of California, and Michael McCullough, of the University of Miami, looked at the effects of regular gratitude. Once a week, a group of participants in their study wrote down five things for which they were grateful. After two months, this group reported feeling more optimistic, happier, and having fewer physical problems, when compared with the control group. To turn gratitude into a habit, try these activities:

• Keep a gratitude journal, writing down five things for which you are grateful every evening or morning (see also pages 246–247).

• Every day, find someone to whom you can say thank you, whether that is a family member, friend, coworker, or a stranger who helps you through the day.

• Once a week, think of a kindness that you can do for someone to whom you are grateful. This kindness can be as small as fetching a coworker a coffee or as large as mowing a neighbor's lawn.

• If you are feeling stressed, sad, or overwhelmed, think of five things for which you are grateful.

Creating a gratitude jar

A gratitude jar can be for personal use or shared with family or coworkers. Wash out an old jar, then decorate it with ribbons, stickers, or wrapping paper. Leave a pen and slips of paper beside the jar, ready to be used. Every day, write down something or someone you are grateful for. If you are sharing the jar with family or coworkers, name names so everyone will know they are appreciated. Remember to pay attention to the small gestures, which all add up to making us feel valued. Once a week, once a month, or just on Thanksgiving, open the jar together.

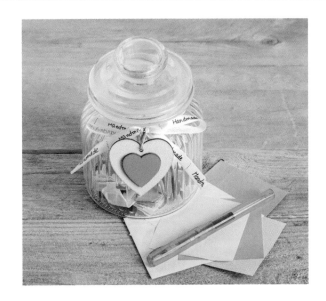

CREATIVITY AND JOURNALING

Creativity is a popular form of self-care for emotional wellness. There is a vast array of different ways in which you can be creative. While some methods require a few existing skills or knowledge, there are others that are accessible for anyone to try. Journaling is both a form of creative self-expression and a vital, constructive tool for managing and healing emotions.

Coloring

There used to be a time when coloring was viewed as purely a childhood activity, but it has become much more mainstream and acceptable for adults to color, too. In fact, the world of coloring books for adults has become big business. Sitting down with your pens and pencils and indulging in a bit of coloring can be highly therapeutic. It is a chance to unleash your creativity, explore colors, try your hand at art, and just enjoy yourself.

It is not just hearsay: One research study has found that coloring can be a therapeutic form of emotional self-care. This is because it is a mindful activity and can soothe a stressed mind. There are lots of adult coloring books available these days, as well as digital downloads that you buy online and print. If you need inspiration, take a look on YouTube, where colorists frequently share videos and record their coloring sessions.

Zentangle

Another way of exploring your creativity and soothing your mind is to try Zentangle. This is a form of art, often produced in black pen on white paper, that involves drawing structured patterns, or tangles. There is a whole series of different patterns to learn, which can be drawn on small square pieces of paper, called tiles, or drawn together as larger designs.

The Zentangle patterns are all easy to learn as they are made up of simple combinations of hand-drawn lines, curves, and dots. You do not need to be good at drawing or have expensive equipment to try it. Focusing on drawing in this way can become a mindfulness exercise. As you concentrate on what you are drawing, anxieties and worries are pushed to the back of your mind. Many people find it both relaxing and rewarding.

Mixed-media art journal

Exploring mixed-media art ideas is another option for unleashing your creativity in a fun and unstructured way. A mixed-media art journal provides you with a place to explore your creativity and, like written journaling, it can be a great way to unload and express yourself.

One of the benefits of a mixed-media art journal is that there are no rules or set methods to follow— it is down to you what you would like to create. Popular methods include painting (watercolors or acrylic), drawing, using pastels, creating textured prints and surfaces, making patterns, or collaging with materials such as paper, magazines, or ephemera.

If you are not sure where to start, browse the Internet for ideas or look up mixed-media art videos online. There are tutorials you can follow, or you can just play with art materials and see what you create.

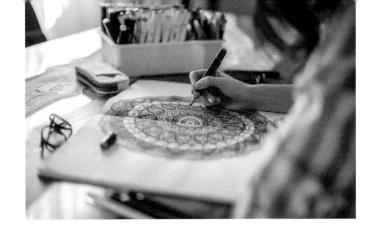

Hobbies

Hobbies are a great form of self-care, as they are all about doing things you love and enjoy. It is good to incorporate plenty of time into your life for yourself and the things you take pleasure in, giving you the opportunity to boost your emotional wellness at the same time. When you indulge in hobbies, you immerse yourself in the activity at hand, be it reading, sewing, crochet, or fossil hunting. It is natural to find yourself losing track of time, being absorbed by the rhythm of the craft, and temporarily switching off from the stress and worry of everyday life.

If you had an old hobby that you used to enjoy in the past, such as horse riding or cycling, try it again. Some skills are never lost and it may simply be a case of rekindling your love for the activity. Or set yourself the challenge of discovering a new hobby. There is nothing to be lost from trying out new activities, and you may find something that really resonates. Look for local activity classes or trial sessions, where you can go along and try several different options. Of course, do not spend loads of money on equipment or supplies before you are sure it is definitely for you. Alternatively, look online for activity videos and see if you can find something that appeals to you. A new skill might be just what you need to boost your self-care!

Journaling

Keeping a journal can be a useful way to record emotions, thoughts, challenges, goals, and successes. Regular journaling encourages mindfulness and self-awareness. Writing encourages us to examine our emotions, but the act of writing can also be a release of pent-up thoughts and worries. Journaling is a helpful tool for working through emotional challenges. We can note down triggers and responses. As we write, we may suddenly recognize negative thought processes that we had never previously noted. As the months go by, we can flick back through the pages to examine progress. Above all, we can write down all the things we are proud of. We can make journaling part of a daily gratitude habit (see pages 244–245). Here are a few tips on how to start journaling:

• Use a pen and a notebook, which form a more immediate and freer connection between thoughts and the page than typing on a computer or phone.

• Decide how long you will write for, with somewhere between ten and twenty minutes a good start. Set a timer on your phone for five minutes before the time is up.

• Is there something in particular that you would like to write about? If not, start with writing about how you feel today. Is there anything you want to achieve or you feel worried about?

• Let your pen and your thoughts flow. Do not censor or judge yourself. Remember that you are writing for you and you alone.

• When you have five minutes left, read back through what you have written. Do your words reveal anything about your own emotions? Do your words trigger a memory? Write down your response to your own writing. If you would like to set yourself a goal, note it down.

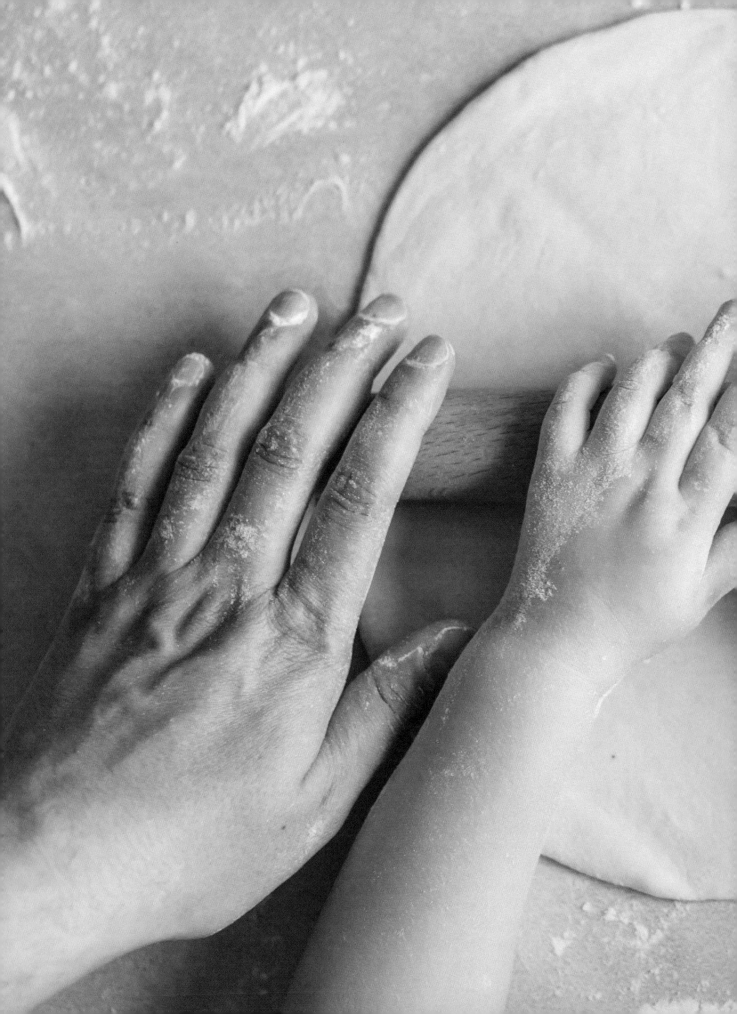

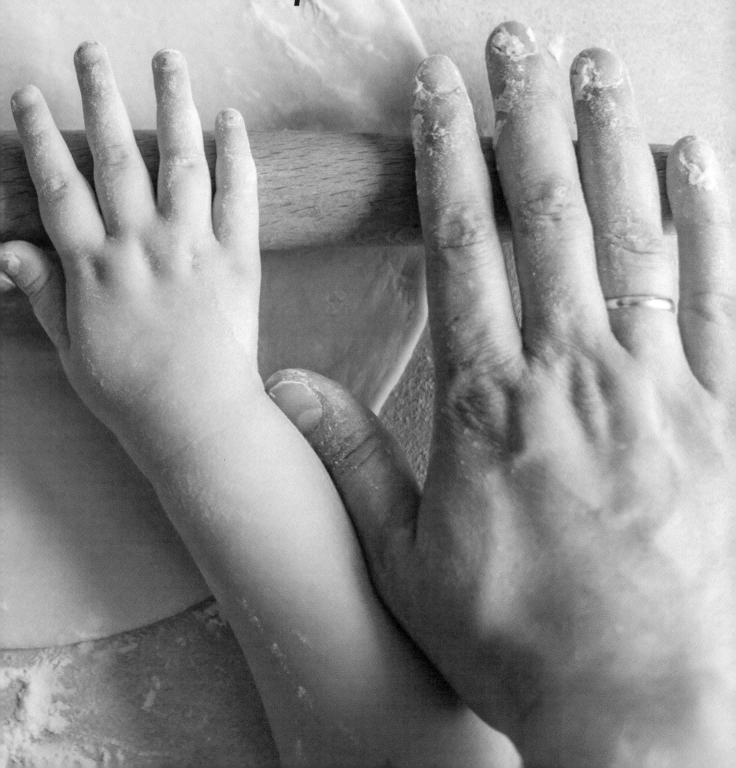

PART FOUR

Work–Life Wellness

THE IMPORTANCE OF WORK–LIFE WELLNESS

Work–life wellness, or work–life balance as it's sometimes known, is a term used to describe the importance of establishing mental and physical wellness at work and at home. The vast majority of us have to work in order to earn money to support ourselves and our families, but we still have personal lives and commitments beyond work.

Finding balance

When either our work or home life becomes stressful or overly demanding, the balance is lost and this can affect our physical and mental health in a detrimental manner. Common problems caused by poor work–life balance include stress, anxiety, poor sleep, lack of concentration, feeling overwhelmed, not being able to keep up with usual commitments, fatigue, exhaustion, depression, and headaches.

Work–life wellness doesn't have to be balanced 50/50, like a seesaw, as realistically our lives aren't perfectly organized in that way, but some degree of balance is necessary in order for us to function well and live happily.

In order to achieve a state of work–life wellness, the key is to feel content and satisfied. Ideally, you need to be happy with who you are, what you're doing, and the decisions you're making. You need to be able to cope with the demands of your working life so you're not stressed or at risk of burnout, and still be able to cope equally well with your personal and family commitments and responsibilities.

Work–life wellness is as important to you as it is to your family, friends, and employers. When you're happy and content, you're more likely to have better physical and mental health, healthy lifestyle habits, and time to look after your needs and those of your family. At work, you're more likely to be productive,

more committed, able to think creatively and make fewer mistakes. You'll enjoy the work you do and the achievements you reach and are less likely to need time off due to illness. It's a win-win situation for both you and your employer.

Healthy workplaces

In recent years there's been greater emphasis on the importance of work–life wellness and a recognition that employers need to promote healthy workplaces, as stress is one of the major causes of employee absence. Ideally, all managers and workplaces should play a role in helping employees reach their potential and achieve a good work–life balance.

In a healthy workplace, an employer helps by:

• Training managers to notice when someone might be feeling stressed or have a poor work–life balance.

• Encouraging employees to have regular breaks during the day.

• Regularly reviewing everyone's workloads and ensuring they are fully achievable and realistic.

• Increasing support for parents and carers, so they are better able to manage work and home commitments.

• Encouraging stress-relieving activities, such as relaxation classes or lunchtime exercises.

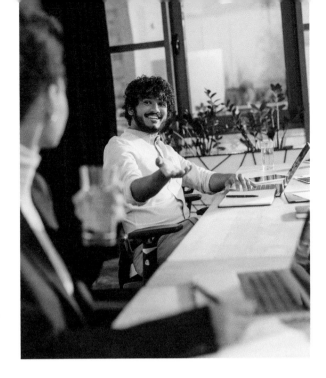

• Asking employees what could help improve their work–life wellness.

• Encouraging a culture of openness, so that everyone feels comfortable and able to speak up and be honest if they're feeling under too much pressure.

• Offering remote and flexible work schedules.

If you're applying for a new employment role, it's worth researching the ethos of the company and finding out how employees tend to be treated and whether the firm has a healthy workplace policy.

If your work has always involved long hours and a demanding environment, then it's sometimes hard to see the stress that this is causing. Every now and again it's good to take a step back and try to see the situation from a different perspective. Ask yourself:

• Are you working unreasonably long hours for no extra pay?

• Are you constantly under pressure?

• Do you struggle to have enough time to enjoy your hobbies because you're working too much?

• Do you worry about work when you're at home?

• Do you feel like you don't have enough time to eat or sleep properly?

• Do you fall asleep as soon as you get home?

• Are you missing out on your kids' important milestones because you're always working?

• How do you feel—do you feel fulfilled by your work, or do you loathe it?

What to do if your work–life wellness is out of sync

If you've answered yes to one or more of the questions above, then perhaps it's time to work on improving your work–life balance. Think about what aspects need to change and consider how to make these changes possible. Perhaps you need to cut down on your hours to save your sanity or be able to spend more time with your family. Where possible, speak to your employer and see if they can accommodate your needs; maybe more flexible hours are available or they could change the work you're doing so that you get home earlier. It's not always easy to make improvements and sometimes they have to be implemented over time, but where your health and wellness are concerned, a change can make a real difference.

HEALTHY RELATIONSHIPS

Healthy relationships are an important part of your health and wellness. If you've got a healthy relationship, you're more likely to feel happy, contented, and satisfied with your life, as it's full of mutual love and support through the ups and downs. You may feel good about who you are, have more confidence and self-esteem, happy in the knowledge that you have someone on your side.

Nurturing your relationships

While some relationships seem to be inherently healthy from the start, others may take more time to nurture and grow, and all may go through periods of highs and lows.

Signs of a healthy relationship include:

• Trust and understanding

• Respect and honesty

• Care and emotional support

• Equality

• Good communication

• Shared values

Developing and building a healthy relationship with a partner, friend, family member, or work colleague is important, as support, friendship, love, and connections are vital for us as humans. If issues do occur—and they often do—one of the keys to sorting out problems is clear and honest communication. Be prepared to admit when you're wrong and take steps to make things right. Be respectful of each other and learn to compromise, so each of your needs can be met and you both get an equal say.

If a relationship has become stagnant or mundane, find more time to spend with the other person and make sure they feel appreciated, cared for, and loved. It's important to have your own interests, hobbies, and friendships, but make sure you spread your time equally. Having shared interests can help you bond and spend more time together.

How to spot a toxic relationship

A toxic relationship is one in which you feel unhappy, constantly drained, and on edge. It's not a pleasant experience to go through and can seriously affect your wellness, but ironically, when you're in a toxic relationship, it can sometimes be hard to know that you are. The repeated negative behaviors can take over, so much so that you may even come to accept them as normal. Someone detached from the situation, who's looking in from the outside, may be able to see the red flags immediately, but when you're in the midst of the situation, you can easily become blinded to reality and fail to realize things are as bad as they are, especially if things were OK to start with.

There are some signs and symptoms to watch out for that could indicate that a relationship might be toxic. They include:

LACK OF SUPPORT—in a healthy relationship, you support and naturally want each other to succeed,

Healthy relationships are full of positive communication and infused with kindness and compassion.

but in a toxic relationship there's a complete lack of support. You don't feel encouraged when you do something and feel like your needs are ignored and belittled.

CONTROLLING BEHAVIOR—in a toxic relationship, the other person will try and control your behavior, perhaps from jealousy or lack of trust. You may find that they constantly want to know where you are, what you're doing, or who you're with, when it should be perfectly normal to be able to do something on your own.

JEALOUSY AND RESENTMENT—if another person seems to be constantly jealous of you and what you're achieving, it can lead to increased toxicity and feelings of resentment, neither of which are pleasant to be on the receiving end of.

NEGATIVE COMMUNICATION—healthy relationships are full of positive communication and infused with kindness and compassion, but with toxic relationships the communication is negative, critical, and hurtful. Being on the receiving end of this can eat away at your self-esteem and confidence.

DISRESPECT—in a healthy relationship, other people respect you and value your worth. In a toxic relationship, the respect can vanish, leaving a gaping hole of disrespect. This may materialize into behaviors such as not bothering to stick to plans you've made together or disrespecting your opinions.

Crystals to help toxic relationships

SUNSTONE—sunstone has vibrant, uplifting energies and can help lift dark moods and discomfort in relationships. It can help you find the confidence to break free and the strength to persevere. Hold sunstone or keep a piece in your pocket at all times.

CHRYSOPRASE—keep a piece of chrysoprase in your pocket. The energy of chrysoprase gives hope, optimism, independence, self-worth, and acceptance of who you truly are.

LEPIDOLITE—wear or hold lepidolite to promote release from toxic situations. This crystal helps with transitions, so its energies will support you as you move to become more independent.

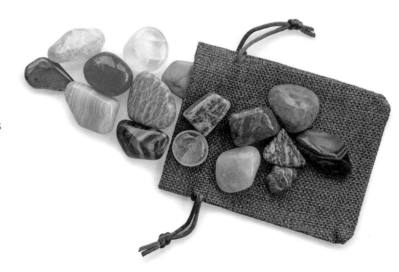

SETTING BOUNDARIES

All relationships, whether with friends, family, or even work colleagues (see page 282), need to have boundaries. Boundaries are important for you and your self-care, so that you can ensure you get the time to yourself that you need. They're also important for other people, so they respect you, know what is and isn't acceptable, and how best to interact with you.

When you don't have boundaries, there's the risk that problems can occur in relationships—such as one person demanding too much time, not respecting your feelings, or a so-called friend contacting you only when they want or need something.

Although it might seem tricky to establish boundaries, it's well worth persevering with them as they can make relationships a lot healthier, happier, and more fulfilled. Plus, they can highlight toxic relationships that are dragging you down, and which are perhaps better left behind.

How to set boundaries

Use these practical steps to guide you in setting boundaries with your friends and family.

Evaluate your relationships
Start by evaluating your relationships and think about how, where, and why you need to put boundaries in place. Is a particular person demanding too much of your time? Are you uncomfortable around certain people? Do you wish you had more time to spend with other people, those who make you feel happier? Or are you fed up with someone else being too "helpful" and trying to make your decisions for you?

Think about what improvements you'd like to make
So, what changes would you like to make to improve these issues? For example, would seeing a friend just once a week, rather than several times a week, make things easier for you? Do you need to remind a friend that while you appreciate their help, you are capable of making your own decisions?

When you're thinking things through, it might help to jot down notes about what you're aiming for.

Communicate
Boundaries are only going to work if other people know about them, so communication is key. This is the part that can be the most difficult, as you may worry about how others will feel—and that's a perfectly normal reaction. They may not know you've been struggling or feeling uncomfortable, and talking about it can bring up difficult feelings.

However, you need to discuss what's bothering you; expressing your needs and feelings makes your friendship honest and healthy. Talk to them calmly and openly and explain exactly what the issue is. Stick with it and remember you're doing this for a good reason, and that, in the long run, the intention is good and it will help you both.

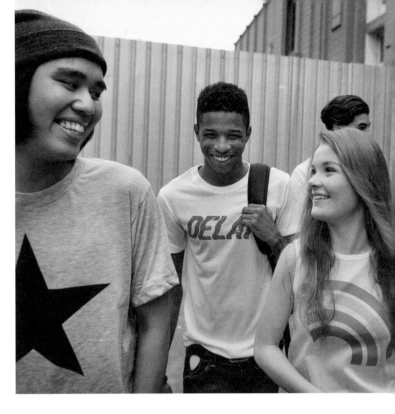

Give them time

If your boundary idea has come as a shock to the other person, give them time to ponder on it. Some space from each other can help you both get things in perspective and provide a clean slate from which you can start afresh. Be there for them if they want to clarify things further, but avoid getting caught up in endless discussions where nothing gets resolved, as this will only add more stress.

Accept a breakup

Setting boundaries can highlight problems in relationships that can't be solved. If there are feelings of emotional manipulation, or passive-aggressive behavior, and the other person is not amenable to discussing boundaries, be prepared to accept that the friendship just might not be right for you. It's not unacceptable to break up and move on from friends—your self-esteem, self-worth, and happiness matter, and it could open the door for better things. Of course, it can be a lot trickier with family, but for your own well-being, you might need to accept that it's better if you don't see them so frequently.

Start afresh

Once you've established your new boundaries, start afresh and maintain them. Don't be tempted to give in and let your standards slide, as this will only encourage previous bad habits to rear their heads. You've gone to the trouble of raising your concerns and discussing boundaries, so stick to them. If your friends "forget" the new boundaries, calmly remind them exactly why they were needed. If they are true and worthy friends, they'll understand.

Be flexible

Be aware that boundaries can change over time, so make sure you don't get too caught up in being obsessive and rigid with the boundaries you set. Accept that people and situations can alter, and be prepared to reevaluate things in the future if necessary. Don't, however, let other people force you to adjust your boundaries if you're not happy to do so.

Maintaining healthy boundaries can be challenging, but stay firm and stick to your decisions. If you have any doubts or niggling worries, remind yourself that your emotional health and well-being are important and that you feel happier and more in control with boundaries in place.

Maintaining healthy boundaries can be challenging, but stay firm and stick to your decisions.

COMMUNICATION

Communication allows you to express yourself and listen to other people. To build social relationships, share your experiences, and enhance your support systems, clear communication is crucial.

Good communication is a skill that can be built on and developed. Being able to communicate more effectively can boost your self-confidence, improve your relationships, and help you feel better about yourself. It's a form of self-care, as sharing your true feelings can help release bottled-up emotions. As well as spoken words, good communication involves body language, facial expressions, and posture, from all parties involved.

How to express yourself

It's not always easy or straightforward to express yourself, especially if you aren't used to talking about yourself. But when you've got someone on your team or in your support system who cares and will take time to listen to you, it's well worth trying. It can really help lift burdens and boost your emotional wellness.

Communication
Here are some tips to help you learn to express yourself effectively:

• Be assertive—be calm and relaxed and try to have positive body posture.

• Explain things as clearly as you can.

• Think before you speak—consider how someone else might take what you say.

• Express your emotions appropriately—don't get angry or confrontational.

• Don't get defensive if the other person expresses a view or opinion that's different to yours.

Listening to other people
Communication is a two-way process—it involves talking and listening. In the same way that you'd like people to listen to you, other people in your support network will appreciate you listening to them, too.

Listening will help build and strengthen your relationship.

You can improve your listening skills by:

• Being patient—let someone else take their time speaking and don't interrupt them.

• Giving them 100 percent of your attention—turn off your phone and focus on the other person.

• Being neutral and open to listening—don't be judgmental about someone else's views or experiences, even if they differ from yours.

• Being prepared to just listen—sometimes a person might simply need someone to listen to them, without having advice or input.

• Showing empathy—show that you're listening, and that you care, by using verbal and nonverbal acknowledgments.

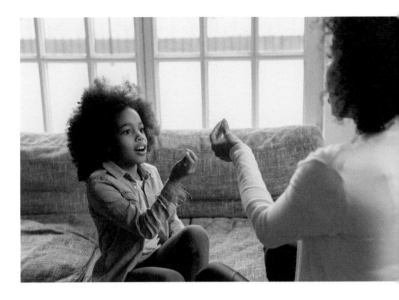

• Acknowledging their feelings—if someone has strong feelings, acknowledge them so they know you're listening and taking them seriously.

• Being encouraging—if someone is feeling low or down, be encouraging toward them; it's not always easy to open up and talk.

Online communication

These days, a lot of communication is conducted online. Although some people find it easier to type emails or messages rather than talk to someone, this form of communication comes with its ups and downs.

When you're communicating online, you lose the ability to see the other person's facial expressions, reactions, posture, and body language. This can sometimes make it tricky to convey a true picture of how you're feeling, and the real meaning behind some words and sentences can be misread, misjudged, or lost completely.

Of course, emojis can go some way to express how words are intended, but they still don't replace the ability to actually see an individual's body language or reaction.

It's important to bear such issues in mind when you're communicating online and try to be even clearer in the language you use and the way you express yourself with the written word. For example, if you're telling someone about how you feel, you may have to write this down more explicitly, explaining exactly how something or someone made you feel.

Coping with conflict

If your communication breaks down and conflict occurs, it can trigger strong emotions, disappointment, and hurt feelings. If handled inappropriately, the conflict can rage on and cause ongoing resentment and fractured relationships.

However, by learning to cope with conflict more effectively, you can help to resolve it.

Communication is key when you're dealing with conflict. As much as you may feel hurt, annoyed, or upset, try to remain as calm as possible. Being calm will help you to understand someone else's verbal and nonverbal communication more effectively. Being in control of your emotions also helps you communicate with the other person without intimidating or challenging them.

It's hard to remain calm in the face of conflict, but it's a very useful skill to learn. If necessary, you can save and offload your true emotions later, either to someone else that you trust or to yourself through techniques such as journaling.

Sometimes conflict can also be eased by adding a degree of humor into the situation. It's important that you judge the situation first, though, as when used inappropriately this could escalate things.

Being able to resolve conflict provides an opportunity for growth. You can learn from your experiences, feel confident in your actions, and build a stronger relationship with the person concerned.

IDENTITY AND THE MIND

Our minds are the forerunners of our speech, actions, choices, and the way that we personally experience and interpret the world. They can be a cauldron of seething thoughts, worries, memories, and plans. The times of greatest confusion, obsession, turmoil, and preoccupation are all experienced within our minds. But they also have the capacity to be a landscape of clarity, simplicity, and peace, making us who we are.

Clarity of mind

Learning to care for our minds with sensitivity, understanding, and mindfulness, we also learn to care for everything that is born of our minds. A mind rooted in calm clarity, understanding, and stillness finds its embodiment in every word, gesture, and choice in our lives. Learning to befriend our minds, we discover the possibility of finding ease in every area of our lives.

When our minds are overfull, burdened with unnecessary thoughts and preoccupations, they propel us through our lives with haste and agitation. When we learn to find spaciousness within our minds, we approach the world with a deepening care and calmness.

A central part of meditation practice is devoted to understanding the nature of our minds, simply because they play such a pivotal role in our lives and our capacity to find well-being. It is possible to embrace our minds with awareness—to sense on a moment-to-moment level the arising and passing of thoughts, images, and mental states. Our minds are no obstacle to deep understanding and compassion— the obstacle lies in the unconsciousness or lack of awareness that leads us to be lost in clouds of confusion. In meditation we explore the possibility of bringing a sensitive and clear attentiveness to our minds, just as we learn to bring that quality of attention to every other dimension of our lives.

Kindness toward your mind

In times of great inner chaos and turmoil in our lives we can regard our minds almost as enemies— untrustworthy and the source of pain. There are moments when our deepest and most noble intentions to cultivate loving kindness, generosity, and openness seem to be sabotaged by the compelling and habitual thoughts and fears that take root there.

Unpredictability appears to be part of our minds. Moments of calm and peace are overtaken by bursts of preoccupation and obsession. The state and quality of our minds often seems to be beyond our control. We wish to be present, spacious, and clear, only to find ourselves floundering in dullness or clouds of confusion.

It is tempting to blame our minds for the turmoil and agitation we can all too easily find ourselves lost in. But the first step in developing clarity of mind is to let go of the blame and begin to approach our minds with interest, investigation, and sensitivity.

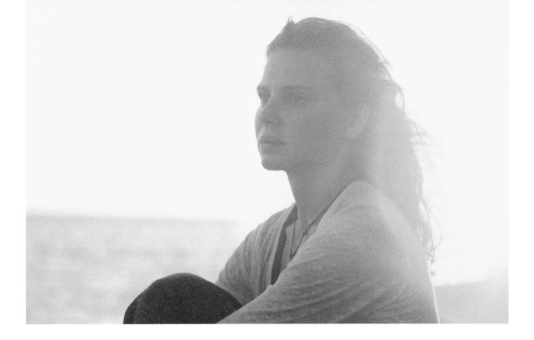

Meditation and your mind

Meditation is not antithought, nor is it a means to suppress the mind. Just as the mind can be the source of some of the most destructive acts and conflicts in our world, so too can it be the source of some of the greatest insights and creativity. The divisions and separations that scar our world will also be healed through our ability and willingness to find peace and understanding within our own minds.

Acknowledging the power of the mind for both chaos and stillness, a meditative practice can teach us that:

• We can find simplicity and cultivate the capacity of our minds for insight, investigation, and stillness.

• We discover we can accept thoughts as thoughts alone, which rise and pass just like everything else in our lives.

• We can think with clarity, learn to investigate the places of confusion that beleaguer us, and nurture a mind of peace.

A calm mind is not intrinsically a mind that is devoid of thought. If meditative depth were dependent upon the absence of thought, it would be irrelevant to our lives. Learning to investigate and understand our minds, we enhance our capacity to think and reflect with clarity. We discover the wisdom of releasing much of the identification and holding that agitates our minds. We learn to let go of many of the futile avenues of thinking, judgment, anxiety, and obsession that do not contribute to our well-being. A mind that is deeply rooted in calmness is an ally in our lives, the source of effective, clear action. Approaching our minds in a meditative way, on a moment-to-moment level, we see more clearly the impact of the mind upon our bodies, hearts, and all of the relationships we form in our lives. Meditation teaches us to listen to our minds, to reject nothing, and to discover the freedom of not being entangled and lost in the world of interpretation and judgment.

In meditation we bring a clear, sensitive attention directly to all of the activities of our minds.

A CLEAR MIND

The first step in cultivating a mind of calmness and clarity is to know the nature of our mind on a moment-to-moment level, to cultivate a mindful intimacy with it, exploring it in all its movements and activities. We discover that our mind is not a static, uninterrupted entity. It is an ongoing process of arising and passing thoughts, images, memories, plans, moods, and responses.

Finding peace

We receive the world through our sensory doors, and our minds perceive and interpret those impressions. The inner world of association, memory, comparison, emotion, and evaluation is set in motion. It is helpful to see the changing nature of our mental processes, as this is the first step in forming a mindful relationship to our minds. As we learn to be increasingly present within those mental processes, we discover we are not helpless, not sentenced to an eternal inner life of floundering, reactivity, and powerlessness before the force of our minds. We are able to introduce into the life of our minds the qualities of investigation, serenity, and simplicity. These are the qualities that teach us how to let go of confusion and complexity and realize the capacity of our minds for clarity, understanding, and creativity.

We discover, too, that the mind is not always constant—that the space and stillness between thoughts can learn to sense the arising of thoughts and be increasingly attuned to some of the states of mind that can, if unnoticed, govern our relationship with every moment in our life.

If our minds are at peace, we discover increasing depths of peace everywhere in our lives. If our minds are balanced and receptive, we are no longer prone to being lost in the multiplicity of events that are part of all of our lives.

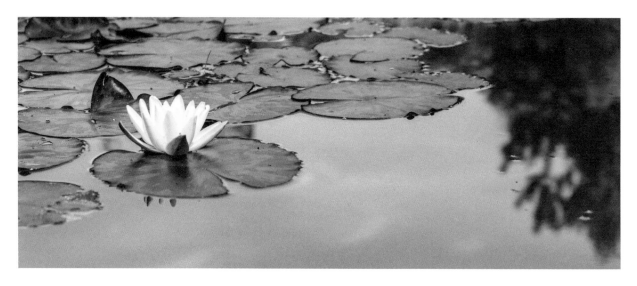

We discover increasing depths of peace everywhere in our lives.

Guided meditation: noting

• Find a posture in which your body can be relaxed and upright. Take a few moments to settle into that posture, finding a deep sense of ease within your body. Let your eyes gently close. Bring your attention to rest within your breathing, focusing your attention either on the area of your upper lip and nostrils or on the rising and falling of your abdomen with each breath.

• As you rest your attention in your breathing, begin to sense all the moments when your attention is drawn to whatever is occurring in your mind. Fantasy, memory, planning, judgment, daydreaming, rehearsing—make a simple note of whatever is occurring so you can see clearly where your attention is lingering in the world of thought. Note it calmly, clearly, and then return your attention to your breathing.

• You may find that you are present only with a single breath before your attention is attracted once more to activity in your mind. Just breathe that breath fully, sensing its beginning and its ending. If your attention is once more drawn to a thought or series of thoughts or images that have appeared in your mind, again just make a simple mental note of that activity.

• Return once more to the next breath. Sense that each time you return your attention to your breathing that you are letting go of complexity and entanglement.

• There may be moments when you are not aware of the movement of your attention from your breath and into a thought pattern. Suddenly you wake up as if from a dream, realizing you have been lost in a thought or fantasy. Don't judge those moments, just make a simple mental note—

"Thinking, thinking"—and return to the next breath. Don't be tempted to try to figure out where the thoughts are coming from or what underlies them. Let your breath be an anchor and also a mirror, reflecting all those moments when your attention leaves your breath and goes to your mind.

• Know when your attention is present within your breathing and when your attention is present within thought. Be equally attentive, with calmness and sensitivity, to each of those moments. You may discover that when you bring a conscious attention to a thought, the thought simply dissolves and disappears. This is fine—don't try to hold on to anything. Sense the disappearing of the thought and again bring a wholehearted attentiveness to your breathing.

• Sense the possibility of seeing a thought as a thought, arising and passing, appearing and fading away.

• Sense a breath as a breath, arising and passing, appearing and fading away.

• Let yourself rest in calm attentiveness, aware and clear within the life of your mind. As your attention deepens, you may discover that your thought processes begin to calm and slow down. You may sense a growing capacity to see thoughts more clearly. You may discover a growing stillness that does not rely upon the absence of thought but is tangible within the presence of thought.

• Cultivate calmness and clarity of mind in each moment.

• When you are ready, open your eyes and come out of the posture.

WHO AM I?

There are countless meditations that devote themselves to the simple question: "Who am I?"

We can go through our lives carrying within us an array of assumptions and images about who we are, and that our sense of "self" is essentially formed by whatever we identify with—our bodies, thoughts, emotions, opinions, and experience. We are prone to describe ourselves by all that we identify with in the moment, saying or believing, "I am sad/happy/a failure/lovable/unworthy . . ." Many of these descriptions have a long history that becomes increasingly solid over time.

A sense of "self"

Just as we are prone to freeze our sense of "self" within the confines of these assumptions, so we tend to enact a similar process with others, identifying them by their bodies, minds, opinions, and appearance. We feel that we are one "self" living in a world of many "selves" that we compare ourselves to, which can cause many anxieties if our self-image is lacking in confidence.

Our images of our "self" can deeply debilitate us, hindering creativity, growth, and our capacity to explore new horizons in our hearts and lives.

Yet with awareness we begin to understand that all of our notions about "I" and "you" are perhaps not so solid as they first appear to be. Our sense of who we are undergoes countless changes within a single day. The "I" that was so downcast at breakfast can be exhilarated by lunch; the "self" that enjoys success can look very different to the "self" that fears failure. So while it is important to feel confident in who you are, it is equally important to recognize that we aren't static beings that have to be, feel, or do the same each day.

Meditation and the "self"

There is a profound freedom in not holding any appearance to be the absolute truth of who we are.

Meditation is not concerned with cultivating a more "perfect self," improving "self," or arriving at a final conclusion of who we are. It is concerned with liberating our hearts and minds from the confines and limitations born of identification and holding. In meditation we learn to bring a gentle and inquiring attention to all the changing faces of "self" as they appear and fade away in our day. Moment to moment, we learn to question and to let go. Inviting the question "Who am I?" into our lives and hearts, we learn the art of inner freedom.

Openness of heart and depth of understanding are to be found.

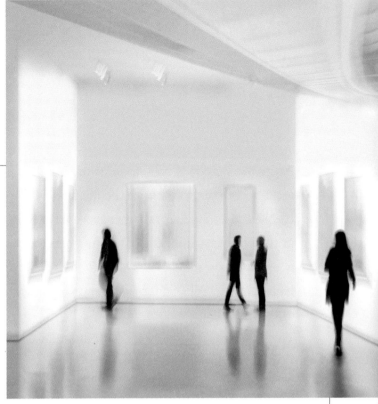

Guided meditation: Who am I?

• As you begin your meditation, settle into a posture of calm balance and allow your body to relax and be still.

• Gently close your eyes and for a few moments bring your attention to your breathing to steady and calm your mind.

• When you feel sufficiently calm and balanced inwardly, turn your attention to the thoughts, concepts, and images that arise, linger, and pass in your mind. Sense how many of those thoughts carry in subtle or glaring words the sense of "I": "I want," "I like," "I need," "I am." Don't judge any of those thoughts or images, simply sense the way that the "I" attaches itself to them. Be aware of a tendency to build a sense of "self" around a passing thought or image. Sense the way that a kind and investigating attention brought directly to any of those thoughts or images loosens the glue of the identification.

• Notice when particularly compelling thoughts, memories, or images arise how an equally strong sense of "self" appears with them and becomes defined by whatever has been taken hold of in the mind.

• Sense whether it is possible to see a thought as a thought and an image as an image, and not as an absolute description of yourself.

• If you sense the phrase "I am" appearing in relationship to any of those thoughts, turn the words around and ask yourself, "Am I?" Notice when there are strong emotions present in your mind and heart, feelings of anger, fear, anxiety, or resentment. Sense in those moments how strongly the sense of "I" appears, how you define yourself by the emotion. Again, in the face of "I am," ask yourself, "Am I?"

• Notice when your attention is drawn to a sensation in your body that may be painful or even slightly uncomfortable. Again, sense the tendency to identify with that sensation—"my knee," "my back," "I am in pain"—and be aware of the fear or agitation that is born with the identification. Explore the possibility of probing beneath the concepts and seeing a sensation as a sensation rather than as a personal description.

• Sense how the "I" never stands alone but is defined by whatever it is identified with. Sense how the identification solidifies everything we take hold of. Bring a willingness to question all of the descriptions and images. Be aware of how learning to question, investigate, and let go frees our hearts and minds from the confines of all the descriptions. Thoughts, feelings, and the sensations in our body will continue to appear, yet they will also pass with greater ease.

• Cultivate the willingness to question "Who am I?" in the face of everything that appears in your inner world, moment to moment. When you are ready, open your eyes and come out of the posture.

AWAKENING YOUR LIFE

An awakened life is one in which the confines of habit are challenged through interest and attention. Habit leads us to see life through the eyes of images and assumptions; awareness teaches us to see each moment, event, person, and ourselves anew. Habit binds us to the past; awareness awakens us to the present. Habit inclines us to dismiss many of the simple activities and events of our day as being insignificant or unworthy; awareness is free of hierarchies of value, deeming every single moment and activity of our day as being worthy of our wholehearted attention.

Freedom from habit

In all of the moments of our lives that are governed by habit, we live only on the surface of existence, disconnected from its depth and richness. Lost in habit, we deny ourselves the capacity to approach each moment with a beginner's mind, the capacity to see anew and to be taught by life. Awareness dissolves habit and gives birth to openness and a deepening connection with all life. It teaches us to probe beneath the surface of all things—our conclusions, opinions, images, and assumptions—to take nothing for granted in this life. Rather than believing we "know" someone, ourselves, or all that we can learn from any moment in life, awareness teaches us to rest in a deeper "not knowing" and questioning. This is the home of wonder, learning, and mystery.

Habit appears to relieve us of the need to be present, enabling us to attend to multiple tasks at the same time. We can wash the dishes while rehearsing our day. We can appear to listen to another person while planning our next encounter. We can walk while entertaining our favorite fantasy. Habit equally appears to relieve us of the need to deepen our understanding of ourselves or of another person. If we conclude someone is boring, irritating, or obnoxious and freeze them into that assumption, we may feel no need to probe our own reactivity nor seek to find a greater tolerance, acceptance, or patience within ourselves. If we hold an image of ourselves as being a failure, inadequate, or always right in our opinions, we may also feel no urgency to probe our own conclusions and self-images and find inner transformation. Habit disconnects us from the moment-to-moment realities of our lives and leads us to live in a world created by our thoughts and images. Awareness connects us, seeking to discover the possibilities of each moment. With awareness and wisdom we come to understand that none of our images can ever describe the truth of ourselves, another person, or anything we meet in our life.

Habit engenders dullness and sensitivity, and awareness engenders vitality and depth. In search of peace, completeness, and understanding, we increasingly treasure vitality and depth, and learn to gently probe the areas of our lives, inwardly and outwardly, that are dulled by habit.

Awareness connects us, seeking to discover the possibilities of each moment.

A daily practice: awakening our lives

Reflect upon your life and all of the activities you frequently engage in, sensing where habit is most strongly present. You might see habit being the governing force in some of the simple actions you undertake—how you wash your dishes, cook a meal, drive your car, or walk to work. You might see that it is within the repetitive activities that are part of all of our lives that we are most prone to becoming habitual and mechanical.

Choose just one or two activities and commit yourself to undertaking them as if for the first time.

For example, as you wash your dishes, sense all of the sensations and movements involved—the touch of the water on your skin, your hand touching a glass, the movement of your arm.

Sense if there are people in your life who have in some way been dismissed from your heart because of an image or assumption you hold about them. They may be the people you find yourself avoiding, the person in your neighborhood store who is hardly seen through lack of interest, or someone who has in some way offended you. Make a commitment to meeting that person, seeing and listening to them with a fullness of sensitivity and attention, as if they were your dearest friend or as if this was both the first and last time you would ever have the opportunity to know that person. Sense what happens when you are willing to probe beneath your images and conclusions.

Each day make a simple commitment to bring a fullness of sensitivity and interest to just one area of your life that you sense is governed by habit.

Sense how the commitment to awareness has the power to dissolve habit in a moment, allowing a new depth and sensitivity to emerge.

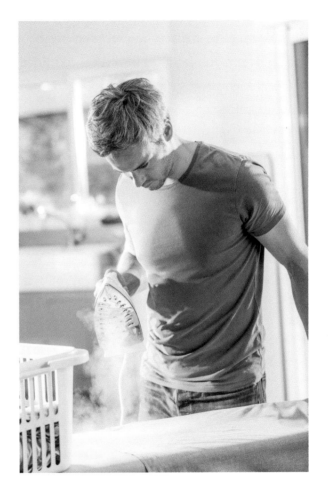

SUPPORT SYSTEMS

It's normal for life to have its ups and downs, and for you to experience times that are more challenging and difficult than others. To help you on this roller coaster, it's beneficial to have support systems in place. Support systems consist of people you trust, who are good at listening, and to whom you can turn for help if you need it.

Good friendships bring meaning and connection to your life, and they help you gain a vital sense of belonging. Some friendships are long-lasting, with people you've known for years and are still in touch with, while other friends come and go. As you journey through life, it's only natural for friendships to fluctuate, as people grow, change, and move on.

Relationships for well-being

The people you surround yourself with can have a huge impact on your well-being. Negative people can be toxic and bring you down, but people who share common interests and have similar values to you can benefit you in many ways. They can lift your mood when you're feeling down, know how to make you smile and laugh, and be the people with whom you celebrate your successes.

While some people thrive on having a large network of friends and acquaintances, when you're looking to establish a solid support network, quality over quantity tends to work best.

You may have family that is supportive, but it's good to have people in your life beyond family whom you can call on. Support systems can include friends, neighbors, mentors, colleagues, or other people you know and trust. It's good to have people in your support system that have different skills and strengths, so you don't rely on the same person all the time.

Support systems offer care, advice, and help when you need it, but they also provide joy, pleasure, and friendship. It's not just one way: Support systems function and survive best when they're mutually beneficial, so make sure you help and support one another.

How to create support systems

Support systems don't just happen overnight; they develop with time. With the right skills, you can create valuable support systems.

Get to know people
Make an effort to get to know people. Start with those you're already acquainted with, such as neighbors, work colleagues, people you see regularly

at clubs or the gym, or who you say hello to while walking your dog. Talk to them, take an interest in their views, skills, hobbies, and lives, and get to know them better. They will, in turn, do the same.

Join new groups or activities
Expand your friendships by joining new groups or activities. Find activity, hobby, or sporting groups

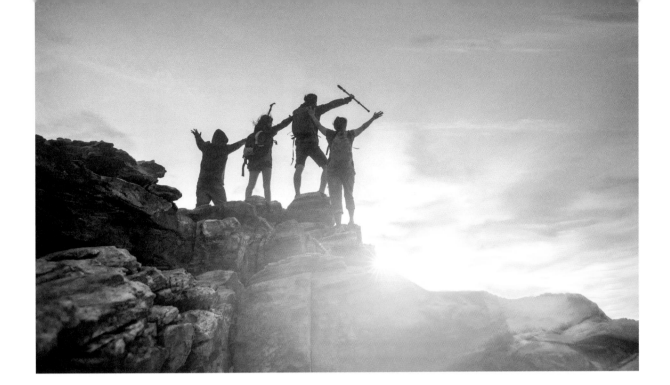

where you'll share common interests. Or try volunteering for a cause that you're passionate about.

Organize social get-togethers

When you've made new friends, organize a social activity or get-together so that you can get to know them better. For example, meet for a coffee, or go for a walk. Sometimes individual friendships can deepen away from the wider shared group.

Be positive and open

Be positive and open and try to see the good in people. Be tolerant of others and don't get annoyed if their behavior or views are different from yours. Instead, ask them to explain why they think or act the way they do. This doesn't mean you have to put up with offensive behavior or views, though.

Keep in touch

Make an effort to develop and nurture connections by staying in touch regularly, be it through phone calls, texts, emails, or seeing each other in person.

Learn to be a good listener

Support systems thrive when you listen to each other. Dedicate time to listening to other people, whether they simply want a chat after a busy day, or they need to offload their worries and concerns.

Confide in others

Learn to open up and confide in the people you trust. No one will offer you help if they don't know that you need it. Confiding in each other builds and strengthens support systems.

Support others

Show you care by being there to support other people when they need help. Offer support in any way you can. Support systems are most successful when you help each other.

Persevere and gather the right tribe

It's not always easy building your support system, or your tribe of connections, but keep trying. If you eventually find that someone doesn't turn out to be who you thought they were, don't be afraid to let that friendship go. Negative and toxic people will only bring you down. Start again and look to meet other people, or strengthen the bonds you have with existing members of your support group.

Above all, persevere. We all need support systems and, however hard it may seem to build yours, it's well worth it in the long run.

ASKING FOR HELP

Asking for help is not a sign of weakness or failure. On the contrary, reaching out is a sign of strength and means that you're taking control.

There's only so much that you can deal with on your own, and support from other people can make a world of difference. Your friends and family won't want you to be suffering alone—and if it was the other way around, you'd want to help them, rather than see them struggling on their own. If you've already got a self-care support system in place, you'll have people around you that you know and trust and can reach out to when you need to. If you don't have anything like that yet, there are groups of people you can turn to for help, such as community support groups, neighbors, charities, religious leaders, or spiritual counselors.

If they aren't able to help you directly, chances are they can guide you in the direction of someone else, or an experienced organization, that could help.

How to ask for help

It's not always easy or straightforward to ask for help, especially if you're feeling out of sorts or in a difficult place emotionally. It's important to try to remember that you're not alone, that you deserve support, and it's not a sign of weakness to ask for it.

Some of the ways in which you could ask for help from friends or a member of your support network include:

• Phoning them

• Meeting for a coffee and discussing your issues

• Arranging to go for a walk with them and talking about it while you walk

• Inviting them to your house to chat about it in private

• Sending someone you really trust an email in which you write down your needs

• Chatting to them online

• Using an online instant messaging system with a trusted contact

If you find it difficult to immediately open up and express your needs and concerns verbally, a method such as chatting online or emailing might be easier. Just be aware of how you express yourself through words—online communication can sometimes lose the intended context without body language. If necessary, you can always use an online or email method as the first port of call and an easier way to open up, then switch to meeting up with the other person or talking together on the phone.

It's important you feel comfortable when you're asking for help, so choose the approach that resonates most with you.

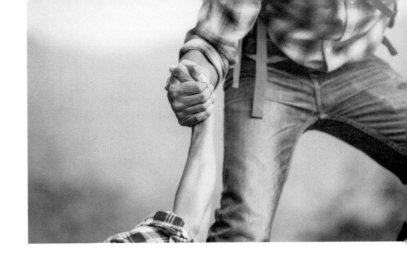

How to know when to ask for help

Sometimes when you're in the midst of everything and in a dark place, it can be hard to know exactly when you need to ask for help.

However much you practice your own self-care routine and regularly manage to achieve your self-care goals, sometimes it's not enough. When you're leading a busy life, working and socializing hard, burnout can occur. Burnout doesn't always happen suddenly: It can slowly and steadily creep up on you and catch you unawares.

As a rough guide, if your self-care routine doesn't seem to be as effective as normal, you're feeling disconnected from yourself, you're struggling with things, or you're feeling like you can't cope in your usual way, it's time to ask for help.

Seeking professional help

There are times when your self-care alone isn't enough and neither is asking for help from friends or family. If you feel that your mood has taken a serious dip, you're not coping well with life, or are suddenly very depressed, you need to seek advice from a medical practitioner.

It's by no means unusual for mental and emotional health problems to need the expertise of a health-care professional. Seeking help isn't a bad thing, and neither is it a sign that you're incapable of coping. It's brave, and a sign that you care about your wellness and want to make positive changes to get better.

It can help to take someone else with you to a medical appointment, both in terms of support and as an additional listening ear. It can sometimes be tricky to take in all the advice and information that you're given if you're feeling unwell.

It may be that you need extra support in the form of medication, treatment, or therapy, or perhaps you may need to be looked after as an inpatient for a while. As the wellness continuum model demonstrates (see page 17), pure medical care is necessary sometimes and plays a crucial part in health and wellness. Medical care can help you move forward to a point where you can begin to add in self-care routines and ultimately take over with pure self-care when you're feeling stronger.

Reaching out is a sign of strength and means that you're taking control.

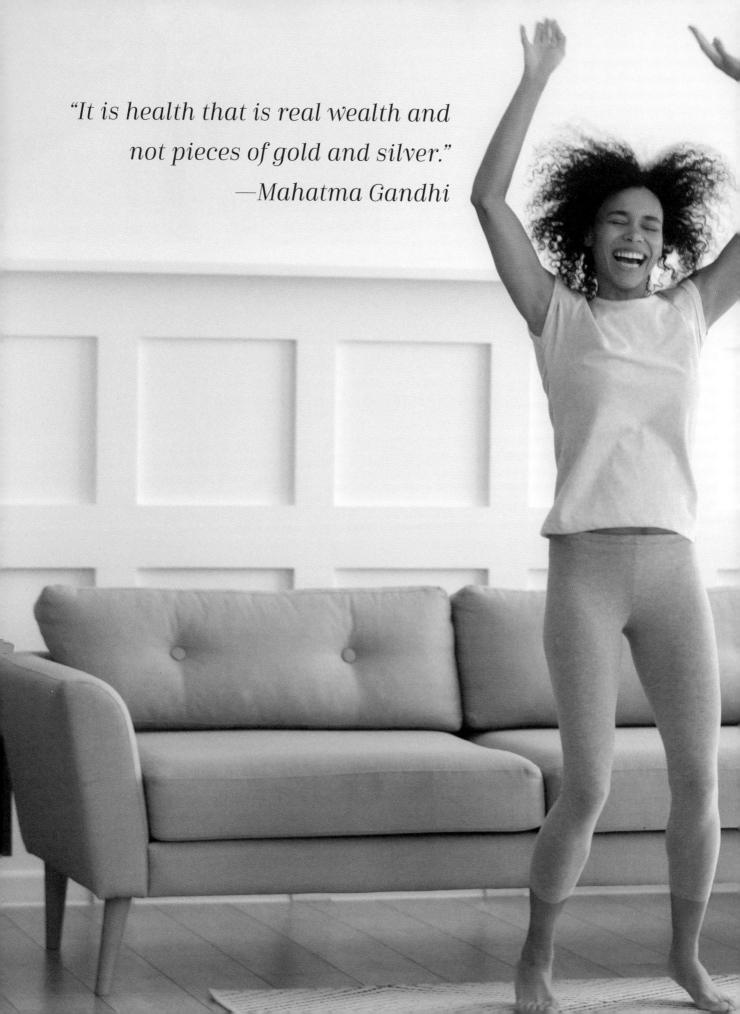

*"It is health that is real wealth and
not pieces of gold and silver."*
—Mahatma Gandhi

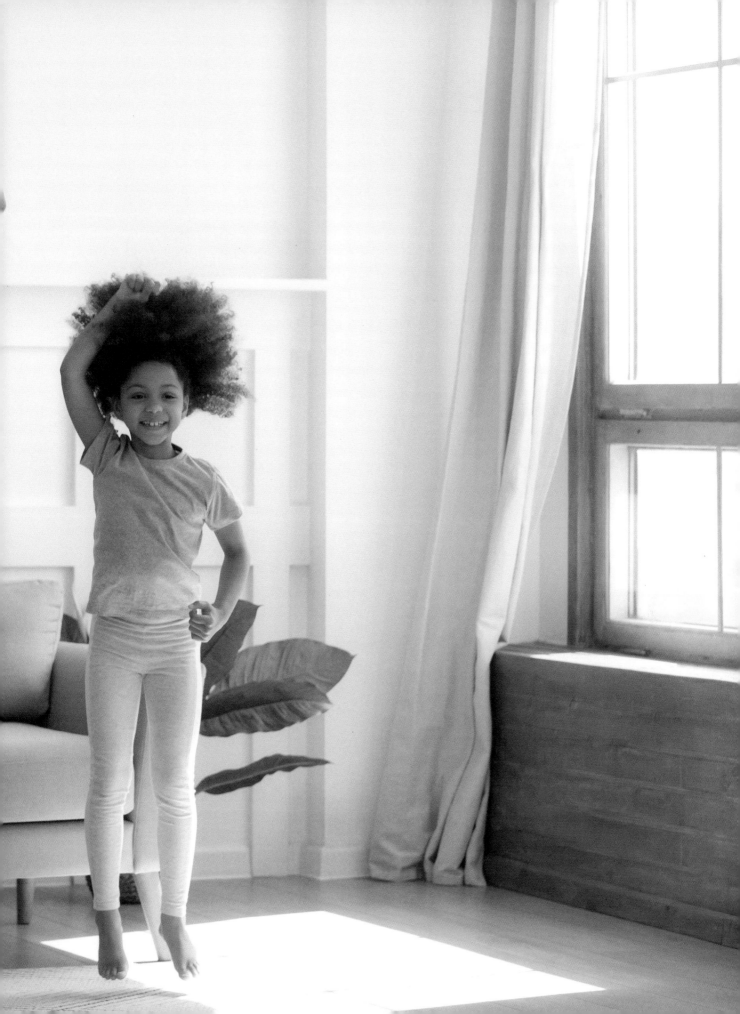

FINANCES

One aspect of life that can sadly be the cause of much stress and worry is money, yet some money woes can be eased by managing what you do have in a better way. By learning some practical money management skills, you can get a better handle on your income and expenses and reduce the amount of stress financial issues cause you. It's great for your peace of mind as well as your overall wellness.

Budgeting is a useful technique to use to help manage your money. In essence, budgeting simply involves keeping track of all the money you have coming in each month and all the money you need to pay out. Creating a budget helps you become more aware of your income and expenses and lets you see at a glance where your money goes. It helps you make better decisions about whether you have enough income to afford certain things, and allows you to ensure you've got enough money for everything that needs to be paid.

How to create a budget

To get started with creating a budget, you'll first need to determine how much you currently spend. Gather together all your statements and bills and make an accurate list of how much you spend each month on costs such as:

• Rent or mortgage payments • Utilities • Food • Broadband and phone • Clothing • Entertainment • Travel • Pets • Credit cards • Insurance

Be aware that there may be some bills that you have to pay only once or twice a year, such as your car insurance, and others that might change slightly each month, such as utility bills. Plus, there'll be times when you have unexpected bills, such as auto repairs or vet bills.

Next, make a note of your monthly and annual income. In an ideal scenario, your monthly bills and expenses will be less than your monthly income. If they're not, then this is a very good reason why a budget could help you!

If your income is less than your expenditure, then you need to look at ways to cut down on your expenses. The longer you spend more than you have, the more debt you'll accrue. Perhaps you can shop at a different store, buy generic groceries, cut out your daily coffee, or swap utility providers to save money?

If your income is more than your expenditure, then you're already in a good position, but budgeting each month could improve things even more.

Now you've got all your figures, it's time to set yourself a budget for each month. Make a plan of how much you need to cover all your bills, but still allow for extras when required. Write your targets down so you clearly know your budget aims. Do this at the beginning of every month, then during the month keep track of your income and expenditure, so you can see how you're faring. It helps to keep you motivated and allows you to make slight adjustments if you need to due to unexpected expenses.

Write your targets down so you clearly know your budget aims.

At the end of the month make sure you've recorded all your bills and expenses and look carefully at how you've done. Did you manage to stick to your budget or did you veer off course? If you went off course, why did it happen, and is it something you can rectify next month? Don't beat yourself up if you've not stuck to your budget rigidly; just accept that these things happen. Pick yourself up and start again next month.

How to set SMART financial goals

Setting yourself short- and long-term financial goals can boost your motivation and make budgeting more successful. Short-term financial goals might include wanting to save more money, pay off your credit card, save for a vacation, or pay for home improvements. Long-term money goals could include being able to live comfortably when you retire, being able to support your kids through college, or buying a property.

When you're setting yourself money goals, make them SMART: Specific, Measurable, Achievable, Relevant, and Time-bound.

By learning to manage your money more effectively, you'll feel more in control, comfortable, and confident that you can afford the lifestyle you have. Setting yourself goals will keep you on track and focused, and help you live and save within your means.

SPECIFIC GOAL	What do you want to save money for?
MEASURABLE GOAL	Can you break your goal down into measurable stages? For example, if you want to save $450 per month, that is just $15 per day.
ACHIEVABLE GOAL	Goals can be reached only if they're achievable within your means.
RELEVANT GOAL	Something that you know fits into your existing budget.
TIME-BOUND GOAL	When do you want to achieve your goal?

MONEY MANAGEMENT: SAVING

Successful money management involves knowing how and when to save money so that your financial situation works in the best way possible for you. There are various ways in which you can save money and make your earnings go further.

Savings accounts

It's always good to have a savings nest egg, as you never know when you might need to dip into it. Having a separate savings account works well, so that the money is separated from your general income and isn't used accidentally. Saving just a few dollars a week can add up considerably over the year. Try setting up a direct debit to make an automatic payment to your savings account each week or month, so that you've got no excuses and won't forget to follow through. Plus, make a pledge with yourself to touch the money you've saved only if you really need to. It doesn't help if you keep dipping into

it for nonessential items—a savings account is best left for important issues that arise.

If your bank offers the option to have several savings accounts, you could open a couple and designate each one to a specific need, such as savings for health care, vacations, or vet bills. Some people find it easier to allocate set amounts to each type of savings fund rather than have everything lumped together in one.

The interest on savings accounts can vary, so look for one that gives you the best deal.

Negotiating better deals

If you've paid the same amount for your car insurance, broadband, phone, or utility bills for years—give or take the usual annual rise in fees—you might be able to negotiate a better deal. It's worth spending time once a year shopping around for better deals that could save you money. A good time to do this is when your annual insurance products are up for renewal, as this can serve as a useful reminder to ensure you're getting the best deals elsewhere, too.

Look online or call a few companies to see what deals they could offer you for insurance or utilities. Sometimes it's best to switch to new companies that

offer better deals, but you could also use their quotes as leverage to negotiate with the companies you are already with. If you've been a loyal customer of theirs for some time, they may not want to lose you, so it's often possible to negotiate a better deal. If they won't budge on their quotes, then that could be a sign to go elsewhere.

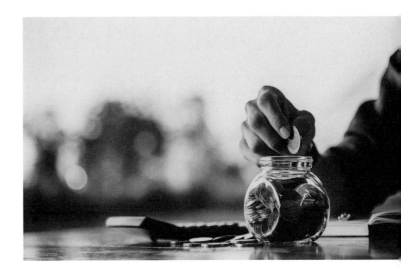

Saving money on shopping

If you've always bought branded goods, the chances are you're paying more than average for items, so think about whether you could save money by opting for store brands and generic items instead. In the case of food and drink, store brands are often similar and you soon adapt to any taste differences; you may even find that you prefer the taste of store brands. If you never try them, you'll never know.

You can save money on bills, food shopping, or other expenses by regularly looking out for discount offers or coupons to use. In some instances, you may be able to stack multiple coupons together and use them in one purchase for an even better discount. There are lots of forums, websites, and online social groups that focus on saving money and feature all the latest deals, so it's worth checking them out and signing up to get alerts.

Cash-back schemes

Some credit card companies offer cash-back schemes or their own points-based schemes whereby you can save money on your shopping or earn money back for purchases.

There are also various websites that give you cash back for shopping at certain sites. They work on an affiliate marketing basis—they get paid to direct shoppers through to other sites—but there's generally no cost involved for you, so it's worth doing. The amount you'll get back varies considerably, so you need to check out the rates before you click through. In some cases, for bigger purchases such as vacations or insurance products, there may be bigger savings or cash-back earnings available.

The interest on savings accounts can vary, so look for one that gives you the best deal.

MONEY MANAGEMENT: SPENDING WISELY

Learning to spend wisely will help you keep in control of your finances and prevent your spending from getting out of control. It's a process that goes hand in hand with successful budgeting and saving money. When it comes to spending wisely, the aim is to spend within your means and not go over your budget. This can of course be easier said than done, but for your health and well-being, sticking to a spending budget does help.

Track your spending

Your monthly spending is likely to consist of a range of different expenditures, such as direct debits for credit cards and bills, standing orders for mortgage payments or rent, plus other recurring payments for insurance, health care, water, and electricity bills. On top of that are all the other purchases you make throughout the month, be it expenses such as coffee or lunch, one-off payments on vacations and travel, gas for your car, or food for your pets.

Unless you look at your bank account or credit card statement regularly, it's very easy to lose track of exactly how much you spend each month. That's one of the reasons why it's also easy to spend more than you expected. Rather than have a nasty surprise when your bills arrive, it's better to take control and know exactly how much you're spending and what it's being used for.

Over the course of a month, set yourself the task of writing down everything you spend, on your credit card, debit card, standing orders, and in cash. Every single expense counts, be it coffees on the way to work, lunch and snacks, train and bus tickets, gym membership, food shopping, presents, cinema visits, clothing, or treats.

Write the details in a notebook, or create a simple template that you can use to record the transactions. When you're out and about, keep your receipts or make a note of money spent on your phone, then update the details at the end of each day.

When you get to the end of the month, add up each separate type of purchase that you've made (how much you've spent on coffee, meals out, travel fares, social activities, nights out, and so on).

Some people find it beneficial to stick to spending cash.

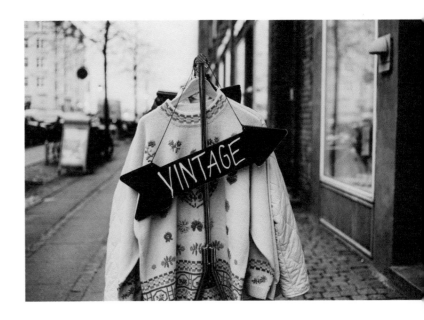

Analyze your spending

Now you have a record of your spending habits over the course of a month, it's time to analyze it. There will be regular payments you need to make each month, such as rent, mortgage, or electricity bills, but what other expenditure stands out? Are there any aspects of your lifestyle that you've spent a lot on over the course of a month?

The results might be eye-opening! When every tiny amount is written down and recorded, it puts your spending habits in perspective.

It's very easy to lose track of exactly how much you're spending when you use contactless payments or simply swipe a credit card to buy, and it's easy to forget how the small everyday purchases add up.

When you look at the reality of your monthly spending, consider if there's anything you could cut down on, especially if you want to save money. Could you prepare your own meals to take to work, negotiate a better phone deal, or walk more instead of taking a cab? A few simple tweaks and changes could make a significant difference.

Becoming a wise spender

In order to become a wise spender, you need to set yourself a budget and stick to it. Get into the habit of allocating yourself spending money each month as part of your budget. You could use it for meals out, cinema trips, or for buying yourself a treat. Any money that you don't spend each month can form a rolling budget or be added to your savings account.

Some people find it beneficial to stick to spending cash rather than using a credit card, as it can make you more accountable and aware of exactly how much you're spending. It's so easy to use a credit card and not take note of how much you've spent, so seeing the actual amount of cash left can be a stark reminder.

One method that can make this work effectively for you is to allocate cash to specific envelopes. For example, put $75 into an envelope marked "treats" and $200 into one marked "food." This helps to separate out your cash spending and ensure you don't accidentally spend it on the wrong category.

FINDING SIMPLICITY

On a daily basis we face an ongoing barrage of messages that endeavor to convince us that having more, becoming more, doing more, and possessing more are the pathways to happiness, fulfillment, and security. All of the great spiritual traditions deliver a somewhat different message, suggesting that genuine happiness lies within our own hearts and minds and can never be truly secured through the multiplicity of possessions, identities, and achievements we gather.

Simplicity in action

Genuine simplicity does not depend upon the absence of activity or engagement.

In our lives we act, make choices, and move through a world that needs our attention. The activities we engage in, when undertaken with awareness, communicate and embody all that we value and respect.

Our aspirations are realized through action and expression. Our choices and acts have the power to communicate a profound calmness, compassion, integrity, and connectedness. A meditative life does not depend upon retreating to the nearest monastery or cave, but learning to be present in all the activities of our lives with awareness and balance. The countless activities that make up our days are not obstacles to peace or stillness.

Undertaken with mindfulness and sensitivity, they become the places in which we learn to deepen the calmness and peace we treasure. The wisest people, who have been central in bringing about the greatest social, political, and spiritual transformations, have been people of engagement and action. Moved by compassion, understanding, and care, they have been fully present in their communities, relationships, and world. Their inner core of balance and understanding has found its expression in the choices and activities they have dedicated themselves to. In a life that often seems overfull, with little ease or downtime, we may come to believe that we have to postpone a deep spiritual life until we reach a point where life asks less of us. Yet a meditative life doesn't demand that we forsake the world, but that we forsake postponement. We can bring simplicity and stillness to our lives in the midst of activity.

We can bring simplicity and stillness to our lives in the midst of activity.

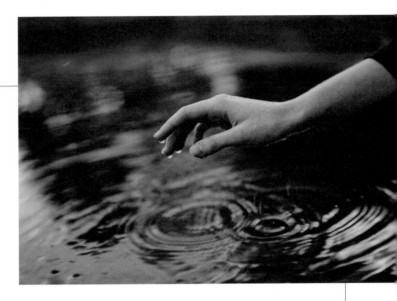

A daily practice: simplicity

As you move into your day, take with you the intention to notice all the moments when no specific activity demands your attention. They might be moments traveling to or from work, breaks in your working day, or a lull at the end of the day in which nothing demands your engagement.

Sense what happens in your mind and body in those moments. Be aware if you are carrying an inclination to immediately fill that space with something to occupy your attention. There may be an urge to pick up a book, turn on the radio, make a telephone call, or search for food.

See if it is possible to restrain the immediate impulse toward busyness or distraction and to simply rest in that moment. Initially you may find that these spaces of "nothing to do" feel moderately uncomfortable or carry with them a sense of there being something missing. Bring your attention to your body and mind to simply explore the landscape of that sense of unease, without judging it in any way.

Reflect on how you might feel at home in stillness, in "non-doing." Initially, the simplicity of stillness and "non-doing" may reveal the complexity and busyness of your mind. Pay attention to the thought streams that arise in those moments rather than being pushed by them into new cycles of busyness.

You might experiment with adopting the lulls in your day as times when you commit yourself to stillness and simplicity. They can be moments in which you befriend your mind and body, learn to let go of some of the busyness that drives you, and discover the deep sense of ease and resting in the moment that may be available to you. Instead of focusing upon what appears to be missing, bring your attention to what is present. The capacity to connect with your mind, body, and present moment is available to you.

You may discover that your capacity to feel at ease in stillness and simplicity brings with it a greater sensitivity and awareness. Let stillness and simplicity be regular companions in each day, a source of renewal and creativity.

Take some moments to reflect upon your life and sense where it is cluttered by objects that no longer serve you well. What are you holding on to, out of anxiety, that you no longer need? Sense whether letting it go would create more spaciousness in your life.

Reflect on what your mind most frequently dwells on. Sense whether the spaciousness of your own mind has been undermined by preoccupations, fantasies, goals, or desires that do not contribute to your well-being. Is it possible to let them go?

Reflect on your life and sense where it may be possible for you to create a greater simplicity. What would you be asked to let go of?

Sense how many of the richest and deepest moments of happiness in your life have been moments of great simplicity. Reflect on what it would mean for simplicity to be a dedicated theme in your life.

WORKPLACE WELLNESS

Being aware of your self-care at work and taking action to boost it is important to create a better sense of wellness in the workplace. You're likely to spend a considerable number of hours a week at work, perhaps under stress or working to strict deadlines and targets, and this can take its toll on your health. The environment you work in, your seating or standing position, and the physical and mental effects of the work can all have an impact on your wellness.

Some employers have become aware of the important role that workplace wellness plans can play and have begun to implement changes to help employees. Research has found that by looking after employee well-being, employers benefit from reduced sickness rates, better work productivity, and increased resilience.

Whether or not your employer has such a plan in action, there are practical steps that you can take to ensure your personal well-being at work is a priority and that you're looking after yourself as well as possible.

Office plants

Having fresh, green, healthy plants in an office—whether small plants positioned on your desk, or larger plants in pots on the floor—could help you feel better at work.

They bring an element of the outdoor natural world inside, and green can be a calming color to have around. Research has shown that incorporating plants into the design of the workplace can boost productivity levels. What's more, plants create a cleaner environment by helping to remove indoor toxins, making the space healthier to work in. There's also evidence that plants positioned at strategic points may absorb noise in the office, which is useful in an open-plan setting.

Hydration

For your physical health, drinking plenty of water throughout the day is essential. If your workplace has a water fountain, make use of it! Or take your own water bottle to work and refill it throughout the day. Some insulated bottles will help keep water cool.

If you get bored with drinking water and would like some variety, bring slices of fruit to work and put them inside a water bottle to add some natural fruity flavor. Aim to drink eight glasses of water daily for optimal hydration.

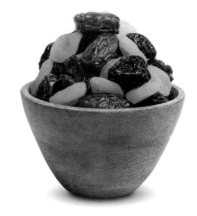

Dried fruit

Workplace posture

How you sit can have a positive or negative effect on your body and in turn affect your health and well-being. Your human resources department should be aware of workplace ergonomics, and any working equipment should be appropriately tailored. As a guide, if you're sitting at a desk, your computer monitor should be positioned at eye level, so your head looks straight at it without you tilting your neck. Office chairs supplied by your employer should support your back; if your back or shoulders tend to slouch while sitting, you may benefit from having a lumbar support on your chair to encourage your upper back to remain straight. For the best position, aim to keep your feet flat on the ground while you're sitting, and pull your shoulders back so your back is flat against the chair.

Movement

If you spend a lot of your working day sitting at a desk, or being in the same position, taking time to move around will be beneficial. You could balance out all the sitting by walking to work in the morning, or by getting off the bus a stop early and incorporating a short walk into your morning routine. At work, consider taking the stairs instead of the elevator and, where possible, have short breaks in which you stretch, stand up, and walk around.

If your work situation allows it, you could swap a conventional desk for a standing desk, as this could help reduce postural issues and stiff joints.

Break reminders

If you get so absorbed in what you're doing that you tend to forget to take a break, try a reminder app. Apps can be downloaded onto your work computer or your phone and can be set up to remind you to take a break at regular intervals. Ideally, try to get up and away from your desk every hour.

Fresh air

Being stuck inside working, especially in a busy office, can get stuffy and hot. Where possible, try to get some fresh air during the day, either by opening a window or taking a quick walk outside. Fresh air can help you clear your head and improve your productivity.

Snacks

If sugary and fatty snacks are common in your workplace, avoid them by taking in your own healthy treats. A slice of cake every now and then is fine, but not every day! Healthier food will help prevent the sudden highs and lows of energy that are caused by a sugar rush.

TIME MANAGEMENT

Effective time management is crucial in a work environment where you're juggling multiple priorities and tasks. If you're going to get everything completed successfully without ending up stressed and exhausted, you need to know how to manage your time, prioritize responsibilities, and learn when to say no to unreasonable requests.

It can take time to find the best way for you to manage work tasks and balance your self-care needs, but it's worth persevering until you get it right. Good time management involves giving yourself realistic, achievable goals, setting boundaries, and knowing when to take breaks.

Setting boundaries

Healthy work-related boundaries help define how you work and guide your relationships with colleagues, managers, and clients.

Boundaries are crucial, as they determine your physical and emotional limits. You can use boundaries to protect yourself from taking on too much work, dealing with unreasonable requests, or getting too involved in office politics. In order to be healthy, a work boundary needs to be flexible and open to change as situations and circumstances evolve. You need to be able to control your limits, but not obsess about them remaining rigid forever.

Setting healthy boundaries at work can sometimes seem tricky, as you don't want to upset your colleagues or how they view you. But if you communicate clearly and ensure your boundaries are mutually beneficial and supportive, everyone should be happy.

If you're not sure how or where you need to set boundaries, take some time to think about the actions, situations, and people in your workplace that make you feel uncomfortable, irritated, or stressed. Then think about what changes could be made to make you feel better and more comfortable. Talk to any other people involved to get their point of view (they may well see the situation in a completely different way) and come to a mutually acceptable way of dealing with it. Good communication is essential in order for boundaries to work.

Taking breaks

Taking breaks is vital for your health, well-being, and self-care. Your workplace should include set break times within the working day, as you are legally entitled to these. If you're self-employed and managing your schedule yourself, you'll need to be disciplined about setting your own breaks.

Studies have shown that if you don't take breaks, your productivity, mental well-being, and work performance all suffer, so doing so is good for both you and your employer.

It's also important to step away from the computer screen regularly, as too long spent in front

Don't be tempted to stay sitting at your desk during your break—this doesn't count!

of a screen can lead to eye strain or headaches. In fact, experts suggest it's beneficial to look away from your screen every 20 minutes. As you look away, fix your eye on something else approximately 20 feet away for at least 20 seconds. This simple act could help reduce the strain on your eyes.

Don't be tempted to stay sitting at your desk during your break—this doesn't count! Get up,

stretch, move your body, and get a change of scene.

A proper time-out away from your desk gives you the chance to incorporate healthy self-care habits into your daily routine: for example, eating a healthy lunch, going for a walk outside in the fresh air or a jog around the block, having a five-minute mindfulness or meditation session, or even fitting in a quick ten-minute power nap if you need one.

Time management tips

Use these practical time management tips to help you learn to organize your time more effectively and ensure you complete all the essential tasks you need to do.

Be organized
Write lists so you're clear on what you need to do. Prioritize tasks so you get the most important things done first. Do them one at a time and enjoy checking them off your list when they're completed.

Allocate your time
Manage your time effectively by allocating specific amounts of time to certain tasks or activities. For example, allow for working, socializing, spending time with family, exercising, taking part in hobbies, and relaxing.

Set deadlines
Set yourself deadlines for when things need to be completed. Make sure they're realistic—it's not helpful to put yourself under excess pressure.

Be flexible
Accept that not everything goes to plan and interruptions do occur. Add some extra time in your schedule that allows you to be flexible if you don't get everything done as planned. Be kind to yourself!

Delegate
Don't try to do everything yourself. Where possible, delegate tasks to other people—whether that's work colleagues, friends, or family.

Be assertive
Learn to say "no" to unreasonable requests—and mean it. You can't take everything on, whether it comes from work colleagues, friends, or family.

Plan time for yourself
Make sure you designate time in your schedule for yourself each day, so you can relax, look after your own needs, and enjoy doing the things you love.

Set finishing times
Set yourself finishing times and stick to them. This is especially important if you're self-employed and don't have a specific end point to your day.

OPPORTUNITIES FOR LEARNING

The benefits of learning should never be overlooked. You're never too old to learn something new. In fact, as part of your self-care it's worth seeking out opportunities for learning.

Studies have found that developing skills or knowledge can play a positive role in aiding well-being. Learning something new can boost social qualities such as confidence, self-esteem, optimism, and a sense of purpose. It can also provide new directions to your life, unexpectedly open doors, and improve social connections—helping you meet people, make new friends, and increase your social support network.

Learning doesn't have to be hard work, nor does it have to take place in a classroom. It can take many forms—vocational, artistic, physical, or musical. Some things can be learned on your own, through reading books, listening to podcasts, or watching videos, while others are best learned in a group or on a one-to-one basis. Be open to, and look for, new learning opportunities in your life; you never know where they'll take you.

Learning opportunities at work

Learning new skills related to your job could broaden your horizons in the workplace. It could even provide a route to a new career pathway or promotion. If your employer offers work-related courses, consider signing up or ask if there's anything available that you could do. If your supervisor could do with a prompt, seek out relevant courses yourself, then propose something that you'd like to do. It will make you seem proactive and keen, as well as creating a great opportunity for you.

Adult education classes

There are always plenty of evening and adult education classes available in local neighborhoods, often held at high schools or colleges. The courses frequently run parallel to school semesters, so look for details being advertised near the start of each semester. Other places to look for learning opportunities include arts centers, theater groups, community centers, and via independent craftspeople.

Adult education classes can take many forms. Physical classes help hone your exercise skills and improve your fitness. Art classes can unleash your creativity and give you the chance to explore new forms of expression. Cooking classes help you improve your cooking skills, understand what constitutes a healthy diet, and discover new dishes to try. Technical classes can teach you new skills. Literary classes introduce you to different authors and deepen your connection with books. Health classes teach skills such as first aid or offer tips and insight into living a healthy lifestyle.

Online courses

If your free time is limited due to work and family commitments, an alternative option is to do an online course. Many of these are professionally run and offer just as good a learning experience as taking a course in person. Plus, they often have interactive elements, too, such as forums or online sessions with other students, so you still reap the benefits of social interaction with the instructor and the other students.

Some online courses can be completed at your own pace, which might fit in better with a busy schedule, while others need to be completed during a set time period. Courses can be paid for or free to participate in.

To find online courses that would suit your needs and interests, search the Internet, check the websites of local schools, or ask online groups for ideas about what might be on offer. Ask friends or work colleagues if they've taken any courses online recently; getting a personal recommendation is always useful.

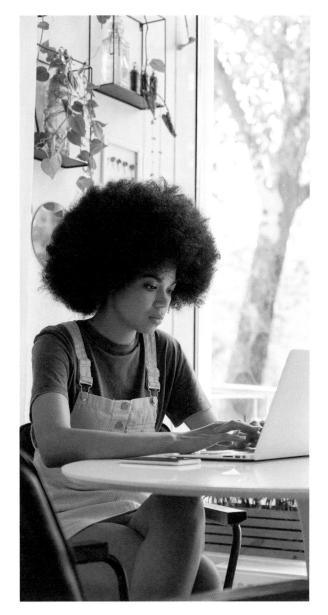

Volunteering

Another option that can provide valuable learning opportunities is volunteering.

There's always a variety of charitable groups and organizations looking for help from volunteers, either on a regular or occasional basis. Volunteering your time to help with a cause that means a lot to you can offer good social opportunities as well as a chance to grow and learn.

You can volunteer to help local, national, or even international organizations; volunteering abroad can double up as a vacation or educational trip, although you do need to take the cost of travel and accommodation into consideration.

Sometimes employers enable employees to take an occasional day to volunteer with a local cause—ask your human resources department if there are any opportunities available. If not, perhaps it's something you could suggest for the future?

SETTING GOALS

Setting goals is a great way of giving yourself a sense of meaning and purpose. Goals can be used in any area of your life, from physical well-being—challenging yourself to eat healthier food or exercise more regularly; to emotional well-being—learning to love yourself more or boost your confidence; and to social well-being—making a new friend or getting a new job.

By setting yourself goals, you give yourself something to aim for and achieve. Goals can keep you interested and engaged, especially if you have mini milestones along the way, and it's great to be able to celebrate when you eventually reach them. Studies have shown that if you want to make a change in your life, setting yourself a target will make you more likely to achieve it.

When you're setting yourself wellness-related goals, it's helpful to have a mix of different aims that are achievable at different points in time—for example, daily, weekly, monthly, or long-term goals. It's good to have one or two long-term goals, but having too many might make them seem too far away or out of your reach, and you don't want to end up feeling despondent about your chances of achieving them.

How to set goals

When you're setting goals, start by deciding exactly what it is you'd like to achieve. It needs to be something you really want, as well as something that you're excited about and will stick to. It doesn't have to be a huge goal; in fact, it's good to start small and then work up to something bigger.

Be realistic and take into account aspects such as your existing commitments and energy levels, and ensure it's something you can currently see yourself being able to achieve.

Write down your goal. Describe exactly what you'd like to achieve and why. Committing it to paper firms up your decision and increases your chances of sticking to it. Telling somebody else about it also helps to hold you accountable.

Plan how you're going to reach your goal. What steps do you need to take? If necessary, do some research into how best you could work toward your goal, or ask a friend for help. Depending on the nature of your goal, you may find it easier to break it down into several smaller steps or stages.

Think about any obstacles or issues that might occur and consider ways in which you could deal with them. Planning in advance for potential problems can make it easier to deal with them if they do arise.

As you work toward your goal, maintain a positive attitude and check off the smaller milestones as you reach them. If you need help along the way, ask your friends, family, or support network.

If life throws you a curveball and your circumstances change, don't be hard on yourself or abandon your aims completely. Just reset your goal, adjust it as necessary, and resume working toward it.

When you reach your goal, celebrate your

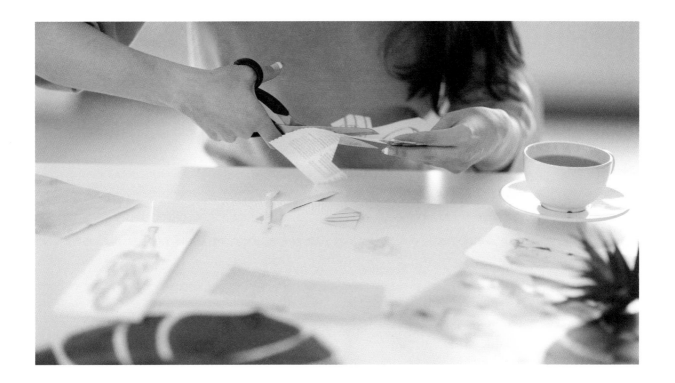

It's good to start small and then work up to something bigger.

success! Feel proud of your achievements and your perseverance, and enjoy the moment with friends. Once you've achieved your goal, you'll know how good it feels and how motivated having that target has kept you, so you might want to consider setting yourself another goal.

Create a vision board

Some people find goals easier to aim for if they can visualize the end result. That's where creating a vision board comes in handy.

A vision board is literally a visual representation of your goal or aim. If your goal is to save enough money to go on vacation, your vision board could have pictures of the location you'd like to go to, and images of the things you'd do while there—swimming in a pool, visiting historic landmarks, or relaxing on a beach.

A vision board doesn't have to just be made up of images; you can also add words or sentences describing your goal and how you'll feel when you achieve it. You can create a board the old-school way—by cutting out images and sticking them on a board—or draw one up digitally.

However you choose to put together your vision board, the idea is to hang it up somewhere you'll see it frequently. That will help keep your goal visible and in your mind, and motivate you to continue to strive for it. If it's something you feel awkward about other people seeing, or if you live in a shared house or apartment, you could always put it inside a cupboard or a drawer where only you will see it.

IMPROVING YOUR WORK–LIFE BALANCE

If your work–life balance is feeling slightly off-kilter and your physical or mental wellness is suffering, it's time to do your best to rectify the situation. Thankfully, there are plenty of practical ways in which you can improve the balance and try to get your home and work life back on track.

Stick to your hours

If you have a very busy or stressful job, it's tempting to work overtime to try and catch up or get everything completed. Although this is fine once in a while, going over your set hours on a regular basis can have a detrimental effect on your wellness. Aim to stick to your set hours as much as possible, especially if you don't get paid extra for overtime. It will do you good to switch off from work.

Be honest when you're struggling

If you're struggling with an excessive workload or extreme demands, no one will know unless you speak up and be honest about it. It's in your employer's best interest to try and come up with a way to resolve the problem and help you cope with the work, and it could make a big improvement on how you feel and your overall ability to perform at work.

Work smart

Adopt the habit of working smart by prioritizing the tasks you need to do and breaking them up into small, achievable chunks. Make a plan for the day of the things you need to do and, if relevant, when you need to get them done by. Where possible, try and stick to your schedule and avoid getting caught up in less productive activities or sidetracked by unexpected emails.

Separate work from home

Once you've left work, try and leave all thoughts of it behind and focus on your home life. Of course, separating your work life from your home life can be tricky if you work from home. Ideally, in a home-working situation it's good to do your work in a room that isn't in the general thoroughfare of your house—use a spare room upstairs or a room with privacy. If you can't do that, then make sure you clear up all your work equipment and paperwork at the end of the day, so that your home space can revert to being a nonwork location. That way you'll also hopefully be less tempted to do any more work or check your emails in the evening. Nonwork time should be dedicated to you, your family, and friends.

It's always useful to understand exactly what rights you have in your place of work.

Separate home from work

In the same way, it's important not to let home or social-related issues swerve into your work. This isn't always easy if you're having a difficult time, but when you go to work try and leave any other issues you're having at home. Dwelling on things during the day could have a detrimental effect on your ability to concentrate and function at work. Instead, try and be mindful and be in the present; you can deal with everything else when you've finished work.

Understand your rights at work

It's always useful to understand exactly what rights you have in your place of work. If it's a long time since you signed your contract, check back and give it another read. Find out what working hours you should be doing, what sick pay you're entitled to, and how much vacation you can take. If you're unsure or have any concerns about the working practices, speak to someone from your human resources department for advice.

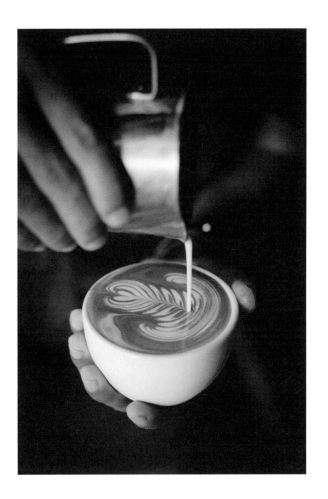

Make changes

If you're really unhappy with any part of your work or home life and nothing seems to be helping, consider whether you need to make changes. Perhaps the job is no longer suitable for you or your relationship isn't working. Change is really hard to deal with, especially on your own, so seek help from friends, family, or work unions and investigate the practical changes you could make to improve things. At the end of the day, your health and wellness matter and there's no point continuing to do things that are making you unhappy or ill.

SPATIAL WELLNESS AT HOME

Health and well-being involve more than just physical and emotional health—your sense of well-being can also be strongly affected by spatial elements. Studies have found that the surroundings you live in can enhance your well-being and have a positive impact on your mood and perception of happiness. So it makes sense to create a living environment that makes you feel happy, safe, stable, and secure.

Your home is your personal domain and it's a place to which you should be able to retreat and where you can feel comfortable, nurtured, and relaxed. In many ways, your home is an extension of your identity—how you decorate it, the furniture you own, and the accessories on display all reflect your individual interests and traits.

There's a lot that you can do to influence and control your sense of spatial wellness and well-being at home, and it's definitely worth investing time and effort into making improvements if you feel a sense of imbalance in this area.

How to improve spatial wellness at home

Your social wellness can be helped by living in a place that you feel safe in. You may not be able to change the wider external environment around you, but you can play an active part in ensuring that your home feels safe and nurturing when you're inside it.

If you currently don't feel safe at home, think about changes you could make that could improve this. For example, would changing the locks, adding window locks, having a burglar alarm fitted, adding

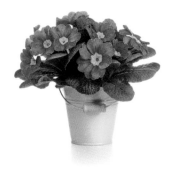

a fire and carbon monoxide alarm, or fitting a new, stronger front door improve your perception of safety and security?

Make a list of the changes you're keen to make, then rate them in order of priority. If you're short on funds, you may need to choose the most appropriate and affordable option, rather than trying to do everything at once.

If you live directly on a road or your front door opens straight in off the sidewalk, you might feel exposed or a bit vulnerable as people pass by. To make you feel safer, you could fit slatted blinds in your windows. These are a modern alternative to net curtains and are practical, as you can angle them in a way that ensures people can't look in, but you can still see out and still have a good level of light coming in.

Your home is your personal domain and it's a place to which you should be able to retreat.

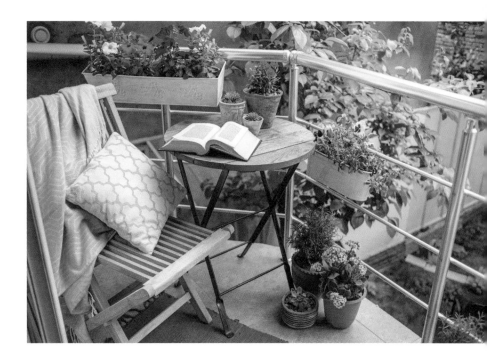

If you have a garden, backyard, or small area of outdoor space at your home, using walls or fences to mark out the boundaries of your space can increase feelings of safety and security. If your neighbors can see right into your property and you don't feel comfortable with this, consider putting up higher fences, adding panels of trellis to the top of existing fences, or planting trees, climbing plants, or shrubs to naturally fill the gaps.

Before making structural changes, such as putting up higher fences or altering existing walls, make sure that they are yours to alter—you don't want to find yourself dealing with neighbor disputes!

It can be tricky making improvements if you're in a rental property or house share, when the changes aren't fully under your control. If you have strong concerns about lack of safety and security, such as apartments not having intercom systems or the locks not being as secure as they could be, speak to the landlord or rental agency and see if they would consider making—or allowing you to make—the improvements.

Moving to a new home

Uprooting yourself from a familiar living environment can understandably disturb your sense of stability. This is especially so if you move frequently due to work or study and keep having to get used to new properties and living arrangements.

Even though having to move might be beyond your control, you can create a sense of stability by having familiar possessions and decor in your home. The building and location may be different, but surrounding yourself with favorite items, photographs of loved ones, and memories of happy times, as well as artworks that make you feel good, can help your feelings of positivity and aid your perception of stability.

Keeping communication channels open with friends and family and staying in touch regularly can increase your personal sense of well-being and keep you grounded, even if your living arrangements feel shaky and unstable.

IMPROVING SPATIAL WELLNESS

Improving your spatial wellness at home also involves creating a healthy living environment. Research studies have shown that homes that are untidy, unclean, and unkempt are more likely to be associated with physical and mental health issues, such as allergies, stress, and even depression. In contrast, if you live in a clean, tidy, and organized home, you're more likely to feel happy, healthier, and positive.

Think about how your home makes you feel. When you step through the front door, do you feel relaxed, calm, and happy to be back? Or does the sight of piles of ironing, dirty dishes, and untidiness make you want to leave again? If it's the latter scenario, now's the time to rectify it. It's your home and you have the power to control what it looks like and how it makes you feel.

Cleaning your home

If you're not a fan of housework, you're not alone! It's a task many people detest, but in order to have a clean home, doing some housework is essential. Dust is renowned for building up in a seemingly never-ending manner, and if you have children or pets, keeping floors and surfaces clean may seem like an endless task.

The key to preventing the idea of housework from becoming overwhelming is to break it down into smaller, more manageable chunks. For example, tasks such as vacuuming the stairs, cleaning the kitchen, cleaning the bathroom, and dusting certain rooms can be done individually, rather than all in one long slog. Some people find that tackling a little bit of cleaning every day works for them, while others favor doing it on certain days.

However you choose to organize your time and fit chores into your week, write yourself a cleaning schedule to keep yourself on track. Building tasks into your regular schedule and doing them at set times means they're more likely to become a habit. And if you've got other family members or housemates on hand to help, delegating tasks to them will also help relieve the pressure! As the saying goes, "many hands make light work."

If you really don't like cleaning, or have only limited time available, consider hiring someone to do it for you. It doesn't have to be an expensive investment and it can help reduce any stress you have about getting it all done on your own. Find a local cleaner by asking for recommendations from friends or neighbors—you may be surprised by how many people you know have their own cleaners!

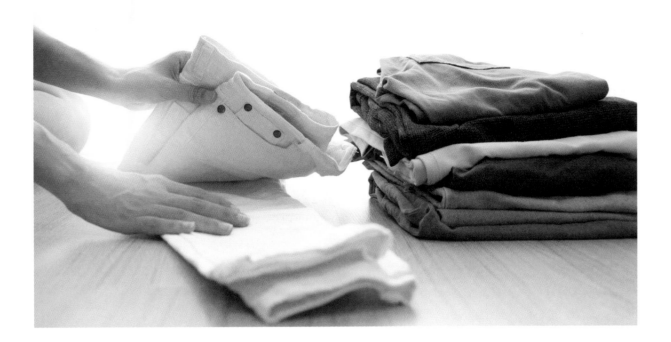

Organizing your home

In the same way that cleaning your home can have a positive impact on your well-being, so too can organizing it.

Clutter can have a damaging effect on your sense of well-being, mood, and even your relationships. It may affect your social life, too, if you're reluctant to invite people to your home when it looks untidy. With a bit of care and attention, a disorganized house can be transformed into a clutter-free haven.

Take time to examine your house and reflect on the good and bad points in each room. Look for particular areas of clutter and untidiness that need to be sorted. For example, are your kids' toys scattered all over the floor in your living room, do your kitchen cupboards need to be reorganized in a better way, or are your closets overflowing with clothes?

If you live in a shared house and aren't able to tidy or reorganize shared rooms, instead focus on any spaces that are purely yours, such as your bedroom or your food cupboards in the kitchen.

Devote time to tidying and reorganization. Don't try to do everything at once; tackle one task at a time. If you've got stuff that you just don't need anymore, be ruthless and donate it to charity or sell it at a yard sale.

In the case of items that are untidy but needed, such as kids' toys, look for ways you could contain them better. Invest in storage containers, pieces of furniture that have hidden storage solutions (such as a blanket box or divan-style bed with drawers built into the base), and put those items away out of sight.

Reorganized cupboards can make finding things much easier, so take out all the items and carefully decide what needs to go back in and what can be donated or put elsewhere. In the case of kitchen or bathroom cupboards, use storage pots to organize similar items, such as packets or boxes, so that you can find items more easily.

Once you've tackled your problem areas, work at keeping them tidy and encourage your partner or kids to do so, too. Adopting a policy of "one item in, one item out" could help you control the items in your home and keep clutter from getting out of hand.

SELF-CARE CHECKLIST

PHYSICAL WELLNESS	MONDAY	TUESDAY	WEDNESDAY	THURSDAY
Go to bed at the same time each night.				
Drink eight glasses of water throughout the day.				
Practice mindful eating.				
Every day, do 10 minutes of an exercise you enjoy.				
Cook a healthy meal.				
EMOTIONAL WELLNESS				
Spend 10 minutes meditating each day.				
Write down five things that make you happy.				
Turn negative thoughts into positive ones.				
Spend 30 minutes reading or being creative.				
Focus on your breathing.				

SOCIAL WELLNESS

Take a five-minute break at work and go for a walk or have a stretch.				
Phone, email, or text a friend with whom you've not connected recently.				
Spend 10 minutes tidying and organizing your home.				
Enjoy spending time with family or friends.				
Set yourself a goal and a plan to save money.				

FRIDAY	SATURDAY	SUNDAY

Improve your self-care habits

Each week try to add a new self-care habit to your routine. It will provide you with more variation and help you develop new healthy habits.

• Walk or cycle to work instead of driving.

• Look at your monthly expenses and see what savings you can make.

• Get to know an acquaintance better—talk to them and listen to what they have to say.

• Start a gratitude journal and record the things that you're grateful for.

• Try cooking a meal with ingredients you wouldn't normally use.

• Give yourself a foot massage.

• Create an area of sacred space where you can be still and unwind.

• Try a new hobby or creative activity.

• Focus on being kinder and more compassionate to yourself and others.

• Discover new opportunities for learning.

• Pamper yourself with a new skin-care product or a manicure.

• Make a cleaning playlist of your favorite songs so you can play it when you're doing the housework.

• Learn to say "no" to unreasonable requests.

• Make a list of happy and uplifting music to play if you're feeling down.

RESOURCES

FOR TIMES OF CRISIS

Samaritans and the National Suicide Prevention Lifeline

1-(800)-273-TALK (8255)

http://www.samaritansusa.org

https://suicidepreventionlifeline.org

Crisis Text Line

Text HOME to 741741

crisistextline.org

HELP WITH ADDICTIONS

Alcoholics Anonymous

www.aa.org

475 Riverside Drive

11th and 8th Floors

New York, NY 10115

The Recovery Village Drug and Alcohol Rehab

www.therecoveryvillage.com

633 Umatilla Blvd.

Umatilla, FL 32784

Smoke Free

https://smokefree.gov

Substance Abuse and Mental Health Service Administration

1-800-662-HELP (4357)

www.samhsa.gov/find-treatment

COUNSELING AND PSYCHOTHERAPY

American Art Therapy Association

https://arttherapy.org

4875 Eisenhower Ave., Suite 240

Alexandria, VA 22304

American Counseling Association

www.counseling.org

American Psychological Association

www.apa.org

750 First St. NE

Washington, DC 20002-4242

American Psychotherapy Association

www.americanpsychotherapy.com

2750 E. Sunshine St.

Springfield, MO 65804

National Alliance on Mental Illness

www.nami.org

FLOWER REMEDIES

Bach Flower Remedies

www.bachremedies.com/en-us

Nelsons, 21 High Street #302

North Andover, MA 01845

Flower Essence Society

www.flowersociety.org

P.O. Box 459

Nevada City, CA 95959

MEDITATION AND MINDFULNESS

American Meditation Society

www.americanmeditationsociety.org

490 Chancellor Dr.

Edwardsville, IL 62025

Heartfulness

www.heartfulnessinstitute.org

International Mindfulness Teachers Association

www.imta.org

JOURNALING

Center for Journal Therapy

https://journaltherapy.com

3440 Youngfield St., #411

Wheat Ridge, CO 80033

QIGONG

Qigong Institute

www.qigonginstitute.org

617 Hawthorne Ave.

Los Altos, CA 94024

National Qigong Association

www.nqa.org

YOGA AND PILATES

International Association of Yoga Therapists

www.iayt.org

P.O. Box 251563

Little Rock, AR 72225

Yoga Alliance

www.yogaalliance.org

1560 Wilson Blvd. #700

Arlington, VA 22209

Pilates Method Alliance

www.pilatesmethodalliance.org

1666 Kennedy Causeway

Suite 402

North Bay Village, FL 33141

United States Pilates Association

unitedstatespilatesassociation.com

PERSONAL TRAINING

National Aerobics and Fitness Trainers Association

https://naftafitness.org

28170 N. Alma School Pkwy, Suite 201

Scottsdale, AZ 85262

NUTRITION

Academy of Nutrition and Dietetics

www.eatright.org

120 South Riverside Plaza

Suite 2190

Chicago, IL 60606-6995

American Nutrition Association

theana.org

211 West Chicago Avenue, Suite 217

Hinsdale, IL 60521

Canadian Association of Natural Nutritional Practitioners

www.cannp.ca

Dietitians of Canada

www.dietitians.ca

AROMATHERAPY

Alliance of International Aromatherapists

www.alliance-aromatherapists.org

3758 E 104th Ave. #36

Thornton, CO 80233

Aromatherapy Registration Council

https://aromatherapycouncil.org

National Association for Holistic Aromatherapy (NAHA)

www.naha.org

Pacific Institute of Aromatherapy

www.pacificinstituteofaromatherapy.com

HERBALISM

American Herbalists Guild

www.americanherbalistsguild.com

P.O. Box 3076

Asheville, NC 28802-3076

The Herb Society of America

www.herbsociety.org

9019 Kirtland Chardon Rd.

Kirtland, OH 44094

ACUPUNCTURE

American Academy of Medical Acupuncture

https://medicalacupuncture.org

2512 Artesia Blvd.

Suite 200

Redondo Beach, CA 90278

MASSAGE

American Massage Therapy Association

www.amtamassage.org

500 Davis Street

Suite 900

Evanston, IL 60201

MAKING CONNECTIONS

American Red Cross

Find out if the Red Cross needs local volunteers

www.redcross.org/volunteer/become-a-volunteer

Meetup

An online resource for finding local events and organizations

www.meetup.com

VolunteerMatch

Search for volunteering opportunities in your local area

www.volunteermatch.org

FURTHER READING

PHYSICAL WELLNESS

2,100 Asanas: The Complete Yoga Poses
Daniel Lacerda
Black Dog & Leventhal, 2015

Aromatherapy for Self-Care: Your Complete Guide to Relax, Rebalance and Restore with Essential Oils
Sarah Swanberg
Rockridge Press, 2020

Complete Massage
Neal's Yard Remedies, Victoria Plum
DK, 2019

Plant-Based Nutrition
Julieanna Hever, Raymond J. Cronise
Alpha, 2018

RHS Grow Your Own Veg & Fruit Bible
Carol Klein
Mitchell Beazley, 2020

Science of Yoga: Understand the Anatomy and Physiology to Perfect Your Practice
Ann Swanson
DK, 2019

Shape Up With Pilates
Lynne Robinson
Kyle Books, 2020

The Complete Book of Essential Oils and Aromatherapy
Valerie Ann Worwood
New World Library, 2016

The Encyclopedia of Essential Oils
Julia Lawless
Red Wheel, 2013

The Little Black Book of Workout Motivation
Michael Matthews
Oculus Publishers, 2018

The Pilates Bible
Lynne Robinson, Lisa Bradshaw, Nathan Gardner
Kyle Books, 2019

Yoga for Everyone: 50 Poses For Every Type of Body
Dianne Bondy
Alpha, 2019

MENTAL AND EMOTIONAL WELLNESS

Good Vibes, Good Life: How Self-Love is the Key to Unlocking Your Greatness
Vex King
Hay House, 2018

Happy: Finding Joy in Every Day and Letting Go of Perfect
Fearne Cotton
Spring, 2018

Mindfulness: An Eight-Week Plan for Finding Peace in a Frantic World
Mark Williams, Danny Penman
Rodale Books, 2012`

No Mud, No Lotus: The Art of Transforming Suffering
Thich Nhat Hanh
Parallax Press, 2014

One Zentangle a Day
Beckah Krahula
Quarry Books, 2012

Practicing Mindfulness: 75 Essential Meditations to Reduce Stress, Improve Mental Health and Find Peace in the Everyday
Matthew Sockolov
Althea Press, 2018

Take a Moment: Activities to Refocus, Recentre and Relax Wherever You Are
MIND
Michael O'Mara, 2019

The Book of Joy: Lasting Happiness in a Changing World
Dalai Lama, Desmond Tutu, Douglas Carlton Abrams
Avery, 2016

The Little Book of Mindfulness: 10 Minutes a Day to Less Stress
Dr. Patrizia Collard
Gaia Books, 2014

When Things Fall Apart: Heart Advice for Difficult Times
Pema Chödrön
Shambala, 2016

WORK–LIFE WELLNESS

12 Rules for Life: An Antidote to Chaos
Jordan B. Peterson
Allen Lane, 2018

Atomic Habits: An Easy and Proven Way to Build Good Habits and Break Bad Ones
James Clear
Avery, 2018

Everything is Figureoutable
Marie Forleo
Penguin, 2019

Getting Things Done: The Art of Stress-Free Productivity
David Allen
Penguin Books, 2015

How to Win Friends and Influence People
Dale Carnegie
Vermilion, 2004

Mental Health and Well-being in the Workplace: A Practical Guide for Employers and Employees
Gill Hasson, Donna Butler
Capstone, 2020

Mindset: Changing the Way You Think to Fulfil Your Potential
Dr. Carol Dweck
Robinson, 2017

Money: A User's Guide
Laura Whateley
Fourth Estate, 2020

Nonviolent Communication: A Language of Life
Marshall B. Rosenberg
Puddle Dancer Press, 2015

Simply Living Well: A Guide to Creating a Natural, Low-waste Home
Julia Watkins
Hardie Grant Books, 2020

Switch: How to Change Things When Change is Hard
Chip Heath, Dan Heath
Crown Business, 2010

The Chimp Paradox
Prof. Steve Peters
Vermilion, 2020

The Holistic Home: Feng Shui for Mind, Body, Spirit, Space
Laura Benko
Skyhorse, 2016

The Lazy Genius Way: Embrace What Matters, Ditch What Doesn't, and Get Stuff Done
Kendra Adachi
WaterBrook, 2020

The One Thing: The Surprisingly Simple Truth Behind Extraordinary Results
Gary Keller, Jay Papasan
John Murray Learning, 2014

You Are a Badass: How to Stop Doubting Your Greatness and Start Living an Awesome Life
Jen Sincero
John Murray Learning, 2016

INDEX

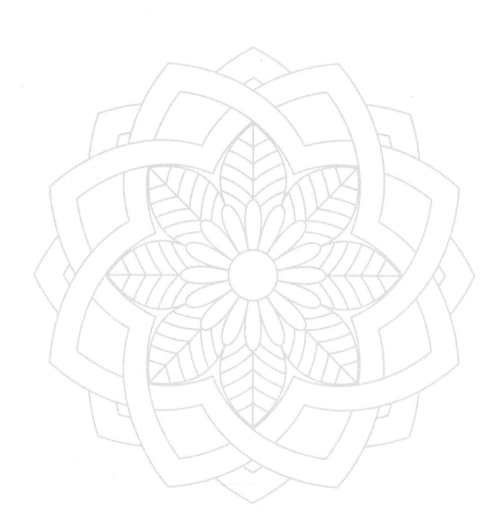